# All Health Politics Is Local

**Studies in Social Medicine**

*Allan M. Brandt, Larry R. Churchill, and Jonathan Oberlander, editors*

This series publishes books at the intersection of medicine, health, and society that further our understanding of how medicine and society shape one another historically, politically, and ethically. The series is grounded in the convictions that medicine is a social science, that medicine is humanistic and cultural as well as biological, and that it should be studied as a social, political, ethical, and economic force.

# ALL HEALTH POLITICS IS LOCAL

## Community Battles for Medical Care and Environmental Health

## Merlin Chowkwanyun

The University of North Carolina Press

CHAPEL HILL

*This book was published with the assistance of the
Lilian R. Furst Fund of the University of North Carolina Press.*

Designed by Jamison Cockerham
Set in Arno, Scala Sans, and Futura Now
by codeMantra

*Manufactured in the United States of America*

The University of North Carolina Press has been a member
of the Green Press Initiative since 2003.

LIBRARY OF CONGRESS CATALOGING-IN-PUBLICATION DATA
Names: Chowkwanyun, Merlin, author.
Title: All health politics is local : community battles for medical
care and environmental health / Merlin Chowkwanyun.
Other titles: Studies in social medicine.
Description: Chapel Hill : The University of North Carolina Press, 2022. |
Series: Studies in social medicine | Includes bibliographical references and index.
Identifiers: LCCN 2021059032 | ISBN 9781469667669 (cloth ; alk. paper) |
ISBN 9781469667676 (paper ; alk. paper) | ISBN 9781469667683 (ebook)
Subjects: LCSH: Medical care—Political aspects—United States. | Environmental
health—Political aspects—United States. | Community health services—United States.
Classification: LCC RA395.A3 C492 2022 | DDC 362.10973—dc23/eng/20211220
LC record available at https://lccn.loc.gov/2021059032

*For*

HERBERT J. GANS

*sociological legend*

*teacher*

*friend*

# Contents

*List of Illustrations  ix*

INTRODUCTION  Localism and the
Ordeal of Community Health  *1*

ONE  New York: Localism, Private-Public Boundaries,
and the Transformation of the Health Care Sector  *14*

TWO  Los Angeles: Two Cheers for Air
Pollution Control: Triumphs and Limits of the
Midcentury Industrial-Ecological Accord  *58*

THREE  Los Angeles: Health Politics
and the Fire Next Time  *96*

FOUR  Cleveland: Health Innovation, Health
Citadels, Health Ghettoes: Progress and
Deprivation in Midwestern Medicine  *140*

FIVE  Central Appalachia: Powering America on
Other People's Bodies: Strip Mining, Environmental
Health, and Human Suffering  *173*

SIX  Central Appalachia: Pork-Barrel Medicine and
Poverty: Devolution and the Problem of Elite Capture  202

CONCLUSION  Localism Is Dead—Long Live
Localism! Or: All Health Politics Is Local*  226

Acknowledgments  237

Notes  245

Bibliography  303

Index  325

# Illustrations

FIGURES

Piel Commission flow chart of New York City bureaucracy
and the "fractitionation of authority"  36

Lower East Side Neighborhood Health
Council–South outreach poster  41

Smog formation in Los Angeles  67

Network of Los Angeles weather stations  69

Simplified rendition of Arie Haagen-Smit's
schematic of smog formation  77

"Warning: The Death Fog Is Coming" pamphlet  81

"Membership Determining Funnel" for Community Health Council  115

Community Health Foundation recruitment pamphlet  147

Local coverage of strip mine mudslides  179

"Citizens to Abolish Strip Mining" pamphlet  183

Pictures of local flooding  187

"Our Hottest Client" (reprint)  192

"The Invisible Power of Coal" (advertisement)  194

Conveying maldistribution  204

Leaflet distributed in Floyd County on
Comprehensive Health Services program  213

Eula Hall and Leon Cooper meeting  215

MAPS

One-mile buffer around Montefiore  25

Two-mile buffer around Montefiore  25

Bronx hospital closures in the 1970s  54

1960 census tracts with 75%+ Black populations before/
after new Watts Health Service Area  102

1970 census tracts with double-digit poverty percentage
before/after new Watts Health Service Area  103

City Hospital and Community Health Foundation sites  145

Segregation in East Cleveland and locations of Cleveland Clinic
and Western Reserve in University Circle/Hough area  153

University-Euclid Urban Renewal Project, Phase II  154

Two Hough-Norwood facilities and the Kenneth Clement Center  165

Historical geography of eastern Kentucky strip mining, 1955  175

Historical geography of eastern Kentucky strip mining, 1975  175

Regional poverty prevalence distribution, Central Appalachia  196

National poverty prevalence distribution  196


TABLES

3.1 Watts First Community Health Council's
demographic composition  114

3.2 Admissions-to-staff ratios at LAC–USC versus
other major California county hospitals  129

3.3 Interdepartmental variation in occupancy by median percentage  130


GRAPH

National coal extraction by method, 1955–75  176

# All Health Politics Is Local

# Introduction

## Localism and the Ordeal of Community Health

In the mid-1980s, the very consequential career of a then anonymous college graduate was just beginning. Frustrated with the ennui of an office life conducting market research—and sensing he had a much larger impact to make—he scoured for an alternative life trajectory. In a periodical called *Community Jobs,* he found something promising enough: an ad seeking somebody who'd "supervise all organizing" in an "area which is 95 percent black." If he took the job, he'd "recruit and train lay leaders" and use "public action skills" for the good of struggling neighborhood residents. The graduate applied, the civic potential of the job making up for the 50 percent salary cut. And when he learned that he got it, he quickly acquired an "old, beat up" Honda Civic, put most of his life's belongings into it, and drove away, from New York City, through Pennsylvania and Ohio, headed to another metropolis in the Midwest.[1]

On his arrival, a cluster of long-standing neighborhood organizations took in the young graduate and threw him into training: crash courses in the art of one-on-one persuasion and of corralling often disparate groups of people toward achieving common goals. The work sometimes meant going neighborhood to neighborhood ascertaining residents' complaints about inadequate trash pickup or persuading enough people to show up at a local government agency to express discontent.

The graduate's mentors came out of a tradition only a degree removed from the 1960s. Reared in the philosophies of community organizing guru Saul Alinsky's Industrial Areas Foundation (IAF), they put their faith in knowing one's environs intimately, then embracing the grit and grind of arduous local-level, block-by-block work. They sensed that their new mentee was a quick study with natural talent, and they put him right to work on several campaigns: removing asbestos in public housing; creating better job training programs for city youth; and fighting garbage disposal companies who located dumps in racially segregated and economically depressed areas. Reflecting on it years later, he'd recall that local organizing of the sort he did "teaches as nothing else does the beauty and strength of everyday people" and their capacities to shape "an articulable agenda for community change."[2]

The young graduate-turned-organizer, of course, was none other than Barack Obama, who'd become the forty-fourth president of the United States twenty-five years after he started out in Chicago. Those early days became the leitmotiv of his historic 2008 presidential campaign, whose anchoring theme was local community organizing for national political change. Long before he became Number 44, Obama was attuned to the adage, popularized by Democratic Party titan and Speaker of the House Tip O'Neill, that "all politics is local."[3] By that, O'Neill meant that the micro trickled up and influenced the macro just as much, if not more, than the other way around. O'Neill would know, having witnessed firsthand the dynamics of American federalism in his three decades in Congress, spanning the mid-1950s to the mid-1980s, and having lived through epoch-making shifts in civil rights, party realignment, labor politics, and the welfare state.

For historians, "all health politics is local" has become a guiding analytic light. The historian Thomas Sugrue has elaborated on O'Neill's insight, arguing that "the persistence of local government autonomy, even amidst the expansion of national government power, has had profound social consequences."[4] His analysis demonstrates the perennial influence local politics has had on the shape, implementation, and long-term fortunes of national policy making and on the broader zeitgeist. Recent accounts of the development of Massachusetts' Route 128 and California's Orange County suburbs affirm Sugrue's conclusions, demonstrating how the worldviews and political behavior of residents in each place contributed to the national ascendance of color-blind liberalism and New Right politics, far before their later emergence in the form of such familiar entities as right-wing think tanks, Ronald Reagan, and the Democratic Leadership Council.[5] Others have shown that broad national narratives miss local dynamics that deviate from them. One major study of government spending in Atlanta, Philadelphia, and Detroit, for example, concludes that common depictions of the pre–New Deal 1920s as one of constricted government activity are fundamentally wrong.[6] An emerging generation of scholarship on the War on Poverty—with which this book engages—shows that it is the local level that ultimately shapes the execution and the fate of ambitious national social welfare initiatives.[7] So does a wave of work on the civil rights movement that upends heroic accounts centered on federal legislation, national organization, and charismatic leaders and instead turns scholarly attention to on-the-ground, day-to-day organizing and smaller legal battles in a variety of small locales.[8]

An older generation of policy scholarship—exemplified by two planning scholars, Peter Marris and Martin Rein, in their underappreciated *Dilemmas of Social Reform*—also took this approach. The duo researched it during the mid-1960s, at the height of the federal War on Poverty as policies and programs were rapidly deployed at a dizzying pace after President Lyndon Johnson's famous call for an "unconditional war on poverty."[9] *Dilemmas* focused on youth job training and delinquency prevention programs that'd been absorbed into the federal government. Marris and Rein followed the antipoverty cash nexus to Chicago and New Haven, Boston and Oakland, and Philadelphia and Newark, among other locales. And along the way, they watched how programs created at the top actually worked when implemented on the ground.

*Dilemmas* captured the frenzy of policy making during a politically tumultuous era and chronicled the pressures facing those pushing for social change. It documented not only victories but defeats, too. "No other nation organizes its government as incoherently as the United States. In the management of its home affairs, its potential resources are greater, and its use of them more inhibited than anywhere else in the world," remarked Marris and Rein, reflecting the exasperation that participants of the programs, to say nothing of scholarly observers who tagged along, must have felt. Social reforms, they continued, "which limp into law may then collapse exhausted, too enfeebled to struggle through the administrative tangle which now fronts them, and too damaged to attack the problems for which they were designed."[10]

What Marris and Rein saw wasn't smooth or seamless. There were struggles over what antipoverty programs ought fundamentally to do: stick to improving the skills of downtrodden individuals or try to transform broader social structures wholesale. Antipoverty efforts unfolded amid a dizzying array of forces. Local political machines attempted to hoard the sudden influx of federal funds or, alternately, resented newcomers onto their turf. At the same time, everyday people took advantage of laws mandating lay participation in social service administration, and if they felt ignored, they weren't afraid to raise a ruckus. The programs pulled in participants from across the ideological spectrum. They sometimes cooperated but just as often clashed. Competing imperatives from the grassroots, multiple government agencies at all levels, elected officials, and social service organizations made the War on Poverty, as it was actually experienced, a rather unwieldy daze.

To observe what they did, Marris and Rein didn't just stick to foundation boardrooms or the grand halls of Congress and federal agencies. They also went for what the political historian Ira Katznelson once dubbed the "trenches" of urban civil society, where "the block and neighborhood provided the most tangible experiences and ties of daily life," where social policy was truly received, then remolded and always contested, and where the outcome of Johnson's agenda would often ultimately be determined.[11]

## Health Politics: The View from 30,000 Feet and from 1 Foot

Local politics' durable influence is particularly pronounced when it comes to health politics in the midcentury United States. By "health politics," I refer to political contests and controversies around how to best enact the betterment of population health and ward off threats to it, whether through allocation of more resources; passage of legislation, regulation, and policies; or activism occurring outside formal governmental channels. Yet even as political historians have plumbed relations between the local and the national—and everything in between—major synthetic accounts of health politics more often than not work primarily at the national level.[12] What results is a historical narrative that is fundamentally bird's-eye and top-down, with only occasional downward dips into regional dynamics. The problem extends to the reigning modes of health research—quantitative studies based on large aggregate, nationally representative data sets—that bleed away, as historians Robert Aronowitz and Sejal Patel have shown, granularity in pursuit of generalizable findings that are supposedly cross-applicable, irrespective of local context.[13] But it is the location of stores selling nutritious food; the vitality of a metropolitan labor market; the quality of neighborhood schools; and the level of residential segregation—and a host of other locally variant features—that determine why zip code, income, education, and race—and a host of other "factors"—matter for diabetes, levels of stress hormones, cardiovascular disease, and life expectancy, among others. Such local texture is frequently flattened.

Elision of the local prevents us from seeing how health initiatives were and are affected, abetted, and constricted by regional idiosyncrasies. Here, I take a cue from historian Judith Walzer Leavitt's classic study of Milwaukee, which showed how an unlikely political coalition behind municipal reform at the turn of the twentieth century led the city to undertake novel programs in food inspection, sanitation, and infectious disease control. These particularities, in turn, explained Milwaukee's marked success in lowering mortality during the 1918 flu pandemic when compared to other cities with less robust public health infrastructure and other conditions. The impact of such distinctiveness deserves further exploration in other local settings and time periods.

*All Health Politics Is Local* argues that health dilemmas in the mid-twentieth century were indelibly shaped by local social topography: political machines, neighborhood organizations, racial politics, urban development, grassroots political mobilization, the flow of grants and government outlays, anchor institutions, political-economic shifts, and exogenous and unexpected events. The result is regional detail thicker and more extensive than what one gets working largely at a national level or in a quantitative mode. *All Health Politics Is Local* uses a multisite structure to identify cross-cutting and common themes across places while preserving local uniqueness. It does not claim that any of these sites—taken in isolation or together—are representative stand-ins for either regions or the country at large. Indeed, it makes the opposite case, for *lack* of representativeness, accentuating and exploring qualities unique to each place. Taken together, it adds up to a national account—but one steadfastly anchored in the local, with connections, similarities, and, most important, particularities and contrasts spotlighted throughout.

There is another problem with viewing developments from the stratosphere rather than closer to the surface. The former is an orientation that privileges elected officials, agency heads, scientists, hospital executives, and policy wonks. Such figures no doubt played important roles, and in this account, they have an abundant presence. But all too often those outside of formal institutions are lost in that thicket: everyday residents, patients, users of social services, and activists. What is needed is a holistic account that merges the top-down institutional with bottom-up foment and the day-to-day experiential, that documents interactions between those in formal organizations and those who worked outside of them. To do that requires more than swooshing into a locale, then flying right back out.

Here, what are often ephemeral field trips instead become extended stays. Readers will learn what it was like to be a patient waiting for hours at an overcrowded county hospital; to work in neighborhood health in an area where few residents had ever had reliable and conveniently located medical care; to sit as a hospital executive, wondering if rioters in the late 1960s were coming to torch your facility to the ground; to fear that a rock from a new strip mine less than a mile from your house might come crashing through your roof, causing debilitating injury or death; to be a federal policy operative dispatched to a remote rural hollow and asked to mediate a bitter dispute between rival on-the-ground factions vying for control of funds; to wake up and feel your eyes involuntarily tear up because of smog from air pollution from the city's industrial boom; and to serve as a county air pollution control officer making decisions in the face of scientific ambiguity over what exactly was entering the orifices of local constituents. Experiences like these are lost in predominant national-level approaches, to say nothing of the locally specific features that determine divergent trajectories in various public health initiatives.

If this book's overarching goal is to argue for a shift of perspective, a corollary aim is to historicize localism as a belief system and political practice for improving the public's health. The postwar era saw a surge of local-level health policy transformation. Its zenith came in the 1960s, when health became a centerpiece of the Johnson administration's Great Society, an enormous package of social welfare legislation unprecedented since the New Deal. Its best-known health initiatives were Medicare and Medicaid, which provided government-funded insurance, respectively, for the elderly and the indigent.

But federal programs such as Medicare and Medicaid have overshadowed lesser-known local health initiatives that grew out of the War on Poverty. This was the part of Johnson's vision aimed at society's most vulnerable and marginalized. War on Poverty projects were remarkable, first and foremost, because they provided medical care to neighborhoods that desperately needed it. But they were also unabashedly about local empowerment. They gave everyday people who used the new facilities a say in how they were run, with federal guidelines mandating "maximum feasible participation" of communities in administering new social services created for them. Harnessing localism extended into environmental health. Authorities dramatically widened the scope of regulatory powers available to local agencies wishing to clean up their own, as it were, backyards. Residents imagined their local environments as sanctified turf to be defended by intrusive polluters they thought might endanger them and make them sick.

And yet the embrace and primacy of the local in health was a historical moment unto itself, and I argue that it petered out by the early 1980s. By the last two decades of the twentieth century, local challenges became bound up with larger supralocal forces. If some found local action to be liberatory, innovative, and effective in earlier years, by a certain later date, localist proponents bumped up against emerging barriers and constrictions, many tied to the changing American economy and threats to the welfare state. Thus whereas many of my subjects here agreed with Tip O'Neill, they ultimately modified his quip so that it read, "All Politics Is Local, but That May Not Be Sufficient," even as, following Sugrue, lineages of the localist heyday endured, part of an ongoing negotiation and "uneasy tension between center and locality."[14] Barack Obama recognized these tensions, too. We'll return at the end of this book to a more chastened version of his young self who grappled with the very real limits of localism, even as he never dismissed its huge influence on American life.

Historicizing localism doubles as an intellectual-historical excavation. It interrogates a pervasive foundational concept in health planning: "community health." Then as now, invocations were legion and omnipresent, yet the term was nebulously defined. Viewing the idea's circulation at the ground level allows us to see how specific on-the-ground conditions gave way to different manifestations of the concept. We'll see visions of community health along multiple axes, sometimes discrete, sometimes overlapping. One was community health as a *rhetoric of unity and universalism*. Here, "community" imagined a population as a common unit, and partisans used it to rally fractured constituencies who'd otherwise pursue divergent interests. It stood in tension with another notion: community as *boundary*, denoting a circumscribed population, whether an ethnoracial group, a type of worker, or people living in a particular place. A related vision for "community health" concerned *control*. Here, it meant that a community—however defined—ought to administratively control the health institutions it relied on. That often existed alongside a conception of community health anchored in *geometry and scale*. In the cases that follow, advocates frequently prized small, highly local units as the best way for administering programs designed to maximize the health of those within them, often arguing that the micro and proximal translated into more sensitivity and responsiveness to local health needs. A final permutation of community health differed from the others, which were fundamentally aspirational. This one was *defensive*, counterposing "community" as a self-sufficient and autonomous unit to be guarded against from outside incursion.[15]

## Structure and Themes

To explore localism's influence on health politics in the period after World War II, I examine medical care and environmental health in four places: New York City, Los Angeles, Cleveland, Ohio, and Central Appalachia. These are not haphazard selections. These sites possessed what might be termed milestone qualities. Several were home to the initial War on Poverty health initiatives. Others contained famous private medical centers with tense relationships with both public hospitals and the neighborhoods that surrounded them. Another headquartered the most aggressive air pollution control agency in the country, while one supplied much of the United States' energy at the expense of its residents' health and safety. The substantive reasons for selecting these cases are bolstered by a decent enough paper trail in formal archives, plus critical assists from participants with personal papers and medical institutions allowing access to private holdings.

Together, the stories that I tell illuminate enduring themes in health politics (and never more so than in the present). One of these is the *tension between the private and public sectors* in carrying out broader population health improvement—that is, the lifting of aggregate health indicators writ large and the closing of inequalities in health outcomes among subpopulations, however defined.[16] Here, I follow debates in the social welfare literature that examine private-public dynamics and how the very meaning of the terms "private" and "public" have shifted over time. These changes gave rise to novel organizational forms, such as public benefit corporations or private-public partnerships, to manage new relationships between the two.[17] There are few better domains to examine how this unfolds than health care, where a two-tier system of hospitals had sharpened by the midcentury: on one side were private "voluntary" institutions, so named because they developed outside government auspices and self-consciously rejected operation under them, in contrast to their public hospital counterparts.[18] Yet the two institution types interacted with each other constantly and, in different ways, were forced to be responsive to larger public demands.

Another theme is *decision-making in the face of scientific uncertainty*. I build on work examining how policy makers and the lay public react to crises where scientific evidence remains unclear or simply absent even as an imminent response is needed.[19] What should one do about a disruptive ecological phenomenon, for instance, if evidence about its dangers is only suspected but not definitively provable? How should public health agencies react to new forms of pollution when basics about what they entail—and what the health effects are—remain unknown?

Then there is *racism in medicine*. Here I extend scholarship on racism's historic role in blocking access to medical resources: from discriminatory policies of insurers; exclusion of Black medical professionals from mainstream channels of education and employment; and public subsidies for segregated hospital construction.[20] Much of this scholarship centers on racist ideas in biomedical science and on Jim Crow's influence in diverting streams of national funding to segregated facilities, most infamously in the Hill-Burton Hospital Survey and Construction Act of 1946. Yet racism in medicine existed beyond the South, not just in overt de jure forms, and the civil rights movement and urban rebellions of the 1960s unleashed waves of opposition to it.

These antidiscriminatory efforts often paralleled—and sometimes crisscrossed with—the *democratization of health decision-making*, whereby health professionals cooperated and negotiated with—or sometimes resisted—lay and nonexpert forces, whether common residents' protests, public pressure to explore certain scientific questions, or policies mandating community input into administration. Studies of the often tense encounters between professionals and nonprofessionals have typically centered on diseases—and claims and counterclaims over how medical research is conducted, questions being asked, and explanations and therapies offered. While pursuing similar questions, I move away from the disease orientation.[21] I also engage a prior generation of skeptical public policy analysts who pondered whether constituent involvement in health service planning amounted to toothless and token seats at the larger table; questioned the logistics of selecting representatives; and pointed out that community participation missed the fundamental point, which was shortage of material resources, not citizen inputs. Much of that criticism was on target and remains a needed check to romantic accounts of community politics.[22] It was largely written, however, about participatory planning initiatives in the 1970s, which, even on paper, assigned a much more diluted role to lay participants. This account instead turns mostly to the era of 1960s insurgent politics, when federal rules mandated much more substantive roles. Challenging a profession as historically exclusionary and hierarchical as medicine was no small achievement, particularly when it managed to serve as a major check to power brokers who'd long set the agendas and controlled the institutions relied on by society's most marginalized.

Antidiscrimination and democratization raise the parallel question of *federalism and decentralization*—namely, the challenges that arise when federal funds are shot downward to local governments, often with decreasing oversight of disbursement along the way. This has led to what political scientists and economists dub "elite capture," when local elites self-servingly commandeer resources from the top that are in fact meant for broader redistribution.[23]

A final theme is the *relation between economic transformation and health*. This engages a literature that has examined threats to ecology and human health from growth imperatives and the rise of a mass consumer economy. At whose expense does the capacity needed to drive such economic expansion come?[24]

A word about the mix of cases dedicated to medical care and to environmental health is in order. The mix stems from long-standing debates over the *limits* of medical care availability in explaining large-scale health patterns. These inquiries have examined how much lack of medical care access can explain both glaring between-group health inequalities and total population health improvement. The upshot of the research? Medical care matters less than one would think, with estimates ranging from around 15 percent (typical) to 50 percent (most generous) for explaining variations in outcomes.[25] Knowing that medical care is not the sole factor shifting population health, I add two environmental health cases to the analysis. The totality of these episodes avoids the myopia of a medical care focus while not discounting its importance.

The juxtaposition, in turn, allows for excavation of the historical and persistent tension between medical care and everything else that has come to be encompassed by the term "public health." This "boundary issue," as historians Allan Brandt and Martha Gardner have characterized it, was renewed in the immediate years following World War II with a profusion of biomedical research infrastructure and health care spending, much of it from reconverted wartime resources. It resulted in the institutional and political overshadowing of nonmedical contributors to health, and it revived existential questions about what the public health enterprise even constituted.[26] These questions had their basis in the early Victorian origins of the modern public health enterprise, with some arguing (then as now) for a highly constricted set of functions, mainly restricted to vital statistics collection, sanitation, and, later, basic preventative health services, and others pushing for the enterprise to reach into wider social, political, and environmental domains, including those with no medical care component at all.[27] Throughout this account, medical practitioners routinely wrestled with the limits of medical care, particularly in resource-deprived settings that are a focus of this book. Parallel attention to environmental health further extends the inquiry of how much medical care could or could not alleviate population health problems that many of my subjects came to see as beyond its scope.

The tension between medical care and everything else around it isn't a conundrum artificially imposed on the events and subjects of this book alone. Consider, for example, the following comments from Howard J. Brown and Kurt Deuschle, two physicians who founded medical care demonstration programs in the Lower East Side of Manhattan and the Cumberland Plateau of Central Appalachia, respectively, and later reflected on their experiences and the impact of their work. Speaking in 1969, Brown told his audience: "The problems of health delivery are inevitably tied up with the vast social problems of the ghettos, and it could well be that we cannot solve the problems of [health care] delivery until we have made some major inroads on the problems of poverty and racial unrest."[28] And during an Appalachian delivery project, Deuschle and his colleagues, after chronicling environmental health threats, basic infrastructural deficits, high unemployment, and the effects of "changes in the coal economy," wrote that it wasn't enough to "merely [provide] more health services or larger appropriations from the public purse without formulation of a new and more effective approach." In a community facing as much hardship as the one they were studying, "sickness" was pervasive, "reflected in the members of the society." The solution had to be multifaceted, with resources targeted to "health problems" and the medical but also complemented by "an attack on the social, economic, political, and educational ills if any solutions are to be permanent." "What are the most appropriate public health *and* medical care solutions," they asked, that society needed "to provide for such a rural slum neighborhood?"[29]

## Domain-Specific Explorations in Medical Care and Environmental Health

Beyond a larger exploration of localism, this book contains arguments specific to medical care and environmental health. For medical care, it takes as its starting point that the history of medical care is the history of crisis management, specifically around sustainability, maldistribution, and governance.[30]

By *sustainability*, I mean the ability of health care institutions to maintain the economic resources, personnel, and political support necessary for longer-term survival. Sustainability crises took many forms. In New York City, for example, by the 1950s the once vaunted hospital system saw a shocking decline in the number of American interns and residents who wished to work in it, along with infrastructural degradation. In Cleveland around the same time, City Hospital found itself in debt after years of nonchalant billing practices. Recessionary pressures in the 1970s constrained budgets in many locales. So did rising health care costs alternately attributable to—depending on who you asked—general economic inflation; technological intensification; rising labor and plant expenditures; and widened access to insurance of both public (Medicaid, Medicare) and private varieties, in turn incentivizing price hikes.[31] All sustainability crises led to various fixes, some more successful than others. They included moving city operations to the county level; refinancing debt; the closure or downsizing of facilities; and tighter affiliations of public hospitals with private medical complexes.

The next crisis, *maldistribution*, refers to the unequal distribution of medical care's fruits. All four places contained many pockets passed over by medical care's rapid ascent and expansion. (And in the case of Appalachia, it wasn't just pockets but the entire region.) Given the medical boom after World War II, medical maldistribution was a provocative indictment of Cold War America and the affluent society's glaring internal contradictions, not to mention a blot on the healing professions, whose talents were only available to some. Amelioration of medical maldistribution, via the construction of new facilities, sometimes came from the efforts of professional social reformers, as with initiatives in New York City and Central Appalachia. But more often, it came from charged demands on the state, especially from the bottom up. This was most dramatically apparent in Watts in Los Angeles and the East Side of Cleveland, where commissions investigating the riots of the 1960s uncovered frustration and anger over deprivation of resources. After decades of neglect, that rage led to fear and then responsiveness from elite institutions: governmental bodies and medical institutions alike made enormous infrastructural commitments to people who'd been long passed over.

The final crisis was over *governance*. I define this as the contestation and protest over who ought to call the shots in medical care administration. Governance crises took varying forms. And often they were linked to the crisis of maldistribution. New facilities often came with pressures from laypersons who wanted input into how their new services would be run. They demanded a seat at the table, part of what I've elsewhere dubbed the "medical governance revolution."[32] Occasionally, administrators welcomed these demands. More often, they had no choice, mandated by provisos attached to funding streams, which required community representation that was bitterly resisted. In New York, Los Angeles, and Central Appalachia, the situation made for long conflicts—some

of which were resolved harmoniously, some of which led to uneasy rapproche-
ment, and some of which led to dysfunction—at new War on Poverty facilities
built for areas in desperate need of resources.

The environmental health stories take place in Los Angeles and Cleveland.
In Los Angeles, I examine midcentury industrial and automotive emissions and
the increasing severity of what came to be known as smog in the two decades
preceding the federal Clean Air Act (1970). In Central Appalachia, I look at
surface mining of coal and its deleterious consequences for area residents. These
stories lend themselves to a dyadic structure for a simple reason: one regulatory
effort (Los Angeles) was partially successful, whereas one (Central Appalachia)
was decidedly not.

One question that arises from this comparison concerns public support. A
striking feature of the Los Angeles industrial pollution story was its universalist
quality and officials' emphasis on assembling a broad and disparate coalition
behind its earliest efforts, which ranged from ad hoc citizens' groups to advocates of downtown development to the otherwise conservative Los Angeles
County Medical Association. In Central Appalachia, by contrast, the early years
of surface mining attracted no such coalition supporting strong regulation or
oppositional efforts, much less one containing powerful bedfellows.[33]

Both regions also illustrate how something—be it air pollution or surface
mining—became socially recognized and framed as a "health problem."[34]
Although the health implications of these two cases may seem intuitive or obvious today, that wasn't the case during their early emergence. In Los Angeles
County, scientists and officials debated whether smog was harmful to human
health or merely a highly irritating and unsightly nuisance. And in Central Appalachia, the potential health ramifications of strip mining remained off the radar
of all but laypersons and activists. Scientific inquiry in both cases later con-
gealed, albeit at radically different paces, around air pollution and strip mining.
The difference, however, came in the response. Officials in Los Angeles County
acted even more rapidly than they already had; those in Central Appalachia
didn't. The two cases allow us to see the reasons behind why environmental
health mitigation is vigorously pursued in some cases and largely ignored in
others.

## Localism at a Crossroads

A major goal of this book is to see the recent history of health politics via a
new prism. It's one that doesn't eschew the importance of developments from
on high but brings it together with developments on the ground and all that
comes with incorporating them. This optic sometimes reveals the local roots of

subsequent federal policy. Elsewhere, it shows variation in local implementation of dictates and programs from the federal government. It can illuminate how federal trends, whether the civil rights revolution, the fiscal crunch, or rapid industrialization and consumerism, left different health imprints depending on where in the country you sat. Seeing the local brings into view how grassroots activism of many varieties—from disparate residents with gripes to organized boards of laypersons—engaged in health politics, both inside and outside formal governmental channels. Most important, remembering that all health politics is local shows how persistent dilemmas in medical care and environmental health take on trajectories ultimately determined by features of the local landscape where they unravel.

But there is a second goal here, too: to interrogate localism as a politics and put the reader in the same sobering position as many of this book's subjects. Like the figure who opened this book, they realized the potential of localism and came to see its very real limits. Advocates for democratic health governance eventually had to confront the structural impediments posed by a new fiscal climate, ushered in by New York City's 1975 debt crisis. The architects of Los Angeles County's pioneering air pollution control program could take pride in its efficacy. But they were also humbled by its inability to defy two trends beyond the program itself: an industrial boom and an autocentric culture that spanned local county boundaries. The riots in Los Angeles and Cleveland were a wake-up call. They extracted concessions from terrified officials—in both government and in elite medical institutions—and injected real health resources into long-neglected neighborhoods with people who desperately needed and demanded them. Yet these victories still existed amid deprivation, both before and, especially, after the riots, made all the worse by the fiscal instability of the 1970s. These end results highlighted glaringly the limits of gaining community health nodes in what was, in the last analysis, still a matrix of racialized inequality and budgetary austerity. Similar tensions were on display in Central Appalachia, where a medical concession was won in a rapidly emerging landscape of intractable poverty, ecological degradation, and environmental health risk, fueled by a national growth imperative—and the need to power it—that had no local response capable of counteracting it or mounting an alternative.

Like this book, they all confronted one question: Whither localism?

# 1

# New York

## Localism, Private-Public Boundaries, and the
## Transformation of the Health Care Sector

The 1960s were a peak time for books, across the ideological spectrum, that weren't just *about* policy but ended up making policy themselves, propelled by dazzling rhetoric and powerful narratives about radically changing the world: Walt Rostow's *Stage of Change* (a future of robust growth and no communism); Rachel Carson's *Silent Spring* (an Earth cleansed of man-made poisons), Ralph Nader's *Unsafe at Any Speed* (a business sector that didn't lie about how easily its products could kill you); Betty Friedan's *The Feminine Mystique* (an America free from the ennui of conventional gender roles); and James Baldwin's *The Fire Next Time* (an America without racism). You might say it was the era of the Vision Book.

If you picked up *Prepayment for Hospital Care in New York State: A Report on the Eight Blue Cross Plans Serving New York Residents* in 1961, when it was published, you probably wouldn't think of it as an epoch-defining title. Plodding, redundant, replete with awkward passive constructions, *Prepayment* instead bore all the imprints of dry technocracy. It was the kind of tome nobody read cover to cover and that inevitably spent more time accumulating dust on a library shelf than it did in many pairs of hands. And yet its lead author, Ray Trussell, had written more than a book. Trussell's thinking would remake health care in the nation's largest city.

Within a decade—and not without a lot of resistance—New York City's public hospitals would go from being run by the government to being run by the city's private medical centers, most of them big-monied, elite, and part of fancy universities. It amounted, in short, to the private control of public goods in order to save the latter from decline.

It'd all begun with an obscure policy book—and the man behind it.

## The Fall of Public Hospitals and the Rise of Ray Trussell

For all its deficiencies of presentation, *Prepayment* contained a powerful yet simple idea: insurance premiums—and health care costs, by extension—were rising because of poorly planned, ill-conceived hospital construction whose subsequent high sunk costs were passed on to consumers.[1] More bloat, more premiums, more costs. What was needed was coordination, some edifice to trim the fat and inject rationality into a hospital landscape riven with infrastructural excess. Trussell spoke the language of regionalism: the growing notion that urban planning could use a lot more coordination, communication, and centralization among disparate and unwieldy parts.

It was an idea perfect, in Trussell's mind, for a New York City public hospital system whose crisis of sustainability demanded more leanness and more organization to have any hope of surviving. And as it happened, the same year *Prepayment* appeared, Trussell got the chance to use the city as a laboratory. He promptly exited life as a professor at Columbia University's School of Public Health and entered New York City politics as its commissioner of hospitals, called in to fix the public hospital system. Trussell proposed, then swiftly implemented, affiliation: essentially a subcontracting arrangement whereby the government would pay the city's most powerful academic medical centers to administer and staff public hospitals. Affiliation amounted to the city waving a white flag and declaring that it couldn't run its own hospitals by itself. The New York City media was enthusiastic about the plan, hailing Trussell as a polymathic savior, with the *New York Post* dubbing him "a medical dynamo dedicated to lifting health standards."[2]

The path to being a medical dynamo first ran through a mayoral commission on hospitals, nominally headed by David Heyman, a businessman and philanthropist with a long-standing interest in the city's health services. Trussell dominated it. Formed in 1959, the Heyman Commission consisted of more than three dozen members: a mix of city officials, philanthropists, and, most represented, administrators from medical institutions. It had a simple two-prong charge. Step one: Figure out what problems afflicted New York City's once vaunted system of eighteen public hospitals, more extensive than any in the country, all underpinned by the powerful principle that each was "expected to take in every New Yorker who applied to them for help."[3] Step two: Figure out something to be done.

Step one wasn't hard. The biggest short-term ailment revolved around personnel. By the late 1950s, with few exceptions, most of the municipal hospitals were failing to attract permanent staff and interns and residents. By one estimate, the city now relied on 9,000 volunteer physicians to cover the permanent staffing shortfall.[4] Shortages existed as well for nurses, dieticians, social workers, and occupational, physical, and speech and hearing therapists. To take just one example, in 1960, the city budget had allocated funds for 6,157 nurses, but only 1,756 positions had actually been filled. For dieticians, 252 positions had been allocated, but only 59 were filled, which necessitated the use of temporary employees.[5] The state of the public hospitals' postgraduate programs proved even more dire and embarrassing. In the previous year, no American interns were placed in any unaffiliated municipal hospitals—that is, almost all of them—by the national intern-matching program.[6] In their place was a stream of foreign medical graduates. Concern over their presence was tinged with a whiff of nativism, but there was no doubt that because of training under different standards and expectations, foreign medical graduates often floundered. "Municipal hospitals without medical school affiliations have lost the continuing high level of professional supervision which would make them attractive to interns and residents," Heyman declared at the commission's first meeting.[7]

There was a simple fiscal basis for the personnel problem. In the early 1950s, the Committee on Interns and Residents, the labor union representing just-minted doctors, noted that municipal hospitals had outpaced the national average wage for house staff. Yet by the end of the decade, the wage trend had reversed. On average, monthly pay for interns in city hospitals was $125, compared to a national average of $189 in all U.S. hospitals.[8] Beyond material incentives, public hospitals lacked the equipment, adequate infrastructure, and strong teaching programs offered by private counterparts, mainly university-based medical centers.[9] Talent was ditching the public medical sector: for better pay and for better training.

Personnel shortages weren't the only problem. Relations between the city and private institutions had reached an impasse, with the private organizations thrust into charity roles without adequate compensation from the city. In the late 1950s, Mayor Robert F. Wagner had promised to raise, by four dollars, the per diem amount that the city paid to private so-called voluntary institutions for its patients, though the city admitted that such increases still likely wouldn't outpace inflationary pressures facing the entire medical sector. Something more than ad hoc payments for public patients was necessary.[10]

Then there was bureaucracy. Heyman Commission members regularly criticized the "unnecessary and expensive duplication of services," which contributed to escalating costs and poor coordination.[11] One source of that problem was indiscriminate—and possibly unnecessary—hospital construction, the sort criticized by Trussell in his tome on insurance premiums. How—and if—to build was especially pressing, since the city planned to build several new facilities over the next decade. For Trussell, it was an opening to introduce his principles of rationalization and test his proposal for enmeshing hospitals with private facilities. He raised them during a discussion of criteria to be considered when locating public hospitals. When one commissioner argued that they ought to be placed near where patients actually lived, "for the people will not leave their own community to go to other areas for medical care," Trussell countered. He argued that institutional resources, particularly proximity to private academic medical centers, were far more important in choosing where to build a public hospital than geographic closeness to patients. And he ended his remarks in one meeting by decrying municipal hospitals that were "isolated[,] poorly staffed[,] and poorly equipped" and pushing for eventual systemwide rationalization, even downsizing.[12]

But by "isolated," Trussell really meant "unaffiliated." And for him, the problems that the Heyman Commission had identified all led to one solution: a systemwide set of affiliations overseen by the city. The position was reinforced by the success of an existing pilot affiliation, that between Morrisania Hospital (a public facility in the Bronx) and Montefiore Medical Center, a voluntary institution with ties to Einstein Medical College and Yeshiva University. The affiliation had begun informally in 1955, when a Morrisania administrator had approached Montefiore's chief executive, Martin Cherkasky, and proposed sharing of house staff—hospital residents—between the two institutions. Implemented in 1959, the agreement had Montefiore lending personnel to Morrisania, loaning technological resources, such as X-ray and laboratory facilities, and providing more Montefiore-level training for Morrisania interns, who might otherwise have sought residencies at private institutions.[13] In a meeting devoted to reviewing the pilot affiliation, Cherkasky backed up Trussell's view that the geographic closeness of the two institutions, coupled with the willingness of Montefiore to share its resources, were the key reasons for success.

If scaled up and replicated, affiliations like Montefiore-Morrisania would come with many perks and fixes for the sustainability crisis. Public hospitals could leverage the private facilities' recruiting power and prestige to solve the staffing problem. And they could benefit from private infrastructural resources—for example, the sharing of supplies. Private institutions would receive guaranteed, contractually backed compensation, rather than impromptu payments, for services rendered, whether taking in patients, providing training, or assisting with administration. A system of affiliations at first seemed like a potentially onerous commitment of public funds. But if the city was serious about solving its sustainability crisis, the benefits would far outweigh the costs, the commission argued. It concluded that the city "should vigorously implement the established policy of affiliating as many municipal hospitals as possible with medical schools or with voluntary hospitals having strong teaching programs" and urged "dynamic follow-through."[14] An affiliation was what would ultimately distinguish inadequate facilities, which the city ought to abandon, from ones that the city ought to support.

If the Heyman Commission's vision was a tight network of public hospitals—locked into orderly relationships with private institutions—it raised a thorny political question: What would happen to those that didn't get affiliated? Trussell's answer was simple: those hospitals were pork, and they ought to close. In its final report, the commission wrote that the city ought not override closure if a hospital "cannot be maintained or the facilities are no longer required." And in one particularly biting passage, it cast long-standing local attachments to otherwise faltering health institutions as sappy communitarian sentimentalism that ought to be divorced from dispassionate analysis on how to "provide optimum medical care." "Good medicine," it stated pithily, "is not practiced by bricks and mortar."[15] Planned closures weren't just idle talk. At one meeting, the commission reviewed a list of a dozen hospitals, naming three of them—Fordham in the Bronx, Sydenham in Harlem, and Gouverneur on the Lower East Side—as good candidates for closure.[16] Sparse evidence was frequently offered to justify these choices. When providing a rationale for why Fordham Hospital ought to close, for example, the commission wrote simply "that there was no need for an out-patient service in this location" while providing little evidence on why that was the case. For Gouverneur, "there was little discussion . . . beyond the fact that it should be closed and not rebuilt."[17] These declarations discounted hospitals' immense political symbolism in neighborhoods, a myopia that spurred much of the later backlash around the affiliation plan.

One reason for that tunnel vision was the composition of the commission. Physician-administrators dominated all major committees where consequential deliberations occurred, giving the proceedings an unmistakably rarefied and undemocratic air.[18] The case for affiliation, unsurprisingly, was shot through with a paternalist streak. While framed as mutually beneficial, institutionalized affiliations would permanently increase dependence of municipal hospitals on private voluntary institutions—and at a monetary cost to the city. The surface reciprocity of the relationship masked the two parties' unequal degrees of desperation. Municipal hospitals, with their personnel shortages and infrastructural deficiencies, needed voluntary affiliates much more than the private institutions needed reliable revenue for their charity role, which, at worst, they could simply stop fulfilling altogether. But the Heyman Commission barely discussed mechanisms to ensure that both sides in the proposed private-public partnerships held up their end of the bargain. Except for a brief discussion of whether municipal hospitals would still decide on their own chiefs of staff, potential for conflicts in affiliation went undiscussed. So did the human element. Commission members repeatedly referred to affiliation as a means to acquire more potential "clinical material," in the cold and impersonal parlance of the time. Such phrasing—and the parochialism behind it—would come under attack later in the decade, after several high-profile revelations around unethical experimentation rocked the medical establishment.[19] But in the early 1960s, additional reservoirs of "material" in public hospitals were a selling point to private medical centers and their expanding clinical research and teaching programs.[20] Affiliation promised to make accessing it even easier.

At the same time, not everyone was oblivious to the power of public relations. Trussell himself commented at one point that the schools shouldn't be perceived as "trying to 'take over.'"[21] It was advice he'd more or less forget to follow in the coming years. For now, though, it was full speed ahead.

In 1961, Mayor Wagner accepted the commission's recommendations, and he plucked Trussell away from academic wonkdom and inserted him into the world of city government, appointing him commissioner of hospitals. Along with Trussell came Martin Cherkasky, who served as an "adviser" while maintaining his post at Montefiore. Trussell proceeded to implement immediately the recommendations he had pushed, initiating five affiliations for Lincoln, Bellevue, Harlem, and Metropolitan Hospitals and City Hospital at Elmhurst. He worked with urgency, writing to one high-level city official that not getting the program under way immediately amounted to "a calculated risk" on the city's part. "Frankly, if I were carried into any one of several of our emergency rooms, I would demand to be carried out," Trussell wrote in a memo that pushed the city to release the necessary funds for the affiliation program—and without delay.[22]

## Mounting Patient Discontent

Trussell might be suspected, with good reason, of exaggeration or melodrama. Affiliation, after all, was his pet program. ("I am the father of the whole business," he remarked elsewhere.)[23] But a steady flow of complaints substantiated Trussell's depiction of a crumbling system with low morale and undertrained or overburdened staff. Henry Herman recalled the experiences of his mother-in-law, who'd been struck by an automobile and brought to Kings County Hospital, then denied a request for a bedpan when she needed to use the restroom. "Since these patients are bedridden," he explained, "they have no alternative but to relieve themselves in their bedding and lie in urine and feces." Herman saw his mother-in-law's experience as exemplary of a larger trend: "We all understand that in a City Hospital such as Kings County a patient cannot expect comfort and service that might be available in a private hospital, but why should misery be compounded by presence of some personnel with sadistic tendencies?"[24] Gloria Clay shared her experience at Morrisania, where she'd taken her mother, who'd suffered a stroke. "It took six hours until she was admitted officially and a resident physician looked at her," Clay recounted. "This was an emergency call. It is ironical. She has become partially paralyzed due to this." Clay had worked hard to transfer her mother to a rehabilitation facility but was met with endless delays that she attributed to understaffing caused by inadequate pay for personnel, particularly nurses.[25] Lillian Feigen, herself a nurse, charged that her father had died at Fordham Hospital's emergency room because of a misdiagnosis and failure to notice his ruptured bladder, which resulted in his death just hours after his arrival. For Feigen, like Herman and Clay, her individual experience wasn't an isolated incident but stemmed from systemwide failures. "It seems impossible to competently care for the crowd of patients seen in the emergency room of that city hospital," she concluded.[26]

These incidents suggested a populace that had for some time held the public hospital system in low esteem. If there was an opportune time to push sweeping policy changes, Trussell had found it. Over the next few years, affiliations accelerated, though their character differed from arrangement to arrangement. The one between Montefiore and Morrisania ballooned from a pilot program that had begun with the sharing of a single surgical resident. Officials planned for it to transition from staff exchanges between schools into a full-fledged joint residency program. In addition to house staff, six Morrisania departments— medicine, neurosurgery, obstetrics-gynecology, orthopedic surgery, anesthesiology, and hematology—received full-time chiefs from Montefiore. In July 1962, the city formally committed to a three-year affiliation contract worth $3 million a year. Besides permanent staff, Montefiore shared its X-ray and laboratory facilities and assumed oversight for Morrisania's medical care services. Summarizing the affiliation's progress, its creators declared that "the partnership has become the prototype for similar affiliations between other voluntary and municipal hospitals in the city. Still in its infancy, the plan is only in the development stage. But it is not too soon to report that the infant is lusty and thriving. The affiliation works."[27] And there were plans for the "lusty and thriving" program to grow still more. In October 1963, the city accepted a parcel of land from Montefiore, located near the hospital, that'd be used for a rebuilt Morrisania facility in a few years' time. If fully realized, the joint facility would represent the ideal configuration that Trussell had advocated, one marked not just by institutional affiliation but by geographic closeness.[28]

Another arrangement, between Columbia University's College of Physicians and Surgeons and Harlem Hospital, generated more controversy. Harlem was a hospital in trouble. In late January 1961, many foreign medical graduates intending to join its house staff had failed an exam given by the Executive Committee on Foreign Medical Graduates, barring them from performing physicians' activities. To avoid a problem like that again, Columbia entered an affiliation. It committed to assisting with supervision of future Harlem interns and residents,

who would receive periodic visits from Columbia faculty in the form of regular rounds, conferences, and lectures. Columbia's most important role went
beyond training. It'd now screen potential hires for departmental director and
assistant director positions at the hospital.[29]

Columbia and Harlem's relationship revealed many inherent ambiguities in
Trussell's grand designs. When one took stock of Columbia's ability to determine hiring, the arrangement looked like a power grab by Columbia or a city
hospitals commissioner looking to encroach on a public institution's autonomy.
And Trussell hardly behaved with tact. When members of the Harlem Hospital medical board balked at the level of control that Columbia and Trussell
imposed, Trussell promptly fired everybody on it, replacing it with a temporary group. He bluntly equated the services rendered by Columbia—and his
larger plans by extension—with the "best interests" of Harlem Hospital and
its patients.

Harlem Hospital administrators weren't the only people upset. When Dean
Houston Merritt (himself a member of the Heyman Commission), solicited
opinions on whether to proceed, many Columbia faculty balked, a reflection
of a university whose primary form of community outreach with the Harlem
neighborhood was real-estate expansion and residential displacement.[30] After
site visits to Harlem Hospital, most Columbia faculty were reluctant to commit to a full affiliation on a level similar to Montefiore's. They worried that
affiliations distracted personnel and diluted resources, even if the university
received financial compensation. Others wondered whether a better alternative
might be advocating for a construction of a new city medical school—one not
named Columbia—closer to Harlem. Status consciousness, too, entered into
the conversation. One faculty member, with more than a little condescension,
disapproved of Harlem Hospital's permanent staff, claiming that few would ever
qualify to teach at Columbia.[31] At best, the prospect of affiliation attracted lukewarm support from Columbia. From its vantage point, the action was hardly
necessary, either to raise revenue or to bolster a civic mission that didn't exist.

And yet, Columbia initiated an affiliation at the urging of Dean Merritt and
Trussell himself, a testament to the policy momentum around the concept, even
in the most traditional and parochial of places. But there was another possible
institutional motive for affiliation: public relations. Long embroiled in conflict
with neighboring Washington Heights and Harlem (which would come to a
boil in a 1968 campus protest), some Columbia leaders saw support of Harlem
Hospital as a means of subduing simmering tensions.[32] The university's president, Grayson Kirk, who by the end of the decade lost his post after campus
protests over university-neighborhood relations, remarked as much, writing
that "the University has a measure of responsibility to the neighboring community of which it is a part and from which it derives sustained support."[33] By the

following year, Columbia signed affiliation contracts to provide psychiatric services and create obstetrics-gynecology and anesthesiology divisions at Harlem.

Just a year later, in 1962, Trussell expressed confidence that his plans were going in the right direction. Throughout an address given at the New York Academy of Medicine, Trussell draped affiliation in the language of community uplift. The Department of Hospitals was making "wise long-range decisions in the best interests of the community." Affiliations between municipal and voluntary hospitals could "and should work together for reinforcement and better service to the community." Mount Sinai's assumption of affiliation duties at Greenpoint Hospital represented "outstanding service to the community . . . at a time when the hospital's plight is desperate." The Columbia-Harlem Hospital affiliation, which Trussell had personally played a major role in strong-arming, exhibited "long range potential for community service, training and research" that was "unlimited." In conclusion, the municipal hospitals were "the community's and only the community can make them what they should be."[34] By the middle of the decade, most of the city's municipal hospitals had affiliated, and Trussell's vision seemed to be proceeding unimpeded.

## Resistance to Affiliation

Not everyone shared Trussell's interpretation of what the community really needed and wanted. Undercurrents of opposition to his plans appeared even before the 1962 Harlem Hospital affair. Though Trussell had depicted affiliations as a way of addressing threats to sustainability, they were also part of a larger program of streamlining that also required trimming fat. In promoting it, the Heyman Commission had laid its criteria for who should get cut and why in generic terms, targeting mainly hospitals that were "isolated," not close enough to a voluntary institution or medical school, or that delivered "duplicative" services. Lack of affiliation was equated with redundancy.

Neighborhood activism against Trussell soon took hold. It mirrored similar developments throughout the nation as academic medical centers' power increased after World War II. So-called town and gown tensions could take many forms. In rural America, many general practitioners, as medical historian Dominique Tobbell has shown, feared getting sidelined by medical schools rapidly undergoing specialization.[35] Their solution was to push—successfully—for family medicine to be recognized as a distinct specialty.

But in New York City, the battles were more heated. A fierce defensive localism arose around cherished medical turf. That wasn't surprising. Public hospitals were different from other government infrastructure of the era—Robert Moses's highways, plazas, parks, and bridges, buttressed by the federal urban renewal program—that New York City residents had increasingly perceived as imposed onto them, and they did not engender the same negative connotations.[36] Quite the contrary: many residents cherished their public hospitals, and they let it be known when some were selected for shuttering. Fordham Hospital resulted in the biggest tempest. In May 1961, shortly after Trussell announced Fordham's closure, the Fordham Hospital Alumni Association quickly drafted a report to protest. Written by Charles Scala, Fordham's director of medical education, it excoriated Trussell and the Heyman Commission, targeting above all their insularity. The decision to close Fordham was "deadly," one in a series of "fatal mistakes" stemming from "total divorce from the wise counsel that could be offered by the hospital physicians, the hospital administrators, and the leaders of the communities."[37] Trussell and cronies had staged something just short of a coup, in the alumni association's eyes, working from secretive "preliminary arrangements." "The Board of Hospitals had already unilaterally decided to close Fordham Hospital," it argued, without any kind of open deliberation. There was much truth to the charges. Fordham Hospital, along with Gouverneur and Sydenham, had appeared on the list of planned closures in a Heyman Commission meeting dedicated mostly to the topic, and its members had never sought outside input.

Apart from blasting the opaqueness of the planning process, the report defended Fordham's existence. It pointed to Fordham's heavy utilization rate (88.6 percent average occupancy), consistent accreditation, and accolades for specific departments: a sharp contrast to other facilities that had failed inspections from the Joint Commission on the Accreditation of Hospitals. And while staffing pressures surely existed, Scala argued that Fordham had performed far above par. Noting long-standing struggles to get Bronx physicians to serve in the borough's four municipal hospitals, Scala pointed out that Fordham had, in its most recent count, attracted 36 percent of 481 physicians willing to do so. And unlike other hospitals, it didn't have any problems filling a full intern and resident class. While Scala acknowledged the high number of foreign medical graduates in the program, he suggested that its established training program, with a regular rotation of lecturers from adjacent universities and hospitals, mitigated against any training deficiencies with which they might have arrived.[38]

At the same time, deficiencies were real. The most glaring were in nursing, where Fordham filled only 25 percent of positions, about as low as the 28 percent citywide rate. And Scala admitted, too, to severe infrastructural deficiencies. Both problems, however, needed to be viewed as the outgrowth of trends that went far beyond Fordham. A nursing shortage had long existed, and it had attracted federal attention. The obsolescence of the physical plant, likewise, stemmed from negligence by not Fordham but the city itself, which in 1956 had promised a "complete modernization" that had yet to happen. Declaring

Fordham's buildings irredeemable amounted to a preordained cover story for closure, at odds with the Department of Hospitals' own assessment a few years earlier. The true root of Fordham's ills, in short, was simple: larger forces beyond it and years of city indifference.[39]

In the alumni association's eyes, the motives behind closure were fundamentally political and hardly borne of economic necessity. "Misleading propaganda" fueled the decision—namely, claims about the superiority of affiliated institutions: "The lay public and political officers are not aware of these facts. When they are told—by medical bureaucrats—that all municipal hospitals must be affiliated with a medical school or major teaching voluntary hospital, they incorrectly assume that patient care in non-affiliated hospitals must necessarily be either inadequate or inferior." In one of many searing sections, Scala openly suggested that a regional Bronx power play was afoot, referencing a 1960 overture by Montefiore Hospital to affiliate with Fordham Hospital that Fordham's board had rebuffed. Without mentioning Montefiore's Martin Cherkasky by name, the report pointed out that Cherkasky had become Trussell's special adviser and charged that Fordham's death would pave the way for Montefiore to acquire another remaining city hospital and enlarge its regional footprint.[40]

In short, while claiming to advocate for a broader community, Cherkasky, Trussell, and other advocates of affiliation were doing anything but. Instead, the report continued, they were proving themselves hubristic and "impersonal bureaucrats with little real interest or knowledge of Bronx hospitals; who were content to be guided by figures, statistics and plans, rather than by contact with experienced hospital personnel, interested community leaders, and responsible officials." They constituted a self-interested medical cabal that had "already committed to a secret course of action rather than to a real and open investigation of the problems and solutions; who were more interested in the distribution of money to voluntary hospitals than they were in safeguards for the taxpayers' burden; and who were more interested in 'cute schemes' than they were in good patient care." The brief from Fordham's defenders punched many holes in Trussell's blanket depiction of isolated, unaffiliated hospitals with poor teaching programs and unneeded and redundant services with middling patient demand. Fordham's catchment area, the alumni association estimated, consisted of 600,000 people, and utilization figures suggested people within it were using the hospital.[41]

In the end, the Fordham alumni association's and Heyman Commission's reports were best viewed less as competing factual accounts of the present than competing visions of the future and where the hospital system ought to go next. For Fordham, unaffiliated hospitals, if given adequate resources by the city, could remedy many of their flaws and thrive independently without the support of private institutions. From the perspective of patient care, not making such a

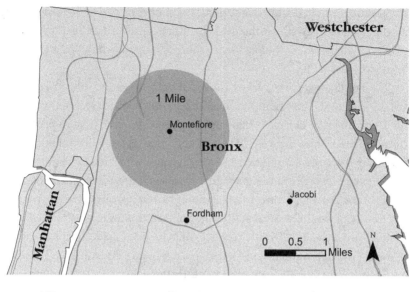

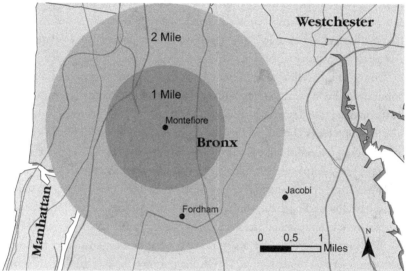

**Bronx power play.** These two images show one-mile and two-mile buffers, respectively, around Montefiore. Fordham Hospital lay in Montefiore's catchment area and led many to claim that Martin Cherkasky and Montefiore's institutional self-interest was a key driver in the Bronx affiliation.

*Source*: Author's cartography.

commitment would disrupt institutional traditions and ties to the surrounding neighborhood. Trussell, on the other hand, saw institutions like Fordham as relics, standing in the way of necessary administrative streamlining and institutional consolidation.

The Fordham report sparked a wave of opposition that blindsided Trussell. In May 1961, 300 unionized Fordham Hospital employees showed up at the Department of Hospitals building in downtown Manhattan to protest the closure. Trussell also incurred the wrath of Samuel Rubin, a member of Fordham's Lay Advisory Committee and a millionaire who'd made his fortune off the Fabergé cosmetics line. Rubin ran full-page protest ads in the city's newspapers. Like Trussell, he invoked community interest, but differently, warning that Fordham would be the first of many public hospitals to go if Trussell continued with impunity: "Drastic changes will have been made, hospitals closed, staff work disrupted and disintegrated, and communities victimized."[42] The ads themselves were striking, consisting of nearly three dozen factoids, many taken from the alumni association report, that recounted the hospital's history and touted its strengths, while rebutting claims that the hospital was in such despair that nothing could save it. They urged readers to deluge the Department of Hospitals with angry calls.

The groundswell against Trussell worked. In an unexpected move, he announced that he would reluctantly leave Fordham open for the time, though he maintained that he did so only because of strong outside pressures. Explaining his decision, Trussell claimed that the community interest had been distorted and hijacked by people like Rubin: "The Fordham thing had got to the point where it was completely irrational. The community was completely confused and up in arms. I just decided there was nothing to be gained by slugging them."[43] Instead of closing, Fordham would remain "on probation," Trussell announced.[44] In 1961, the city announced an affiliation between Fordham Hospital and Misericordia Hospital, a voluntary institution, in what amounted to a compromise between the two initial proposals.[45] Fordham didn't close and maintained most of its autonomy, given Misericordia's relatively minor size compared to other institutions in the region. But it would, in the end, still be affiliated.

## Battlefront Two: Showdown in Queens

A second battle occurred in 1962 in Queens, when the city announced an affiliation between City Hospital at Elmhurst and Mount Sinai Medical Center on the Upper East Side of Manhattan. It attracted an unusual coalition of opponents: neighborhood activists and physicians. Each saw something uniquely wrong about affiliation.

Neighborhood activists viewed affiliations as a disruption of neighborhood autonomy. A largely symbolic lawsuit against Trussell and Mount Sinai, filed by a resident asking for an injunction, argued that Trussell's new powers were granted "without laying down policy and guide lines."[46]

Meanwhile, a group calling itself the Committee to Save City Hospital at Elmhurst, saw affiliations as detracting from a patient-centered mission. Though promoted with benevolent communitarian rationales, affiliations were really about something else: conversion of public hospitals to a "vast laboratory stressing research and teaching with its ward patients (poor and without influence), potential guinea pigs."[47] The fears were hardly ungrounded, given the references to "clinical material" in various meetings about affiliation. If Trussell was claiming affiliation to be in the best interests of the community, these were voices counterclaiming to be the real community, arguing that Trussell's pronouncements carried no such legitimacy. The Elmhurst protestors' rhetoric was compatible with the times, too. Scorching critiques such as Jane Jacobs's *Life and Death of Great American Cities* and Herbert Gans's *Urban Villagers* were inspiring opposition to imperious urban planning and big institutions.[48] The world of medicine wasn't exempt.

Neighborhood protest dovetailed with another bloc trying to stave off Mount Sinai: the 350-plus volunteer physician staff and their medical societies. Whereas the protestors had focused on disruption of institution-neighborhood ties, this group cast affiliations as threats to private physicians' collective power and ability to maintain skill via regular interaction with hospital patients. By swapping in permanent, nonvoluntary, and salaried staffs at newly affiliated hospitals, this argument went, affiliation at Elmhurst (and elsewhere) would divide the city's physicians into two tiers: an employed elite class with access to hospital privileges and those closed off from them. The Elmhurst situation sent the Kings County Physicians Guild into hysterics. Trussell had carried out the affiliation plan in an "almost inhuman" manner, the guild charged, and wished "to deny men of honor, integrity and devotion in the practice of medicine the opportunity to give freely of their services." Affiliation was "forced," and Trussell's powers amounted to "absolutism." The guild perceived affiliation as large-scale state meddling in medical practice, something regional medical societies had consistently opposed throughout the twentieth century, except for regulation of licensure.[49] The most eloquent (and far more temperate) physician-opponent of the affiliation was Lester Tuchman (husband of the much more famous popular historian Barbara Tuchman). He believed that affiliations and permanent staffing would lead to a "two-doctor system, an elite within the hospitals, and an inferior order outside."[50] Tuchman's opposition was also hugely consequential for the conflict at Elmhurst: he served as its chief of medicine and formally opposed the affiliation. In response, Trussell followed his Harlem strategy. He fired the entire forty-two-member Elmhurst board, and Tuchman along with it, in February of that year.[51]

The move enflamed Trussell's opponents and led to a legal challenge to reseat Tuchman and the board. Although a lower court reinstated them in May, by then, much of the opposition had withered. A critical turning point came during a planned walkout of attending staff, when 167 physicians broke ranks and pledged to stay and go along with affiliation. The breakaway group included ten members of the forty-two-member ousted board, which split opposition. Trussell followed by replacing the 130 physicians who'd still refused to accept the affiliation with fresh physicians from Mount Sinai.[52] At Elmhurst at least, affiliation remained very much on track.

## The Lower East Side Exception

A third dramatic conflict occurred on the Lower East Side, sparked by Trussell's announcement that he'd close Gouverneur, the only major public hospital in the immediate area. In doing so, he kicked a hornet's nest, and the subsequent uproar underscored the cultural significance people invested in their neighborhood hospitals.

For many residents, the closure came as not only a shock but a betrayal. For decades, the city had long committed to building a replacement facility for the Lower East Side. That promise followed years of agitation from its famous block-level advocacy groups, some of which dated back to the Progressive Era settlement house movement. Like most other city hospitals at the time, Gouverneur was starting to reel by the mid-1950s. Although personnel shortages posed a problem, the biggest was its decaying plant. Site visits from accrediting agencies commended the enthusiasm and quality of the staff but bemoaned the material conditions in which they worked.[53] Writing about Gouverneur, the Joint Commission on the Accreditation of Hospitals praised the hospital for "render[ing] a valuable and necessary service to the poor of the lower East Side of New York City under difficulties. There are no private patients." But Gouverneur's "ancient structures and facilities need replacement badly," it continued. "The administration and the medical staff in spite of being handicapped by these facilities are doing a worthy job."[54]

In 1954, a renewed campaign for a replacement facility escalated after Basil MacLean, the commissioner of hospitals at the time, abruptly scrapped plans for a new facility.[55] Two years later, the Lower Eastside Neighborhoods Association (LENA) circulated a petition among volunteers who canvassed the neighborhood to obtain 20,000 signatures.[56] The campaign was just one in a flurry of actions to pressure the city for a commitment. Spearheaded by LENA's Health

Committee, its participants made the case for a new hospital by pointing not only to the facility's degradation but to the aggregate socioeconomic status of the neighborhood and the high child-to-adult ratio, which necessitated maternal and child health care. Geographically, the two closest alternatives to Gouverneur were outside the area, northward at Twenty-Eighth Street or southward at Chambers Street, around City Hall and other administrative buildings. And the current Gouverneur building itself, LENA noted, stood outside major bus lines, requiring some residents to make a "long and arduous trip" if they wished to visit. Accentuating this spatial dimension meant envisioning the hospital as a vital neighborhood anchor. "We are deeply convinced that our community needs a new and enlarged hospital to replace Gouverneur, centrally located so as to be easily accessible to the children and elderly people in our neighborhoods," LENA noted.[57] A modern hospital was a solution to the crisis of medical maldistribution on the Lower East Side.

LENA's campaign occurred on the heels of a report by the Hospital Council of Greater New York, which studied Lower Manhattan's population trends to issue recommendations on medical care infrastructure for the area. Its chief goal was to evaluate whether a planned addition of 1,300 general care beds to the area would be better allotted entirely to northward Bellevue Hospital, a much larger facility affiliated with three universities, or spread between Bellevue and Gouverneur. Surprisingly, the council wrote sympathetically about rebuilding Gouverneur. In language remarkably similar to LENA's—that is, the language of community—the council noted that a new hospital would be "a focal point of the community's interest in health and medical care" and "a meeting ground for the physicians practicing in the neighborhood."[58] Together, neighborhood pressure and establishment support convinced the city to revive the Gouverneur project.[59] But despite these rhetorical and monetary reassurances, Gouverneur advocates openly wondered whether the transition would ever occur. In the *East Side News* just days before the end of 1960, George Freedman, director of the New Era Club Lecture Forum, asked: "Is the new Gouverneur Hospital a mirage?" before reviewing a decade of promises repeated, then broken.[60] In early 1961, two events would justify this skepticism. In February, the Hospital Council of Greater New York reversed its position from a half-decade earlier and advocated closing Gouverneur, citing the decline of its residency program, accreditation problems, and Bellevue's availability to absorb patients.[61] In Trussell's first weeks as commissioner, he publicly opposed a new facility but delayed issuing a final word on the closure question until further assessment by his staff. But privately, Trussell had likely made up his mind already, having singled out Gouverneur for elimination during the Heyman Commission's meetings.

Patients reacted anxiously to the limbo. Alejandro Felix's sentiments were representative: "I'm praying they keep this hospital open until a new one is built because I have four kids and Bellevue is much too far. You have to take two buses to get there and I'd have to take all of my children with me because I don't have a baby sitter."[62] In March, LENA organized City Hall protests. And it mounted arguments similar to those at Fordham and Elmhurst. In an impassioned memo to Trussell, LENA leaders argued that problems with the residency program and accreditation stemmed from the city's indifference to a decade's efforts of "calling the City Administration's attention to Gouverneur's obsolete plant." The only thing worse than that negligence was closure and the disruption that would result.[63]

But there was a key difference from the Bronx and Queens battles, too. Advocates for Gouverneur never rejected affiliation. Indeed, they *embraced* it as a solution to the institution's woes, especially as an alternative to closure. Detailing what an ideal Gouverneur might look like, LENA raised the prospect of Gouverneur serving as a "hospital for our local community" and a smaller satellite facility to Bellevue. Far from trying to steer a course completely independent of private facilities like their counterparts at Fordham, Gouverneur's advocates openly wished for stronger affiliations, as evidenced by previous overtures to New York University and nearby Beth Israel Medical Center.[64]

The receptiveness toward affiliation explained the city's willingness to save Gouverneur at the eleventh hour through Mayor Wagner's intervention. The city would close Gouverneur's inpatient services but would expand the outpatient department, turning it into an experimental ambulatory clinic affiliated with nearby Beth Israel and administered by one Howard J. Brown, a former physician for the United Auto Workers' medical care program in Detroit. In 1954, he'd moved to the city and served as the director of professional services at the Health Insurance Plan of New York, a network of clinics heavily used by union members.[65] Brown came out of a New Deal milieu that hatched numerous experiments in medical care delivery across the country, most backed by organized labor. All were part of a vision, as historian Jennifer Klein has shown, of "health security."[66]

Brown had spent much of his career learning about workers' social environments and how that affected their health care usage. Now he took the same ideas to the Lower East Side. When he took over Gouverneur, he swiftly sought to create a two-way feedback loop between it and the surrounding patient population. This was to be no ordinary facility. Gouverneur instead cultivated relationships with Lower East Side social service agencies, using them to inform patients about Gouverneur and to learn about the social context of their health problems. The hospital not only hired employees directly from the Lower East Side but made sure they possessed language ability—Spanish, Chinese, and Yiddish—appropriate for an ethnically diverse Lower East Side population that was 29 percent Puerto Rican, 3.2 percent Chinese, and almost a quarter first-generation immigrants who'd lived in the area for less than five years.[67]

Brown also instituted continuity-of-care clinics, whereby a patient would see the same physician on repeat visits. He achieved this through the hiring of a stable staff consisting of "seven internists, six pediatricians, and two general surgeons," alongside forty part-time physicians.[68] At its best, continuity of care itself fostered closer patient-doctor relations and familiarity.

The early successes were impressive, and Gouverneur's national profile grew. In the *Milbank Memorial Fund Quarterly*, an influential health policy journal, Brown and his associate director, Harold L. Light, described "basic operating principles" undergirding a relationship between larger community and service provider. Medical care couldn't be delivered in a vacuum. Rather, it was to be offered "in a manner which was conducive to meeting the patient's psychological, social and emotional needs as well as his biological ones." Indeed, "the patient functioned as part of a larger milieu—in his own home and in the broader community—and these forces, therefore, must be taken into account if the service rendered was to be meaningful." It meant that patients weren't just passive but "would have, at all times, access to the administrator so that they might voice their views on the services rendered." The most powerful principle would soon prove to be a landmine, for it addressed the question of control and authority. It declared that "the community at large was entitled to a voice in the program and should share in the decision making process wherever possible."[69]

Operationally, evidence suggested enthusiasm for the new Gouverneur. Patient visits were increasing, especially for prenatal care, and there was a 25 percent decline in emergency room visits at nearby hospitals, suggesting that Lower East Side residents were no longer using emergency rooms as a major source for care.[70] The Gouverneur experience stood in contrast to the Fordham and Elmhurst standoffs, which had ended in uneasy detente (Fordham) or staff turnover and firing (Elmhurst). Meanwhile, the newly affiliated Gouverneur was pioneering a more innovative form of medical care delivery.

Into the mid-1960s, New York City officials had rapidly confronted three crises in medical care. Created to address maldistribution, New York City's celebrated hospital system found itself confronting a crisis of sustainability. That led to the institutionalization of affiliations, though hardly without resistance from varying forces opposing Ray Trussell's top-down implementation of the program. But though defused for the moment, this crisis in governance continued to simmer.

## Affiliation against the Ropes

Any era of good feelings around public hospitals and affiliation proved short-lived. In 1964, Mayor Wagner decided not to run for reelection, and a year later,

Trussell stepped down.[71] His successor was John Lindsay, a charismatic and telegenic liberal Republican who understood the power of the pulpit and committed himself to support for social services aimed at the city's most vulnerable. He understood and spoke the language of Black militancy, too, comparing the plight of some of the United States' urban neighborhoods—as were many radical activists—to the plundered nations overseas ravaged by colonialism and underdevelopment. The state of city health care didn't escape Lindsay's ire. During his 1965 campaign, he attacked his predecessor's signature health policy idea—affiliation—and made health care a priority.[72] His campaign materials bluntly assessed Trussell's program: "Nothing has changed today."[73]

Lindsay's blunt criticism presaged a raft of critical reports that appeared during his first term. All spotlighted affiliation's failure to fix the crisis of sustainability that had given rise to the policy. One sensational group of findings came from Governor Nelson Rockefeller's blue-ribbon commission on hospitals, whose lead investigator was Seymour Thaler, a brash state senator from Queens who submitted a shocking interim report in 1966. That year, Thaler had conducted site visits at almost all the municipal hospitals, and he'd found little about the postaffiliation world that was encouraging. At Kings County Hospital, a resident using an electrocardiogram told him: "I hope another more serious patient doesn't come in since there is no other electro-cardiogram available, and we would have to take this one away from this patient."[74] At two hospitals, he heard house staff complain about unreliable blood samples from laboratories. Suspecting problems, the physicians had sent the same blood in separate vials and received two different sets of results. Besides problems with reliable equipment and laboratory technology, the physical plants remained in lackluster, even outright abysmal, shape. At Fordham Hospital, Thaler watched surgeries in three operating rooms with open windows and no other ventilation. Broken locks allowed anybody to enter the swinging doors. Nearby, surgeons "scrubbed up across the hallway 20 feet from the operating rooms and then walked through a main corridor, occupied by visitors and hospital personnel."[75] Besides overcrowding, at another hospital, Thaler and his fellow inspectors found "an enormous accumulation of filth and debris in the basements of two buildings used for patient care," alongside walls with out-of-order water pumps.[76] "The number of needless deaths, to say nothing of the enormously increased misery, is incalculable," Thaler wrote.[77]

But beneath the surface horrors, Thaler suggested, lurked a systematic problem. One episode provided a window into what that might be. Thaler observed an eighty-two-year-old woman who had been admitted to Greenpoint Hospital after falling down the stairs and cracking multiple ribs. Greenpoint transferred her to Kings County Hospital without X-rays, which resulted in a prolonged wait for a repeat of the process. What seemed like a gratuitous transfer from one hospital to another was, Thaler learned, increasingly standard practice. The transfers occurred not by accident or disorganization. They were a regular result of hospitals wishing to rid themselves of patients without insurance or other means of payment by shuffling them to the most taxed of public hospitals. To Thaler—and subsequent investigators—this phenomenon, known as patient dumping, didn't just occur between public hospitals.[78] It actually seemed most commonly conducted by *private* institutions, which dumped patients into the public hospitals with which they were affiliated.

Dumping was just one of many indicators that the affiliations were more often parasitic than benign private-public resource sharing. In the longest section of his report, Thaler argued that use of affiliation money—more than $200 million since the start of the program—lacked oversight. Physicians drew double salaries from both private affiliates and public institutions. Institutions were using affiliation funds to provide "exorbitant" salary boosts to administrators. Many permanent staff supposedly hired for city hospitals didn't show up regularly. And equipment originally purchased for city hospitals sometimes found its way to private affiliates instead. In one case, a heart profusion pump intended for Metropolitan Hospital, a public facility in East Harlem, instead was transferred to New York Medical College's glitzy Flower Fifth Avenue Hospital. In other cases, purchased equipment simply languished, unused and in storage, without explanation. In short, affiliation had become a money funnel, wasteful, and, above all, a means of diverting resources away from city hospitals and to private institutions.[79] What Thaler had observed on his hospital tours were symptoms of a new institutional arrangement that lacked needed oversight.

Thaler's report contained no small measure of political grandstanding mixed with genuine concern. A Queens politico at heart, he chose the most vivid and shocking set pieces to underscore his charge that the hospitals were nowhere near the quality that affiliation was supposed to help attain. And he was hardly immune from selective deployment of data. In one section on the state of internship programs at affiliated hospitals, for example, he noted an anemic to nonexistent rise in interns at Coney Island, Queens General, Greenpoint, Fordham, and Elmhurst, while failing to discuss the dramatic increases that had occurred at institutions like Morrisania and Harlem. Moreover, he probably wasn't the best public face to be mounting an antiaffiliation case. (Five years later, he'd be convicted of trafficking stolen U.S. Treasury bills.)

Still, subsequent findings by other governmental bodies substantiated the overall thrust of Thaler's charges. The final Rockefeller commission report, released later in 1967, noted "inadequate upkeep of physical facilities, insufficient supplies," and "obsolete and insufficient equipment," too.[80] In 1968, New York State issued another report, confirming not only these conditions but numerous "fiscal abuses" that contributed to them. The abuses included sloppy maintenance of inventory, plus the transfer of affiliation money into bank accounts that accrued interest, all subsequently pocketed by the private medical centers.[81] Affiliation, at worst, was a piggy bank for private medical centers, and it was looking like anything but a resounding success. Into the 1970s, given the mounting scandal, it was unclear whether affiliation would survive.

## Affiliation: A Future Uncertain

The two most influential assessments of affiliations went beyond cataloging problems. They instead asked: where to next? One was sponsored by the Washington, D.C.–based Institute for Policy Studies, a left-leaning think tank, and it accentuated the program's exploitative and undemocratic qualities. Written by Robb Burlage, a founding member of Students for a Democratic Society (SDS), the report recommended an end to "omnibus" affiliations, which had been marked by "too much uncontrolled domination by the scattered 'private' and 'academic' sectors of health service." In its place would be a centralized agency, which Burlage called the Metropolitan Health Services Commission, to oversee the municipal hospitals, and, as critical, District and Neighborhood Health Planning and Review Councils. These councils would be made up of residents providing bottom-up policy input—that is, the critical voice of the community—which had been lacking in affiliations up to this point. Burlage's proposal was infused with the intellectual influence of the American New Left—he'd written passages in SDS's founding Port Huron Statement—and its key thinkers' push for "participatory democracy": more decision-making influence by everyday people on the powerful institutions that affected—and disrupted—their lives. For Burlage, that included private medical institutions: unaccountable and autocratic in all the ways that SDS had famously criticized.[82]

Burlage's interest in the New York medical world wasn't just a random curiosity. It grew out of the political storms that greeted affiliation's initial rollout. The Institute for Policy Studies received much of its funding from Samuel Rubin, the member of the Fordham Hospital Lay Advisory Committee who'd been instrumental in the campaign to save the facility from closure and who'd funded newspaper ads on its behalf. The experience had left Rubin obsessed with how power flowed in the New York health care sector. After Burlage's report appeared and received coverage in the *New York Times*, Rubin gave him additional seed money to start a small New York City–based think tank called the Health Policy Advisory Center (Health/PAC), which would monitor and critique the city's health policy, expanding on the original Burlage report. In the winter of 1968, the *Health/PAC Bulletin*, the organization's newsletter, explicitly compared the relationship between the private medical centers and the public hospitals to imperial powers and their colonies, a direct influence of "Third Worldist" revolutionary movements that grew out of two decades of decolonization, plus mounting opposition to the Vietnam War.[83] The analogy was explosive. Affiliation wasn't just corrupt; it was racist and exploited the minority patients who made up a large number of public hospital patients.

Another rhetorically less scorching, but still pointed and critical, report grew out of an investigation ordered by Mayor Lindsay. Chaired by *Scientific American* editor Gerald Piel, the so-called Piel Report appeared about six months after Burlage's. Like Burlage's report, the Piel Report found lingering problems with affiliation and spared no words in saying so. Treatment at municipal hospitals failed to "provide an adequate setting for modern medical care."[84] Unlike Burlage and Health/PAC, however, the Piel Report didn't center unequal power relations between private and public institutions. Instead, it focused on labyrinthine municipal bureaucracy. The Piel Report turned the tables on the city itself, arguing that ossified administrative procedures, irrespective of private affiliates' conduct, impeded effective health provision and implementation of affiliation. Many problems identified still lingered—plants in disrepair, equipment hoarded, fuzzy accounting—and resulted from directives having to flow through a gauntlet of agencies, including the Bureau of the Budget, the Comptroller, the Board of Estimate, and the Departments of Personnel, Public Workers, and Welfare, to say nothing of the ones dealing directly with health. Moving from an idea on paper to an approval to execution within this "fractionation of authority" was glacial. Even bureaucratic fixes designed to respond to problems ended up worsening them and creating more organizational bloat. As the report put it, "[Their] cumulative impact has so hamstrung administration and delivery that, were it not for the activities of many extremely dedicated personnel—heroes of quiet determination—the 'system' would come to a complete breakdown."[85] For Piel, red tape was the fundamental problem. Still, affiliation abuses weren't off the hook, either. There existed "no provision for accountability other than a post-audit of the voluntary hospital's books," and above all, affiliations created disorganized and "divided management"—additional "fractionation"—between two sets of administrators, one from the city, the other from the private affiliate itself.[86] At the same time, according to Piel, affiliations had accomplished one of their earliest goals, to improve staffing shortages at residency programs in a number of city hospitals.

Burlage and Health/PAC and the members of the Piel Commission came from very different political and professional orbits: the first from student radicalism and neighborhood activism, the second from the science and medical establishment. Their different appraisals of affiliation obscured major common points. Both agreed that the current system remained fragmented, lacked accountability, and required a centralized administrative unit. But whereas

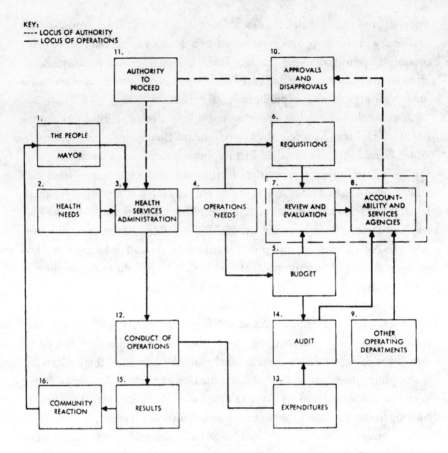

Figure 18. The Present Health
Care Delivery System:
Fractionation of
Authority

**Labyrinthine Bureaucracy.** In this flow chart, the Piel Commission conveyed the maze one had to navigate in the hospital system as it existed in the 1960s. Its members were making the case for a centralized entity that could streamline a number of these functions.

*Source*: "Problems, Causes, Solutions," in *Community Health Services for New York City: A Case Study in Urban Medical Delivery*, ed. Robert B. Parks (New York: Praeger, 1968), 508.

Burlage advocated for an entity that remained within city government, the Piel Commission pushed for a chartered nonprofit corporation operating autonomously outside of formal city structures. This Health Services Corporation would receive city funding and have its officers appointed by the mayor, but a high level of administrative independence would free it from the bureaucratic cobwebbing that the Piel Commission had criticized. An administrator wishing to order equipment for a city hospital would now deal with a single agency's protocols alone rather than a web of other nonhealth agencies that had a hand in expenditure approvals.

A series of supplementary briefs went further than the Piel Report itself and probed the larger context in which reform of medical care occurred. One paper, entitled "Community and Institutional Needs," summarized the state of health services in each of the city's boroughs, noting woeful maldistribution in numerous geographic areas, especially outside Manhattan, which possessed the highest concentration of facilities. But it juxtaposed data on medical availability with larger contextual details, including such alarming health trends as elevated infant mortality rates in high-poverty neighborhoods such as Harlem and the Lower East Side. The interconnectivity of the social and the medical was striking: "High infant mortality rates indicate not only low income, but all the depressing correlates of poverty: high incidence of tuberculosis and venereal diseases; low level of education and income, high crime rates and juvenile delinquency, crowded and deteriorated housing."[87] If the actual Piel Report hewed mostly to technocratic amelioration, these attached briefs questioned—albeit understatedly—the larger social order and its discontents. Here, Piel did converge with Burlage. Both saw health deprivation as rooted in unequal resource distribution at large.

Beneath these observations lurked an indirect question: How important a dent could health services innovation really make amid these challenges outside the medical sphere? And what were the implications for future medical care policy? It was a question that health policy reformers in New York City and elsewhere asked throughout the decade, often without answering via a direct policy response. For the Piel Commission, the closest consideration came when its members discussed, in one supplemental paper, recalibrating relations between traditional medical institutions and their environs. Its members declared that "the health services system must manifest itself deeply in the community. . . . It must become identified with the local community. It must 'explain itself' through information programs that improve community understanding of available services and possibilities for self-help. The interface between the community and its health services must be made as uncomplicated, inviting and efficient as possible."[88] One way to accomplish this was through the creation of smaller and decentralized facilities (not just traditional large city hospitals) that'd "serve a smaller community and, potentially at least, would enjoy a closer involvement in community life." It was exactly what the Gouverneur experiment was attempting to do on the Lower East Side.[89] And it was successful enough that it'd soon go national.

## The War on Poverty and the Crisis of Governance

The Lower East Side experiment unfolded in a New York City neighborhood alongside another one nationally: President Lyndon Johnson's Great Society and its attendant War on Poverty. Johnson's vision had huge health implications. Medicare insured all seniors, regardless of socioeconomic status. Medicaid offered insurance to the medically indigent, providing millions with access to institutions that had previously closed them off. But programs administered from on high weren't the only story, either. Nearly $1 billion went to a mix of programs—job training, housing, early childhood education (most famously, Head Start), and Peace Corps–like initiatives scattered all over the United States—that were largely implemented from below.

Health was no exception. In the opening days of President Johnson's War on Poverty, the federal Office of Economic Opportunity (OEO) got word of Gouverneur's early triumphs and used it as one of a few templates for its neighborhood health centers initiative. (The others were two centers that opened in Mound Bayou, Mississippi, and in Boston, devised in 1965 by Count Gibson and Jack Geiger, two physicians who'd been active in the civil rights movement.) The new federal program soon seeded similar facilities across the country.[90] These centers wouldn't just provide health care, though. They'd also allow patients to be play an active role in it, as part of OEO's Community Action Program. It mandated that any agency receiving its funds, health or otherwise, needed to ensure "maximum feasible participation" of poor laypersons (or representatives of them) in decision-making, typically in the form of community councils.[91] For War on Poverty–funded organizations across the country—whether in health, housing, job training, or whatever else—this led, at least in theory, to the sharing of the helm, and its authority, with new and unfamiliar hands.

For Gouverneur, it meant the creation of the Lower East Side Neighborhood Health Council–South, whose formal mandate was "the review of applications for OEO assistance, the establishment of program priorities, the selection of the project director," plus input into various programmatic issues that might arise.[92] Tests of how much power the council really had would soon lead to conflict. And the Gouverneur experiment's early years, colored by optimism, soon gave way to familiar challenges around governance.

But in its very first days in 1967, the health council focused on organizing work, and conflict would come later. In practice, the activities of lay councils like it varied across the country. Some mainly restricted themselves to little more than take-it-or-leave-it advice given at an arm's distance. But many became more deeply involved, and the Lower East Side health council was one of them. Its first head was Antolin Flores, who'd arrived in New York City from Puerto Rico twenty years previously and came from a long career in tenant advocacy. His two partners included Terry Mizrahi, a community organizer who'd recently graduated from Columbia's School of Social Work, and Martin Rosenberg, a Gouverneur employee.[93]

Day to day, this work of the council extended the efforts of the early Gouverneur and the hospital's forging of links with those living around it. One way was through door-to-door interactions that simultaneously ascertained health problems and connected patients to Gouverneur. Its style had more than a little in common with the methods of community organizers like Saul Alinsky, whose Chicago-based Industrial Areas Foundation had been conducting trainings in similar kinds of techniques for two decades.[94]

One example of community health organizing came in the summer of 1967, when the council carried out a study researched by ten "health aides" from the Lower East Side, all between the ages of eighteen and twenty-two. The survey asked residents how many times they'd visited Gouverneur, what exact services they'd used, how long they'd spent in the waiting room, and whether language barriers had posed a problem. Respondents rated their treatment from Gouverneur's different employees from "very well" to "poorly" and had the opportunity to describe in their own words "how Gouverneur can serve you better."[95] Some of the survey results were very encouraging. On usage of services, most respondents stated that they would visit a hospital rather than stay home. Seventy-five percent also reported that they'd seen a physician in the past year, knew of health care facilities in the area, and "more often than not found them to be satisfactory or very satisfactory," though a "substantial minority" also reported dissatisfaction and little outreach. Only 5 percent had never seen a doctor. And about two-thirds carried a Medicaid card, though one-third didn't and received more information on how to obtain one from the council's health aides.[96]

Although the survey responses suggested that early Gouverneur outreach efforts had paid off, the council's own report was far from celebratory. It declared that "even with its competent medical institutions, parts of the Lower East Side continue to be a breeding ground for some of the worst social problems." Questions on housing issues yielded substantial complaints, particularly about housing quality and landlord abuse. Elsewhere, the respondents pointed to many unanticipated problems, some of which fell outside a narrower, strictly medical, conception of health. Many profiles of residents developed this theme. "Mr. and Mrs. C." were a couple expecting a child. They struggled on welfare and lived in an "unsanitary" apartment where the toilet stood in a hallway outside, part of a building "filled with rats" and housing many drug addicts. An "old and sick" woman, "Mrs. M," lived in isolation, was on welfare, and had "trouble cashing checks." She was lost in the public assistance system, "never see[ing] the same welfare investigator twice," "get[ting] promises but no results." She was "afraid of leaving her apartment" and couldn't convince Gouverneur to "pick her up and bring her to the clinic because it is not an emergency." Isolation was "Mr. Y's" way of life, too. "He has diabetes, epilepsy, heart condition and glaucoma," the report noted. "He cannot get out or around. He says his welfare investigator was no help to him." The story of "Mrs. C" on Pitt Street was the most tragic. A former drug addict, she had gone missing before the health aides could intervene. As the report related, she had "no place to live and no money to buy food and clothing." Her sister had thrown her out, and "she disappeared soon thereafter."

Taken together, the cases formed an argument: health was affected by a panoply of social influences. This was similar to what the Piel Commission had concluded. But that report had been written dispassionately, a data analysis of anonymized mortality trends. The health council's account came from the realm of lived local experience and direct observation. Area residents themselves had linked "narcotics addiction," "welfare," "bad housing," and "poor health" when asked what they thought the Lower East Side's most severe problems were. The council stated the links even more explicitly: "The target neighborhood has one unifying factor—*poverty*!" "Health," it determined, "is broader than the absence of disease particularly in low income neighborhoods. Improved mental, physical, and environmental health is as much tied to improving the conditions of housing and welfare as it is to building new and better medical and health structures."[97]

The health council's work grew, and it concluded that it needed a full-time paid staffer, not just volunteers. It was a decision that sparked periodic governance fights with Gouverneur's private affiliate, Beth Israel, which administered the facility.[98] These battles had roots in how OEO commonly distributed funds to lay councils. Instead of being sent directly to the councils, OEO dollars went to an intermediary. It meant that lay councils' actions ultimately depended on the good faith of a middleman separating them from OEO. On the Lower East Side, that entity was Beth Israel.

On the surface, the council's desire to hire a full-time health advocate didn't suggest trouble. A job ad called for someone who could "maintain existing [communication] with the community and seek to expand ties between individuals in the community, community groups and the Health Council with Gouverneur." But what did "expand ties" entail, and how much authority would Beth Israel and Gouverneur really share with the council and, by extension, the community? The council had reason to answer worrisomely, for Beth Israel's new director was none other than Ray Trussell, who'd landed there after leaving his city post, one where he'd shown little inclination to attain any buy-in from the lay public. When the council identified its choice for the position and

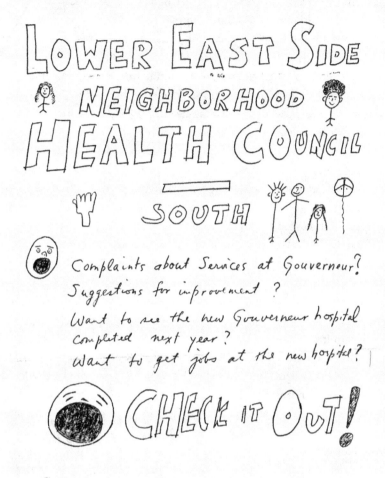

The Lower East Side Neighborhood Health Council - South is a federal
funded agency. Its board membership is made up of community people living

**Lower East Side Neighborhood Health Council–South outreach poster, ca. 1967–68.**
*Source*: In private collection.

asked Gouverneur administrators for additional OEO funds to hire her, Trussell refused.[99]

Trussell's instinctual aversion to lay input wasn't the only problem. So was the health council's actual pick: Gloria Cruz. Cruz happened to be one of the most publicly visible leaders of the Young Lords Party, a revolutionary group modeled after the Black Panthers that fused Marxism and Puerto Rican nationalism.[100] Cruz had become heavily involved with the Health Revolutionary

Unity Movement (HRUM), a health-focused spin-off of the Young Lords. The group had developed a political platform based on the Panthers' ten-point program.[101] It demanded "total self-determination of all health services in our oppressed communities through community-worker boards" and "complete decentralization of health services and their control to meet the needs of our local communities." Apart from demanding more control over health facilities, HRUM called for them to catalyze economic betterment, demanding "complete upgrading and career ladders for all people" they employed. Last, it urged education to "expose all the leading health problems, unemployment, poor housing, racism, malnutrition, police brutality, and all other forms of exploitation."[102] The rhetorical gloss, for sure, was far more explosive than the council's. But fundamentally, the council and HRUM shared core interests in community empowerment: hence, the selection of Cruz.[103]

Unsurprisingly, Trussell balked at Cruz. She likely recalled for him the tempests—in far more revolutionary and radical a form—that'd greeted him in the early days of the affiliation plan. Moreover, calls for "community control" were exploding across the country, including in New York City around public schools. The council fought hard for Cruz as its pick for health advocate and forced Trussell to reverse his veto, but only after an appeal to OEO's Washington, D.C., office.[104]

Securing Cruz's appointment didn't end strife between the health council and HRUM on one end and Ray Trussell and Beth Israel on the other. It'd be the first of many fights. In June 1968, Beth Israel had distributed a family planning program proposal to the council for its input, then proceeded to ignore the council's feedback entirely, making Beth Israel's contact with the council a token gesture.[105] The grievances accumulated. In August 1969, Trussell removed from Gouverneur's OEO annual grant a proposal for employee job training and career ladders, all without ever consulting the council.[106] It was enough to convince the council that it ought to adopt formally HRUM's ten-point program. The following month, fifty members from both organizations forcefully entered Trussell's office after another veto, made without council input, of a Gouverneur-based cancer screening clinic that the American Cancer Society had proposed.[107] Two months later, in November 1969, the council again felt relegated to token advisory status when the Gouverneur directorship freed up and Trussell's handpicked choice, Reinaldo Ferrer, took office over the health council's objections.[108]

A final, explosive turning point came in December 1969, when the health council received a sympathetic letter from Harvey Karkus, a Gouverneur doctor who had openly deplored Trussell's imperious conduct and promptly lost his job. A few days later, in January 1970, 120 people confronted Trussell in protest. A "shoulder to shoulder police barricade," in the words of one account, greeted the protesters. Officers arrested four people, including two workers and Gloria Cruz, all of whom were fired.[109] The actions left the council indignant and created a full-blown crisis of governance. In a letter to Congressman Leonard Farbstein, the council's first organizer, Terry Mizrahi, wrote that "since Dr. Trussell came on the scene, conditions have deteriorated and community and workers have lost confidence in Beth Israel." The firings were "an illegal and immoral act," reflective of a "contemptuous attitude shown throughout."

But tensions developed on the advocates' side, too. Staking a claim to speak for the community was fraught with ambiguities. Many questions arose about the wisdom of the council's choice of Gloria Cruz as the full-time health advocate and, more broadly, its decision to ally with political revolutionaries such as HRUM. A surprising criticism came from Local 1199, the hospital workers' union that represented Gouverneur's employees.[110] Local 1199 was no ordinary union. It historically had been active in opposing racial discrimination in hiring and had more than its own fair share of members with left-wing and communist pasts in the rank and file and leadership. In a letter to Trussell, OEO, and Gouverneur's head of services, Gouverneur's Local 1199 workers described Cruz as a "highly destructive force at Gouverneur" who had "created antagonism among the employees and between staff and patients." She had "tended to exacerbate the situation and increase the existing tensions of the patient and staff." They concluded: "We welcome a community representative who would help us to improve services at Gouverneur but we feel that Mrs. Cruz is not that person. Her past actions indicated she was a negative influence in the area of patient-staff relations."[111] The letter contained several hundred signatures, most from unionized 1199 workers, whom one could hardly characterize as the political tools of Beth Israel.[112]

The health council realized that its alliance with HRUM and Cruz posed problems. It didn't directly defend them but instead deferred to general governance principles. Whatever the foibles that might exist in revolutionary groups, council members argued that Beth Israel's dismissal of Cruz, *their* choice for a patient advocate, breached proper OEO protocol. Process, in other words, was principle. The council received outside support for its view. Ella Strother, a member of a similar lay medical board in Baltimore, had learned of the Gouverneur fracas and wrote to Stephen Joseph, an OEO operative, declaring Trussell's actions a violation of OEO participation mandates. Strother further declared that "for the first time," neighborhood residents were "active participants in a health care system rather than passive recipients of services. Representatives of the residents of the community, functioning as a neighborhood health council or health association, share in policy-making for the center, making certain that the services offered, and the manner in which they are offered, are responsive to the needs of the people in the neighborhood." The health council and Cruz were part of that shift in power and had been treated "shamefully."[113]

But arguments about HRUM's role continued, and they raised important questions over what exactly "community" constituted and the legitimacy of those who claimed to speak for it. In protesting Trussell's actions and the firings, the council and HRUM consistently invoked the "community" notion and their role as a critical conduit between it and a hierarchical medical giant. But how much community cohesion in fact existed? There was little evidence that Local 1199's rank and file were fully committed to HRUM's leadership, after all. "While HRUM claimed its goal was improved health care for the community," an 1199 *Drug and Hospital News* piece read, "it was unable to demonstrate any significant community support."[114]

An OEO employee assigned to the Lower East Side situation, Laura Ackerman, picked up on the community rhetoric's tensions. She blamed the rancor, in part, on the imprecise legislative language—"maximum feasible participation," "direct involvement of the people"—that either side could invoke in its favor. Beth Israel, for example, "[felt] that community involvement is a process wherein non-professional people are given education by hospital professionals concerning health care." For Beth Israel, community participation simply meant outreach and health education. For the health council, it meant those things but shared governance as well. In the words of Ackerman, the council saw "itself as a lay board of directors which understands the health needs of the community and is qualified to have a policy making voice and to act as an advocate for patients."[115] OEO ultimately sided with the council, and it reversed Trussell's actions by reinstating Cruz. At the same time, it required the council to draft a more precise "work plan," cosigned with Beth Israel, to create a formal system of negotiation in the event of future conflict.

On balance, OEO's arbitration was favorable to the council and resulted in a momentary cooling down from the confrontation of the previous years. It was a necessary de-escalation. Combat over governance had exacted a toll on service. A 1969 council survey of patients revealed considerable patient frustration. Some of the complaints about personnel included "carelessness and indifference of medical staff particularly the doctors," "rushed examinations," "lack of respect and concern for feelings of patient and/or patient's family," and "insensitive treatment of patients, particularly non-English speaking patients." This came on top of complaints about long wait times, misplaced charts, a low number of translators, inadequate transportation to Gouverneur, and an overall "inability to relate to the needs of the patients."[116] The new work plan addressed these shortcomings. Although it contained clearer mandates for communication between the health council and the Beth Israel administration, the plan focused on improving health outreach and on creating new preventative health programs, particularly screening for tuberculosis, anemia, nutritional disease, lead poisoning, and cancer detection (controversy over which had resulted in one of the Trussell confrontations). It suggested a renewed focus on medical care itself, rather than community health politics, at least for the time being.[117]

At the level of city politics, potential additional calm came with the founding of the Health and Hospitals Corporation (HHC) in July 1970. The city had chartered the HHC in response to the mounting criticisms over the affiliation. Inspired by the Piel Commission's recommendation for a new "public benefit corporation"—as such entities were now being called—city officials backed the HHC, believing that a single agency devoted to hospitals enabled stronger centralized oversight over affiliations and would prevent the documented abuses of the 1960s.[118] As important, HHC received budgetary independence, managing its finances and avoiding the bureaucratic morass endured by a traditional city agency.

The Health and Hospitals Corporation meant changes in the affiliation landscape. In the case of Gouverneur specifically, Ray Trussell would be removed from the equation. Beth Israel administrators wanted to phase out their affiliation with Gouverneur in a couple of years, after construction was finished on a long-promised new Gouverneur Hospital. The new Gouverneur would come under the direct control of HHC—not of a private medical institution led by the controversial Trussell.[119] In late 1971, the health council shifted its focus to the handover of Gouverneur. It met with HHC chairman Joseph English, expressing hope for a better relationship with HHC.[120] That hope was short-lived. As part of the transition, Beth Israel had designated HHC the sole grantee of federal funds, and when HHC applied to renew Gouverneur's grant for the 1972–73 cycle, it left only vague provisions for the council's participation in governance. The corporation admitted as much, referring only to "contacts engaged in by the applicant with two community groups" before elaborating on "significant problems in relation to community participation."[121] The actions hardly suggested a reversal from the days of Beth Israel. In February 1972, Terry Mizrahi denounced the HHC in a fierce public statement and repeatedly pressed against the decision to include no provisions for involvement of laypersons in decision-making.[122]

The latest fight proceeded on two levels. The council, with the help of Mobilization for Youth (MFY)'s legal services, filed a federal lawsuit that charged administrators at Beth Israel, Gouverneur, and HHC with violating OEO guidelines on community participation and with instituting an "effective revocation" of its role. The involvement of MFY wasn't surprising. Born in the early John F. Kennedy administration, MFY originated as a social service agency devoted to preventing youth delinquency. But soon, thanks to the participation of activists and community organizers, many of them political radicals, its activities had expanded greatly beyond this initial purview and into advocacy for welfare recipients and exploited tenants.[123] The MFY-assisted lawsuit requested that the court mandate the council's participation or else revoke $2 million worth of federal funds that HHC had received for Gouverneur.

While that lawsuit made its way through the legal system, the council filed a separate grant application with the federal government to become direct recipient of federal allocations. The conflict made the major New York City papers, with Ray Trussell remarking to the *Daily News*: "You can't have civil disorder and medical care in the same four walls."[124] On May 23, 1972, the U.S. District Court for the Southern District of New York handed down a decision favorable to the council, issuing an injunction mandating the HHC and Beth Israel to offer it an official participatory role.[125] In his opinion for the court, Judge Morris Lasker similarly concluded that the HHC had contained "no provision for a neighborhood health council," as required by OEO guidelines. "We do find," he explained, "that the law requires either a properly structured board of directors or a neighborhood council to participate in planning and other aspects of the project. Neither is provided for in the grant to HHC." But at the same time, in a nod to the vexing politics of community, the court questioned whether *the council* ought to serve as the long-term community representative. Still, until a "substitute body [was] available," the health council, which Lasker acknowledged had amassed a track record over the years, would have to serve in the capacity mandated by the OEO legislation.[126]

The council had won a lease for itself, fortuitously timed with the September 1972 groundbreaking of a fourteen-story, 216-bed new Gouverneur Hospital that it and generations of Lower East Siders had fought for. To applause, Mayor Lindsay declared that "the delivery of high quality health services should be the number one item on the agenda of America for the decade to come."[127] The high mood existed, however, alongside Gouverneur patients' continued grievances, which appeared in a new official newsletter where patients had considerable space to vent. One nursing aide said she'd "like to see the attitudes of the doctors changed. I think because doctors came from wealthy families. They [have] lots of schooling and they look down on people." Another: "Once, the doctor yelled at a clerk who was making a phone call. He assumed that she was making personal phone calls. Actually, she was making an appointment for a patient."[128] Jennie Sing complained about a five-hour wait. Rafael Carderol stated that "the first thing I would like to see changed is the personnel behavior in this hospital. When asking them questions, they are very nasty which I think is not very right. Like I said I came to the hospital with pains and when I asked the nurse if I could get analgetic because I needed it very badly, she just looked at me and walked away." Two Black workers complained, too, about whether Gouverneur Hospital would remain committed to the idea of hiring more workers from the surrounding neighborhood and wondered whether there existed employment discrimination against Black employees.[129]

But the newsletter, on a whole, carried a hopeful tone. Daniel Wong, one of the emergency room physicians, stated that he wanted to see people "have a feeling of belonging to the hospital." He explained: "I feel that no matter how much facilities we have, no matter how many personnel we have, if you don't have that feeling, it will just be another bureaucratic monstrosity." And the newsletter editorial declared: "If all of us begin to think from the patient's point of view, to start from their needs, we will have the beginning of a magnificent hospital that truly serves the community."[130] More than a decade after Howard Brown's founding of Gouverneur, his original principles seemed to be affirmed in the wake of so much conflict over a crisis of governance. But into the early 1970s, governance battles such as those at Gouverneur would recede in the face of emerging ominous threats to sustainability.

## Historical Contingency and Health Care: The Role of the 1975 Fiscal Crisis

Things seemed auspicious enough in 1970, when the state chartered the Health and Hospitals Corporation to address affiliation's shortcomings and oversee the entire system. Unfortunately, the early years of the HHC were an administrative comedy of errors. The corporation inherited a dated collections system from the city's Department of Hospitals that left it with a whopping $45.2 million deficit in its first year. On top of that, the city had allowed individual public hospitals (and, by extension, their private affiliates) to make personnel decisions autonomously—but with little oversight from the new agency, resulting in another $40 million overrun in 1971.[131] As HHC's first president put it later, such decentralized decision-making had occurred "prematurely," without sound economic footing and before an agreement with the city on its exact financial contribution in tax revenue to the HHC. The resulting debt stalled the agency's operations in its early years, with the HHC forced to implement a one-year hiring freeze that lasted until September 1972.[132]

The affiliations themselves proved a persistent headache. An audit conducted two years after the corporation's formation by the state comptroller's office found that affiliates filed mandated monthly expense reports irregularly and that most ended up spending less than the monthly advance made to them for their services. At best, the spending discrepancy was a sign that affiliates were spending money more efficiently than projected. At worst, it was evidence that institutions were using affiliation to hoard funds for other purposes or, in the words of a comptroller's investigation, creating "a major reserve of unneeded cash." Whatever the case, HHC oversight of the affiliations remained lax, with the amount advanced to private institutions unadjusted to their actual spending. The "contract-required practice of paying fixed advances, unrelated to expense needs, is wasteful of Corporation resources," the city later concluded, pegging the total excess amount at $10.3 million. A review of separate accounts, created by institutions for holding affiliation dollars, showed that many institutions made withdrawals that exceeded how much they *reported* for affiliation operating costs. In response, the HHC created a thicker firewall between funds specifically earmarked for affiliation and those used for an institution's general operations. It required that excess unused funds be placed in interest-bearing accounts designated solely for affiliation expenses.[133]

The greatest difficulties affecting the entire municipal health system weren't internal and administrative, however. They stemmed from wider political and economic pressures beyond it. Signs surfaced years before the city's infamous fiscal crisis in 1975. One involved the unreliability of Medicaid funds. In contrast to Medicare, which provided seniors with guaranteed medical insurance funded by the federal government, Medicaid programs were run by individual states and involved labyrinthine funding streams. The federal government, states, and on occasion large cities and counties worked out what percentage of a Medicaid allocation each would cover. The total Medicaid pie, in other words, consisted of federal, state, and sometimes municipal pieces. In New York, the state legislature forced a 25 percent New York City contribution to the program to help match a federal 50 percent appropriation.[134] This was a recipe for volatility. Any hiccup or alteration in any one leg of funding could disrupt Medicaid budgeting, usually forcing sudden cuts with reverberating consequences. In 1968, for instance, only a few years after New York State's Medicaid program had begun, it announced an alteration to eligibility requirements that eliminated 600,000 people from its rolls. That had a chain reaction: New York City had to ponder cutting hospitalization stays as a temporary solution to the sudden Medicaid revenue shortfall.[135] One estimate by an areawide planning agency guessed that Medicaid revenue could fall by as much as 20–30 percent because of the state's eligibility changes that year.[136]

Federal budget cuts in the era of Richard Nixon, Gerald Ford, and the New Federalism, which greatly shrank federal commitments to state and local governments, added still more pressure to city operations.[137] Just as the city recommitted itself to a series of major construction projects, including dozens of "neighborhood family care centers" modeled after facilities like Gouverneur, the Department of Health, Education, and Welfare announced a wave of targeted cuts. After receiving approval for a budget, two of the city's existing neighborhood health centers learned that they'd be facing a sudden 13 percent budget reduction requiring "existing programs and/or program elements . . . to be eliminated."[138] The action prompted heated comments from Gordon Chase, head of the city's Health Services Administration (a sister agency to the HHC in the process of being phased out). He remarked that the cuts demonstrated "Washington's disdain for cities and for their urban health problems."[139] That was a diplomatic way of characterizing the racist nature of the cuts, given the neighborhoods they affected the most and the changing city demographics resulting from two decades of white exodus. New York City's white population had tumbled from 90.2 percent in 1950 to 76.6 percent in 1970, paralleling trends in other cities across the country.[140]

Shrinking government funds for operating costs made public medical facilities more reliant on third-party insurance payments, whether private insurance, Medicare, or the precarious Medicaid. But of eight neighborhood health centers that the city oversaw, only three consistently drew more than 70 percent of their revenue from such sources.[141] The rest needed government financing. Increasingly, officials believed that service reduction or elimination might be the only option for such facilities without reliable third-party revenue. Health and Hospitals Corporation president Joseph T. English stated bluntly that "the survival of the Corporation's services, let alone their improvement, is dependent upon money"—namely, from governmental sources beyond New York City. English's observation was dramatic yet somehow didn't quite convey the gravity of the problem. The corporation was already on wobbly financial foundations, and the city had promised expensive buildings for deteriorating facilities.[142] These included new facilities in the Bronx (Lincoln and North Central Bronx Hospitals) and Brooklyn (Woodhull Hospital), the delays over which had prompted political restlessness and charges of neglect.

Fiscal pressures and perceptions of inefficacy led to the end of John Lindsay's mayoralty in 1973 and English's time at HHC. But New York City's health care problems were fundamentally structural, not the result of its executives. That became clearer in the run-up to early 1975, when the city learned that it had been cut off from credit markets and was at risk of imminent default. A confluence of forces had resulted in the city's crunch. Above all was loose administration and monitoring of cash flow, prevalent across dozens of agencies and exemplified by the HHC's early years. Because of an insufficient tax base, the city had taken to generous financing of operations with bond sales. It sold a staggering $8.3 billion and $900 million in short- and long-term bond notes, respectively, in fiscal year 1975, an increasingly untenable kicking of the budgetary can that delayed inevitable confrontation of fiscal problems. The breaking point came when banks refused to service city debts anymore.[143]

But the lender strike was symptomatic of a bigger problem. As historian Kim Phillips-Fein has argued, rollbacks in state and federal commitments to large cities had necessitated such borrowing in the first place.[144] This tendency persisted through the crisis itself, with the Ford administration and Congress infamously refusing to support bailouts to New York City. ("FORD TO NEW YORK CITY: DROP DEAD" read an infamous giant headline on the front page of the *New York Daily News*.) Instead, the city got the Municipal Assistance Corporation and the Emergency Financial Control Board (EFCB). For future revenue, these makeshift agencies agreed with financiers to swap out the city's short-term bonds for long-term bonds. The Municipal Assistance Corporation and EFCB then assumed control of city finances, slashing expenditures left and right, while imposing harsh austerity budgets in the hopes of restoring access to credit markets and paying down debt. When additional federal intervention finally did arrive, it came not in the form of aid but as short-term loans with rates pegged at 1 percent higher than Treasury bill interest rates. The cumulative result, historian Jonathan Soffer has noted, "creat[ed] a city in which almost nothing was maintained or repaired for a decade," after a 27 percent workforce reduction and a 75 percent decline in capital spending.[145]

The effects on the HHC, already struggling to gain fiscal and administrative footing in its infancy, were extremely pronounced. Between 1975 and 1980, a net payroll reduction of 17 percent reduced the total corporation workforce to what it had been at the start. Service cuts complemented workforce shrinkage. Between 1972 and 1982, average lengths of stay fell from 11 to 8.3 days, while the total number of "days of care" declined 23 percent. Five years after the crisis, bed capacity dropped by 18 percent. Even so, admissions by 1978 exceeded those in 1975, which indicated an overtaxed and underresourced system having to serve more people with far less.[146] The inability to revert to pre-1975 spending practices under the Municipal Assistance Corporation and EFCB's oversight meant that there was no alternative but to cut services—and then cut some more. This came on top of parallel slashing of the health department budget: "$10 million, or roughly 20 percent," administered in three rapid waves.[147]

The emergency agencies thus impeded one of HHC's very reasons for being: financial autonomy from city administration. By having to submit detailed budget plans for EFCB approval, HHC governance became as constrained as that of traditional city agencies. Far from pursuing its own independent sources of revenue, most of the corporation's financial planning entailed scaling down its ambitions and conforming to EFCB spending targets. In the first fiscal year after the crisis, the new agency reduced expenditures by $45 million to $1.4 billion, only to be pressed by the city's budget office into explaining why it had not carried out an originally projected cut of $65 million. Lack of HHC autonomy extended to minutiae. In the fall of 1975, Mike Holloman, the new HHC president, learned about the agency's subordination to myriad external forces when he found himself humiliatingly haggling with city micromanagers over the purchase of supplies for the long-delayed Lincoln Hospital building in the South Bronx.[148]

## The Consolidation of Affiliation

Encumbrance of HHC autonomy, though, was ultimately secondary to questions about the long-term survival of the public hospital system, and they were thrown into sharp relief by the 1975 crisis. Radically different views about the health care system's future quickly emerged. One camp was represented by Lowell Bellin, the city's new commissioner of health, and another by Ed Koch, then making a name for himself as a U.S. House representative.[149] Together, they privately pondered the possibility of getting rid of the public hospital system altogether, with exceptions for a facility here or there. In Koch's view, the $200 million of unreimbursed charity care provided by the municipal hospitals was a budgetary burden, though he never clearly stated where those patients might then go or what incentives private institutions might have for absorbing them. Bellin speculated that governmental reimbursement of health providers would keep increasing and eventually give way to more and more patients who would "vote with their feet," opting for private institutions over the municipal system. For Bellin, that would take the form of national health insurance, which he took as a given, despite its legislative failure during the Nixon administration. "The process of exodus from the municipals and entry to the voluntaries will be inexorable," Bellin predicted. "If my analysis is correct, then the question looms larger. Will the City remain in the municipal hospital business forever? . . . To what extent can the constituencies of the municipal hospitals . . . slow the inevitable?"[150] Later in the year, Bellin suggested that a large segment of the system—"hospitals with low occupancy and high per diem cost"—should be closed and that the HHC, so long as it refused to consider closure, was helping to "bleed all the hospitals including the viable ones."[151] Bellin's positions reflected a growing suspicion, exacerbated by the crisis, about whether a generous public sector was desirable and sustainable.[152]

The unfolding of the crisis kept talk of gutting the system alive, and Bellin soon aired his views publicly. One counterpoint came from Samuel Wolfe, a Columbia professor of public health. He had spent the earlier part of his career in Saskatchewan, helping to plan Canada's national health insurance program, before moving to Nashville, Tennessee, to set up a community health center. In an assessment of the public hospital system's problems, Wolfe faulted Bellin's belligerence and lack of support for the HHC. But apart from criticisms of Bellin's boorishness, there was more in common between Wolfe and Bellin than appeared on the surface. Although Wolfe didn't suggest that the municipal hospital system itself might be growing obsolete, neither did he argue that things ought to go on as usual. As analysts in other municipalities across the nation would also discover at the time—and as Bellin speculated—there *were* signs that inpatient usage at public hospitals was trending downward. Some of it, as historian Rosemary Stevens later observed, was due to the influx of Medicaid and Medicare, which allowed patients to take newly available dollars to private facilities.[153] Wolfe's analysis of two years of municipal hospital data showed that utilization rates of inpatient beds hovered consistently in the 70 percent range in four boroughs (excluding Staten Island), with a substantial number now used for functions other than health care delivery. Cuts targeted at them might thus have the dual effect of eliminating both redundant (and costly) excess capacity while adhering to budgetary imperatives posed by the fiscal crisis.[154]

For Wolfe, decisions about hospitals, whether about cuts or construction, had to be made after sober and rational inquiry about actually existing needs. Unfortunately, too many decisions made by New York City health care planners had been motivated by institutional self-interest, not dispassionate needs assessment. "It seems very evident . . . that local interests and pressures—often with powerful financial backing—have determined whether or not beds would be created. Whether they would be needed and how they would be used seems to have been another matter," he argued. This was a tactful but charged criticism of the power that affiliations had granted to private institutions. As an example, Wolfe pointed to the imminent completion of North Central Bronx Hospital, a public hospital, in 1976. North Central Bronx had been aggressively lobbied for by Montefiore and Martin Cherkasky, a strong ally of Trussell during the affiliation plan's implementation. Montefiore Hospital not only would serve as North Central Bronx's new affiliate but would also be located right next to it: a spatial configuration that Trussell and Cherkasky had advocated as paramount, one of more importance than even proximity and convenience to clientele. The North Central Bronx–Montefiore affiliation prompted Wolfe to write that "decisions about the creation of municipal hospital beds and the perpetuation of the municipal system of care have been made by spokesmen for the non-public sector over the years." Montefiore's role in locating North Central Bronx amounted to "irrationality" driven by the former.[155]

Just as perceptive were Wolfe's comments on how hospitals fit into larger neighborhood politics. As the neighborhood fights around hospitals demonstrated, residents infused the facilities with enormous political meaning that transcended surface concerns about medical needs. Wolfe elaborated that "a health facility creates jobs, job opportunities, secondary services in the surrounding community, and so on." It wasn't surprising, then, "that people will react with fury and anxiety combined when both their jobs and their health care security are under assault at the same time." It was a reason why "delay in paring down the municipal hospital system" might be wise, "a strategy to assure that caring and compassion be shown to the part of the community that will be affected."[156]

All the developments Wolfe explored—responding to harsh budgetary imperatives, reducing excess infrastructural costs, and navigating neighborhood political context—played out into the 1980s, especially after the 1977 election of Ed Koch as mayor. A year before, the city eliminated inpatient and emergency services at multiple municipal facilities, most notably Morrisania (Bronx), Gouverneur (Lower East Side), and Sydenham (Harlem). Fordham Hospital (Bronx), the center of a nasty standoff over city plans to shut it down two decades earlier, was closed outright this time round. The moves had come, first and foremost, as responses to EFCB demands on HHC. And they did contain some rhyme and reason, targeting the excess inpatient beds that Wolfe had discussed.

At the same time, the *manner* in which the cuts were administered reflected the emerging constellation of power within municipal health care. Fordham had a weak (and unwanted) affiliation with Misericordia, a small voluntary facility. Sydenham was an outlier that had never affiliated and had been eyed by Trussell for closure back in the days of the Heyman Commission on affiliation. Gouverneur's affiliation with Beth Israel had been strong yet wracked by discord and was coming to an end, albeit a drawn-out one. It, too, had come up repeatedly in the early Trussell deliberations about closure. Thus the EFCB and the fiscal crisis offered a pretext for closing or scaling back three facilities that had long been in the crosshairs. The opening of Montefiore-affiliated North Central Bronx in Fordham Hospital's catchment area only reinforced suspicions that private affiliates really called the shots, especially in a time of crisis. Morrisania, although affiliated with Montefiore, was deemed redundant and obsolete with the emergence of North Central Bronx, long championed by Montefiore.

But despite the power plays at work, it was difficult to argue that the closures themselves really generated a shortage of services, rather than simply reshuffling medical infrastructure into more concentrated institutional hands. Gouverneur still provided outpatient care and would now rely on New York University–affiliated Bellevue Hospital to the north for inpatient services. Given the rise in outpatient care demand—the opposite of the decline in inpatient—allowing Gouverneur to focus on this function might well have been a smarter use of resources. The new North Central Bronx Hospital accommodated gaps in services generated by Fordham's closure. And Sydenham, however powerful a neighborhood symbol, was decreasingly important as an actual provider of services when compared to Columbia University–affiliated Harlem Hospital. Warm neighborhood ties and collective memory of Sydenham were inaccurate

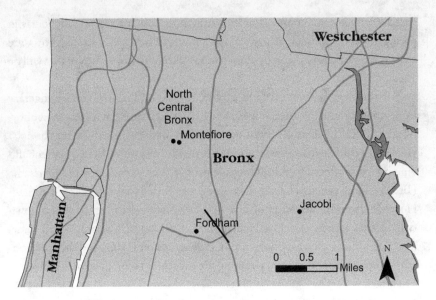

**Bronx hospital closures in the 1970s.** This map shows North Central Bronx and Montefiore together, alongside the closed Fordham and Jacobi, a more distant Bronx public hospital to the east, also affiliated with Montefiore. For many, this spatial arrangement demonstrated Montefiore's consolidation of regional power.
*Source*: Author's cartography.

indicators of how many people depended on it, though such sentiments had been enough to stave off its closure previously. The 1975 Harlem Community Health Survey, conducted by Harlem Hospital, found that Sydenham accounted for only 4.7 percent of hospital care in the Central Harlem area, compared to 25.1 percent for Harlem Hospital. The city's own data showed a low utilization rate, hovering in the mid- to high-60 percent range. Between 1973 and 1978, its daily census fell from 122 to 90 patients.[157]

Still, prompt outrage that had followed closures and cuts demonstrated the political volatility surrounding such moves—the "fury and anxiety" Samuel Wolfe had analyzed—especially when carried out with little consideration of their ramifications for workers. District Council 37, which represented a large share of public hospital employees, threatened to strike in May 1976, citing the closures and systemwide layoffs of 3,150 health personnel, including 1,450 at facilities with services to be trimmed. The strike was averted after an ad hoc panel chaired by state senator Basil Patterson, an influential political figure from Harlem, recommended a thirty-day review of the layoffs. It eventually halved their number while not recommending full reversal.[158]

Residents also perceived cuts as attacks on cherished neighborhood institutions. Even before the EFCB era, budget cuts had always struck an enormous emotional chord. At Gouverneur, one early budget protest emanated with moral outrage. At a demonstration in front of the city's Health, Education, and Welfare federal building, banners were emblazoned with such phrases as "War against Sick People" and jabs at individual department officials.[159] At another 1973 demonstration, Gustavo DeValasco, Gouverneur's new director, declared the cuts an assault on community health: "Those who work against the community will ultimately be unmasked by the community who will sit in judgment. In the time to come, every child in the Lower East Side will know who denied them the right to decent health care."[160]

The language of community recalled the governance struggles of the 1960s. But it occurred in a radically new context: one not of aspiration but, rather, of fiscal doom and gloom. Fights over single neighborhood institutions seemed quaint, less important now that the entire city (and, for that matter, the country) confronted structural upheaval that threatened the very fiscal footing of large swaths of the public sector. That became ever more apparent a few years after the brink of default when budgetary axes fell hard and fell rapidly. In 1978, the city moved swiftly to implement a "hospital closure incentive program" that compensated private affiliates for public facilities' shuttering. The policy allowed them to receive higher Medicaid reimbursements and move resources they'd otherwise spend on a discontinued affiliation to other operations in their fold.[161] And in 1979, an emboldened Ed Koch, far less sensitive to racial connotations of hospital closure than his predecessors, moved forward with plans to close Sydenham. One influential guiding hand in Koch's administration was none other than Montefiore's Martin Cherkasky, whom Koch had appointed as a special adviser on health. At one point, Cherkasky mused about the possibility of shrinking the municipal system by half, either through closures or sales of facilities to private institutions such as his own. As the lead proponent for the construction of North Central Bronx, Cherkasky had recently advocated that Montefiore purchase the public facility outright, a proposal that drew support from some policy makers at the state level, though never came to fruition.[162]

Other hospitals, such as Cumberland and Greenpoint Hospitals in Brooklyn, were eventually closed. Although both were affiliated, neither of their affiliations was particularly strong: Cumberland with a nonacademic voluntary institution, Brooklyn Hospital, and Greenpoint with Mount Sinai, which devoted far more attention to City Hospital at Elmhurst in Queens. Parallels existed, too, between the Brooklyn situation and that in the Bronx, where Fordham had closed and North Central Bronx had opened. For a decade, the city had planned a major new public facility, Woodhull Hospital, for Brooklyn to be affiliated with Downstate Medical School. Although delayed by the city's fiscal problems, when Woodhull opened, it eliminated much of the need for these smaller neighborhood institutions.[163] Thus, by 1983, the two Brooklyn facilities, along with Sydenham in Harlem, had closed.

What remained in the wake of the fiscal crisis was a municipal health care landscape transformed. With the fiscal crisis and a city functioning under an austerity budget for the next decade, it was hard for obstinate public hospitals that resisted affiliation to claim they could get along in a self-sufficient manner. Indeed, in such a context, affiliation appeared much more benign than harsher alternatives such as outright privatization. Far from a mere instantiation of inexorable "neoliberal" ascendancy or an example of public institutions' carrying water for "private interests" on the march, affiliation was one of many paths for a public hospital system struggling to bandage itself in the 1960s, and it was a solution with an uncertain and contested future into the early 1970s.[164] A decade later, it was hard to see any other means of saving public hospitals without the resource-sharing that affiliation afforded. It was the contingency of the fiscal crisis that entrenched it. As Kim Phillips-Fein and Suleiman Osman have argued, such post-1970s shifts originate from multitudes of sources: some premeditated and ideological, launched from the most rarefied global and national levels, others variations in local practices that over time resulted in new modes of governance. For New York City health care, it was, to borrow political scientist Timothy Weaver's heuristic, social transformation "by design" and, later, "by default."[165] The result was a public-private partnership of sorts, scaled down and consolidated in the hands of the city's unique cluster of private medical centers.

Predictably, the transformation had attracted heated protest and opposition, some extremely legitimate—the closures resulted in severe job losses—and some rooted more in a vision of autonomous and self-sufficient health care increasingly untenable even before the fiscal crisis. If one was to object to the new order, it was perhaps most convincing if focused less on the eventual outcome—the entrenchment of affiliation—than on the way it was achieved and the disproportionate influence given to certain movers and shakers such as Montefiore. By the end of the 1970s, it was clear that there existed a health analog to what journalists Jack Newfield and Paul DuBrul famously called "the permanent government," an unelected group of New York institutional stakeholders working behind the scenes and who clutched far more power than elected officials.

Through all the events, Ray Trussell, architect of the affiliations, had faded from the world of New York health politics, having alienated many supporters during his brief—but highly consequential—tenure as hospitals commissioner. When Trussell had announced his retirement from Beth Israel, he'd long been out of city office and exerted little direct influence on current policy makers. His marginalization, and in some quarters, disrepute were not unlike the final days of another flagrantly undemocratic New York planner, Robert Moses. But as with Moses, the foundations laid by Trussell had snowballed long after he had receded from a central position in the spotlight. Ten years after he exited the political stage, his unfinished planning revolution in New York City municipal health care was now complete. He was the most important local health bureaucrat most New Yorkers had never heard of.

In New York City, one man's vision had vanquished other competing ones in a fierce contest that played out over two decades. In Los Angeles, a decade before the affiliation wars, the opposite occurred and in a different domain of health politics: environmental health. There, angry residents, medical societies, the recreation sector, and the government itself formed a coalition to fight threats posed by rapid industrialization in the land of sunshine. Collectively, they yoked the language of community and civic duty with strong demands for air pollution control. Far from protracted combat, the demands yielded partial concessions from some of the worst culprits. Local health politics, this Los Angeles episode demonstrated, need not always be characterized by disunity. It could also yield the language of consensus.

# 2

# Los Angeles

## Two Cheers for Air Pollution Control: Triumphs and Limits of the Midcentury Industrial-Ecological Accord

When I was growing up in Los Angeles, my uncle would visit and never forget to mention how much more breathable things were up north. Smog and heavy traffic remain the most reliable standbys for making fun of the city and frequently appear in films satirizing Los Angeles culture. In Steve Martin's *L.A. Story*, a protagonist pulls off a crowded highway and sees an electronic billboard appearing to give him life advice. Similarly, Michael Douglas's *Falling Down* follows an antihero who finally snaps after sweating in his car while stuck in bumper-to-bumper congestion on a muggy and miserable day and goes on a ballistic rampage through the city. *Demolition Man* features a cryogenically frozen Sylvester Stallone waking up in 2032 only to be introduced by Sandra Bullock to a radically different Los Angeles, one where smoggy air has given way to pristine skies and where orderly processions of evenly spaced autonomous cars have replaced traffic snarls. It's a recurring visual joke.

For those who cling to these depictions of Los Angeles smog, it can come as a shock that the smog problem was once a lot *worse*. Bad as some days can be now, they pale in comparison to the midcentury era, when the local press would write about "daylight dim-outs," residents would instantly wheeze or cry involuntarily if they went outside, and thick blankets of smog covered the region for up to a week. For that improvement, unacknowledged though it is, they can thank the efforts of people like I. A. Deutsch.

Deutsch was an engineer from Chicago who came to Los Angeles in 1946 after officials had gotten word of his successes in controlling smoke from Midwest factories. They wanted to know if he had anything to offer more than 2.5 million residents who were suffering from the thick and foul fog everyone had simply started calling "smog." Deutsch spoke to a gathering of mayors from Los Angeles County, but his message wasn't encouraging. Los Angeles terrain was, well, weird and unique: ocean, flat basin, mountain range. It trapped pollution, and Chicago's example offered lessons of only limited value.

But Deutsch didn't leave the mayors hanging. On the contrary, he showcased—with gusto—various instruments that he'd developed for measuring emissions and analyzing their composition and volume. If Los Angeles wanted to figure out what was behind smog, it couldn't proceed half-heartedly. Engineer Deutsch sounded more like Engineer Patton when he declared that the county would turn over every rock: "We will go to the butadiene [rubber] plant and analyze the gases released in the various operations. We will go to one or more selected oil refineries and test fumes emitted. We will go to smelters, chemical plants and other potential fume producers and find out whether they are spewing offensive irritants into the atmosphere. We will test buses, trucks, automobiles, incinerators and rubbish dumps and determine whether these sources are responsible."[1] Deutsch's fighting spirit became a driving force in an all-out war on smog that would grow to include large swaths of the city: officials like himself, critical figures from the realm of private enterprise, physicians, politicians, scientists, and angry residents. Together, these forces led to Los Angeles County's development of the most powerful air pollution control authority in the United States, one that'd eventually serve as a template for the Environmental Protection Agency almost three decades later. The Los Angeles experience was an object lesson in how to regulate aggressively despite scientific uncertainty about the nature of air pollution, its exact risks, and how to fight it. Local pollution control officials balanced fiercely competing imperatives during the heyday of the California boom, navigating between preserving Los Angeles's industrial growth while protecting residents from the new ecological hazards that growth posed.

## Smog: The Lay Response

It's tempting to view the Los Angeles fight against smog through the lens of scientific triumph: problem posed (by smog), problem understood (by scientists), solutions enacted (by officials). Yet the smog program and its aggressiveness were propelled, first and foremost, by grassroots foment from irate and irritable residents. Over the next decade, they'd continuously exert pressure and prod Los Angeles into action—any action—long before a full scientific account of smog even existed.

It wasn't hard to see why. Blankets of dense emissions regularly enveloped the region, and as early as 1943, the situation had become intolerable. One January day felt like a "gas attack," as one account put it, with the area "engulfed by a low-hanging cloud of acrid smoke" for hours. Another in September led to an "unscheduled" end to daylight.[2] County officials pledged to investigate the causes of these attacks.[3] Some speculated on possible sources of what quickly came to be known as smog: maybe rubber plants, maybe industrial stacks, maybe just traffic. But they could offer no concrete answers on its origins or what compounds were exactly in it. Smog was a term, then, that denoted everything, yet nothing.

Not all attacks were as awful as that day in 1943 that turned the city into a war zone. But even in milder form, smog riled residents, who weren't shy about making their grief known to elected officials in a series of blistering letters. Complaints peaked at the end of 1949 when yet another severe attack resulted in a smog blanket covering the region for almost two weeks. On the eleventh day of the attack, one L. S. Adams asked the county board of supervisors: "How long do you think the patience of Los Angeles citizen[s] will last? My patience is exhausted and I know I am not alone in that. I have the house completely closed and enough of the messy stuff seeps in to make eyes water and cause dizziness."[4] Miriam Yergin complained: "My eyes are smarting, my nose is running, my head aches, my business efficiency is impaired, my health is being ruined as well as my disposition—all because of this blankety-blank SMOG that has hugged this city, almost continuously for the past five months."[5] Raymond Berg begged for more forceful action and talked about his children, who "come home from school with tear-smeared faces complaining that it is hard to see to study because of the eye-smarting, rottenly unclean air." His lungs were "crying out for a fresh draught of sweet, clean air which they have not had for over a fortnight."[6] Fred Mayer had simply had enough and threatened to move. A recent transplant to Los Angeles, he'd delayed a permanent commitment to the area because of the "terrible pollution," "which is blotting out the very sun, and making more than four out of five days a sort of mild hell." The "L.A. 'smog' is intolerable," Mayer concluded, before stating again that he and his family were planning to leave.[7] One particularly ornery constituent replaced "Los Angeles" in a letter with the words "Smog Town," while another composed a poem that went:

That smog is with us day and night;
We get sick enough to die;
It blacks out the lovely, sunny blue
of California's sky.[8]

These complaints all addressed the existential unpleasantness of smog and its quality-of-life threat, but many residents framed smog explicitly in the language of health. For Berg, smog didn't just irritate one's eyes and nose. It was a "death pall," the byproduct of "manufacturers spewing their death-dealing poison out over this vast area and subjecting the now millions of lives to the indignities they have suffered since the first synthetic rubber was turned out at the beginning of the war!"[9] Adams was even more blunt: "If you fellows think that is harmless to health you have another thought coming."[10] A senior named Lynne Swaim asked: "Since when has the ill-health and utter discomfort of people been subordinated for the 'greed' of industry?" For Swaim, that discomfort came in the form of "the blue-gray choking fumes [that] are pressed unhealthily down the people" and the "DAILY HORROR of having [her] eyes burn" to the point where she could "scarcely keep them open and [was] forced to rub them constantly and bathe them with eye drops."[11] This language of death and health from Berg, Adams, and Swaim was striking, appearing almost two decades before toxicology penetrated the popular imagination in the wake of such works as *Silent Spring* and the environmental activism of the 1970s.[12] In the early midcentury United States, health framing wasn't nearly as instinctive. But Los Angeles was an exception in part because it was so exceptional, and a local toxicological lay discourse defined smog as an environmental health hazard from the 1940s forward.

Regarding culpability, residents weren't shy with their speculations. After characterizing the "acrid fumes" as a "menace [to] public health," Dean Beckwith focused on common methods of rubbish disposal, specifically the burning of waste and personal backyard incineration devices.[13] On "backyard burning," F. E. Mills added that "one incinerator can create as much smoke, if burning steadily all morning and afternoon, as a small industry could."[14] Others, like C. F. Harvey, complained about traffic, especially buses, with "exhaust and fumes" that were "just as bad and just as nauseating as it ever was."[15]

Residents were often unabashedly political, too. For many, the problem was a petrochemical industry that prioritized economic growth over residents' welfare. Florence Aberle pointed to Columbia Steel and Bethlehem Steel, noting that the industrial behemoths had fought air pollution controls. She wrote, sarcastically: "Property is valuable & must be saved—but human health is expendable."[16] Ford Sammis was losing patience over sluggishness on the part of officials. He wanted a "clamp down" and declared that "a country which can produce the H-bomb has enough technical talent to find out what is causing smog."[17] Another resident pled similarly: "I beg you to take the drastic steps, which you must have within your power to do, to bring about an immediate improvement, and ultimately, a clean atmosphere to this city."[18] For these residents, smog wasn't just an irritant and wasn't just a health hazard. It was a problem of political power—namely, who possessed enough of it to pollute with impunity.

## Early Air Pollution Policy: Between Consensus and Conflict

In Los Angeles politics, the county was king. In contrast to cities like New York, Los Angeles's mayor was structurally weak, and the most important power lines—over the purse and over regulatory authority—ran through the county board of supervisors. Critics called the body's members "the five little kings," a reference to a total supervisor count that never changed and thus concentrated ever more power—and resource control—even as the county's population kept exploding in the postwar years.[19]

Yet that power could be wielded toward positive ends, too. Despite being accused of foot-dragging, county officials wielded administrative muscle and acted swiftly from smog's early days. After the 1943 attack, the county took its first steps toward emissions control when it formed a "Smoke and Fumes Commission."[20] A couple years later, the county health department crafted an ordinance prohibiting discharge of "any dense smoke or fumes" for beyond three minutes or "charred paper, ash dust, soot, grime, carbon, noxious acids, fumes, gases or other material which cause injury, detriment, nuisance or annoyance to any person or to the public or which endanger the comfort, repose, health or safety of any such person or the public."[21] This was all-encompassing, catch-all, highly elastic language, and it reflected a state of flux in both scientific understanding of what smog even was and the regulatory options available to control it. But the ordinance sent a clear statement: the county would be aggressive and cast a wide net.

A convening of the county's mayors in 1946 was critical. There, Supervisor John Anson Ford got commitment for countywide action. "The cause may arise in Torrance and the effect felt in Altadena," said Los Angeles mayor Fletcher Bowron, referencing two suburbs thirty miles apart to accentuate why the problem of pollution required address by county government. Other speakers joined in underscoring the need to think about smog in region-spanning terms, one to be attacked in a "centralized manner." A parade of mayors, even those from heavily industrial municipalities such as Long Beach and Azusa, all pledged support. Azusa's mayor, Raymond Lamm, reported that residents regularly "had to evacuate the entire north end of our city due to the very serious types of fumes that came in."[22] Residential welfare seemed, for the moment, to trump other considerations, including the economic.

Commitment from the county's cities soon led to a regulatory apparatus. County attorney Harold W. Kennedy outlined the legal basis for vastly strengthening the county's makeshift Office of Air Pollution Control. It rested on two pillars. One was the long-standing constitutional police power granted to states and, by extension, to local municipalities to "promote the general welfare of society" by "regulat[ing] private interests for the public good."[23] The other was an evolving interpretation of what a "public nuisance" was and what could be done about it. Nuisance law allowed the government to regulate pollution even if it could not prove that every individual in a jurisdiction would be harmed by it. The threat of population-wide effects was enough.[24]

Beyond doctrine were actual mechanisms such as joint powers contracts whereby cities would enforce local ordinances that mirrored county codes. It was a sharp contrast from the status quo, whereby Los Angeles's cities had to adopt county ordinances individually, one by one.[25] When it came to air pollution, Greater Los Angeles would proceed as one, under unified county governance. It was an early example of what Christopher Sellers, writing about the suburban response to smog in the area, has called "a new translocal politics, addressing an aerial commons shared by the basin's separate parts," and it made sense, given that smog "served as an alarming reminder that industrial environs like Long Beach or the downtown were far more inextricably bound to suburban enclaves than their residents had imagined."[26]

A new pollution control authority wouldn't just regulate; it'd also research the science of air pollution. And on that front, it had a lot to do. Chicago engineer I. A. Deutsch suggested that Los Angeles's particular topography made it more predisposed to severe smog attacks than other regions. Lessons from elsewhere, then, would only have so much applicability, given the idiosyncrasies of the landscape. Deutsch announced an initiative that'd send field researchers to potential sources of pollution, where they'd systematically collect air samples, explore their composition, and identify "known concentrations of suspected irritants," taking advantage of new equipment developed by the U.S. Army during the war.[27] The goal: figure out why smog was so bad in Los Angeles and what could be done about it.

Then there was the political front. Officials needed to bolster wide political support, particularly from the Los Angeles business class. One method was to frame pollution as a threat to economic health, not just to bodily vitality.[28] At the 1946 convening of mayors, Supervisor Ford noted that while "the cost in injured lungs and mucous membranes is apparent on health and actual death, those factors present another side, equally, perhaps, if not greater in its financial totals, and certainly the cost in aesthetic values."[29] A polluted climate, in other words, was also bad for the business climate, not just for physiological welfare. "We recognize, too," Ford would remark, "that our tourist industry is in very real jeopardy and that the attractions of our distinctive climate, of our seashore and mountains each of priceless worth to all Californians—are at times completely obliterated by this unforeseen by-product of war-time and post-war development."[30] Such a rhetorical strategy exploited long-standing tensions, identified by the historian Paul Sabin, within the private sector in Los Angeles, especially between nonindustrial and industrial factions. Officials thus made particular appeals to firms outside petroleum and other heavy industry, especially real estate, tourism, and entertainment, which all depended on an immaculate outdoor aesthetic.[31]

Industrialists were harder to win over. But early on, county officials cast air pollution control as a civic duty. They cultivated what might be called an industrial-ecological accord. A year before the mayor's conference, the county's H. O. Swartout called for a "spirit of responsibility and co-operation" from Los Angeles's manufacturers. He pointed to early voluntary efforts by factories to control emissions and characterized the worst offenders as declining and "marginal producers" that "frequently complained of losing money and of being on the verge of bankruptcy." They stood in contrast to the "leading industrialists" who cooperated. "Much of the grime that is by some people considered inseparable from industrialization is unnecessary," Swartout optimistically declared.[32]

Swartout's rhetoric of consensus, however, masked potential, if understated, conflicts. In the report where his remarks appeared, he surveyed the emerging industrial landscape of Los Angeles. In each section, Swartout outlined the scale of a potential industrial contributor to smog, espoused hope for a cooperative spirit, but then ended by identifying formidable challenges that might arise with impending regulation. Regulation meant change, and he wrote that the county needed to "recognize that bringing it about will cost every automobile and bus operator money." Elsewhere, when discussing the imposition of a centralized apparatus for regulation, Swartout speculated that those in areas experiencing little to no smog burden might resist the idea of having to pay for escalated pollution controls primarily benefitting others. And, he continued, "If the people of any city owe their livelihood or prosperity to industries, they are likely to resist the idea of having strict ordinances against smoke and fumes—all the more so if they themselves are not great sufferers therefrom."[33] This push-pull between consensus and conflict would color the Los Angeles pollution program for the next decade.

## A New Regulatory Edifice

In its infancy, however, potential political opposition took a back seat to the task of setting up the Office of Air Pollution Control's day-to-day operations. The agency began with a full-time staff of six at the end of 1946. Via a combination of complaints and their own sleuthing, office staff inspected three major classes of sources: stationary points, trains, and diesel trucks, issuing violations when appropriate. Whether to issue a violation was left to the judgment of the initial inspector and, if necessary, special hearing boards and the district attorney's office. In its first year of operation, a total of 1,392 smoke violations were reported, but only five cases ultimately required the involvement of the district attorney. Consequently, the office's early reports radiated optimism. One thanked the railroad industry for its "splendid cooperation" and praised fruit growers who'd installed smoke-abating facilities on their grounds.[34]

This ethos of cooperation continued into 1948, when state legislation enabled the Office of Air Pollution Control to become an autonomous county agency, the Air Pollution Control District (APCD), along the lines conceived at the mayors' conference two years earlier. The law inaugurated a permit system whereby facilities, with APCD oversight, voluntarily installed emissions control equipment, such as fume and dust collectors, gas absorbers, and incinerators (an alternative to the burning of waste).[35] But against potential violators who didn't cooperate, the APCD took aggressive action. One example came when it found fifty-seven dumps "burning rubbish in the open" and closed forty-two of them.[36] Further, the legislation drew no distinction between private and municipal dumps.[37] Private facilities were as open to severe sanction as public counterparts, despite the political conflict that might ensue from targeting business. Still, the APCD sought to adopt as cooperative a course as possible. It allowed the Los Angeles Chamber of Commerce to set up sector-specific committees—for example, one for steel foundries—that proposed new instruments for emissions reduction that the district would then evaluate for efficacy, part of a larger effort by the chamber to accept but also circumscribe the extent of early regulations.[38]

This industrial-ecological accord was always fraught. In its first year, the APCD passed rule 53a. It required alterations to refineries' combustion equipment, limiting sulfur emissions to 0.2 percent by volume from any single source.[39] In a statement to the agency, the Western Oil and Gas Association, the petrochemical industry's chief regional lobbying entity, vacillated between deference and opposition. On one hand, wrote George J. Murray of its public health committee, the area's petroleum facilities would be "able to operate within reasonable tolerances of smoke and gas emissions." But what exactly constituted "reasonable" was another matter. The association—practically within the same breath—invoked the ongoing, and as yet inconclusive, nature of scientific investigation to criticize rule 53a. Murray argued that it had not "been determined that sulphur compounds in concentration of 0.2 percent at point of discharge adds to any extent whatever to the lack of visibility that takes place in this area under certain climatic conditions." Thus, he continued, there was "no indication that setting the limit of sulphur compound emissions at 0.2% will contribute toward the solution of the smog problem any more than would setting it at 0.35%."[40] Was 0.2 percent therefore quite so "reasonable"?

Nevertheless, despite its unease with the agency's actions, the Western Oil and Gas Association wasn't going to put up a fight. Murray vowed "to offer whatever it may toward the ultimate solution of the entire problem for the benefit of the community generally."[41] The response from the American Smelting and

Refining Company was similar. It focused on rule 53's similar zinc oxide limits, arguing that it didn't feel there was "ample evidence" to show it was "more than an insignificant factor in the formation of smog." But then the firm pivoted, promising to play its civic role in the air pollution control effort. "We are in sympathy with your objective to make Los Angeles County a better and more healthful place to live," the company stated, pointing to its voluntary experimental efforts at limiting emissions of metal solids during smelting.[42]

Even if a spirit of civic consensus characterized the first year of air pollution control, the passage of rules with quantified limits created a political powder keg that'd require delicate handling by the county. Explicit identification of compounds, after all, meant indictments of specific industries and, as would shortly be apparent, individual firms. The ambiguity of the relationship between regulators and industry was underscored by a 1948 county grand jury report on nascent county air pollution efforts. Though the report argued for upgrading APCD staff, it was largely oriented toward the needs of industrial firms and took a benign view of them. It disclosed that the grand jury had received "complaints . . . from industry," and it cast aspersions on APCD's current field inspectors, writing that they were "grossly unfit to contact the public" and unqualified to "meet those highly experienced chemists and engineers found in large industry." And yet the final takeaway came right back around to the song of community and cooperation. "Community support," the report concluded, "is badly needed on the local level. Every man's luncheon club and every woman's organization must take this smog problem up in their individual communities."[43] A public statement from the APCD at the end of the year mirrored the grand jury's sentiments. "Much effort," it read, "must be devoted to the education of industry," which "as a whole" would "cooperate to solve their own problems to the point of determining the best method for control."[44]

## The Scientific Puzzle of Smog

As regulatory machinery grew, so did scientific investigation. Science had political implications, especially if it pointed to more specific culprits. The Long Beach Chamber of Commerce recognized as much when it complained that too much enforcement had been "directed heretofore, against industrial abuses" rather than "other factors" that might "contribute to as great or a greater degree" to smog.[45] An initial overarching question was why air pollution in Los Angeles was harder to control and how it differed than that of such counterparts as Chicago and Saint Louis, and soon (and infamously) Donora, Pennsylvania, where smog blankets caused by emissions from industrial plants had sent the region into crisis for the better part of a week in 1948.[46]

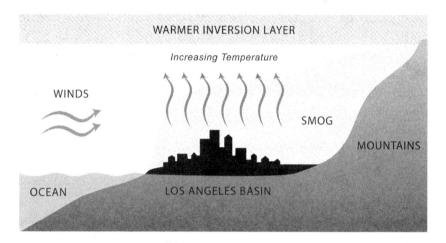

**How smog formed.** Heat resulted in a temperature increase from the surface, form-ing an inversion layer that, along with Los Angeles mountain ranges, trapped smog. Winds were insufficient for full dispersion but distributed the byproducts across the Los Angeles basin.
*Source*: Author's rendition.

One of the first APCD studies, led by a young UCLA meteorologist named Morris Neiburger, explored how quirks of Los Angeles weather patterns and topography contributed to smog attacks. He identified two critical phenomena. One was "inversion," when the air temperature above the Earth's surface steadily *increased*, rather than *decreased*, as was typically the case. This prevented "vertical dispersion" of pollutants that would normally disappear into the atmosphere. Instead, an "inversion layer" of warmer air acted as a figurative floating blanket of sorts, trapping pollution underneath it. Another factor was wind speed and its ability to disperse emissions fully and replace them with "fresh air." When the wind failed to disperse emissions, higher concentrations resulted and were trapped in the Los Angeles basin, which then enveloped the area beneath, cre-ating, in other words, what people were calling smog.

Neiburger's study stressed the simultaneity of the phenomena and elabo-rated on how they worked. In an analysis of data collected during the fall of 1946, he noted that "not one complaint of air pollution was received . . . on days when the temperature *decreased* with height throughout the lower three thousand feet of the atmosphere." Temperature inversion, in other words, was a critical factor on days with higher smog. But temperature inversion was not sufficient by itself.

Magnitude mattered, too. Data from weather stations indicated, in fact, that no complaints occurred on the majority of days with "low strong" inversions. The amount of "advection"—wind that passed through the region—was a critical second factor. Here, Neiburger's analysis showed that on days with a high number of complaints, wind advection dropped *below* the average of 100 miles per day to 20–60, enough to *move* pollutants but not actually disperse them to the point where they were no longer concentrated enough to cause smog. The study concluded "that variations in weather are capable of producing profound variations in the pollution concentration in the Los Angeles basin."[47]

The weather station data also provided new clues about how exactly emissions traveled, even if what exactly all of them *were* remained unclear. Neiburger modeled the trajectory of air currents, noting that in Los Angeles, winds typically began at the ocean. They moved inland by the afternoon, then reversed course in the evening away from the range of mountains surrounding the region before once again moving in an inland direction with a new day, all while fresh wind streams entered from the ocean.

By analyzing air samples at specific points along a trajectory, researchers could determine how long the air had been circulating in the basin, where it had come from, and how much it had "stagnated"—become polluted—along the way. Tracking aldehydes, they discovered connections between high concentrations and low visibility (the maximum distance one could see when looking straight at the sky). The biggest threat to visibility occurred in the morning hours and in areas with "industrial and heavy traffic sources," especially in the southern and eastern areas of Los Angeles. For example, two air samples were collected on September 14, 1946, at 10:30 A.M.: one from traffic- and industry-heavy Vernon, another from nonindustrial regions. Measured visibility of the Vernon sample, "which by then had spent nineteen hours over the southern part of Los Angeles," was very low, at one mile, compared to eight miles for the second.[48] Los Angeles's mountain ranges played a critical role, too, trapping a regular supply of air from the Pacific Ocean and recirculating it in the basin throughout the day. Taken together, Neiburger's study had identified preliminary links among the natural and the social. Temperature inversions, slower winds, sluggishly circulating air, movement through areas with heavy traffic and industrial sources, and mountains around the county perimeter: all had contributed to the periodic smoggy days of the past few years.[49]

Another advance came from a 1947 investigation by Herman Roth and Engelbrekt Swenson, two scientists at the University of Southern California (USC). Whereas Neiburger had focused on macro-level meteorological influences, the USC researchers turned to the micro-level and "irritant aspects of atmospheric pollution." Specifically, they examined the physiological effects of varying formaldehyde concentrations and moderators such as a person's age and

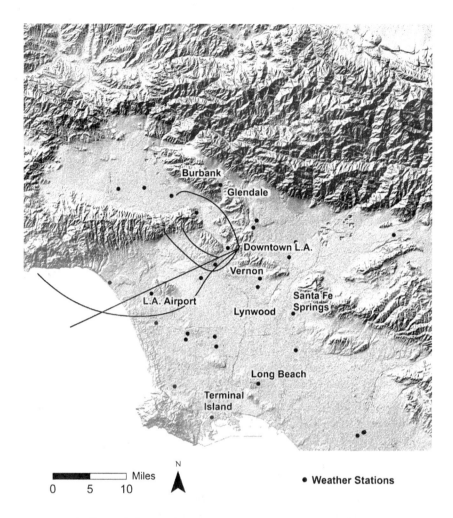

0    5    10 Miles    N

• **Weather Stations**

**Network of Los Angeles weather stations, represented by dots.** Morris Neiburger and James Edinger used them to discern wind patterns and how these patterns circulated pollution throughout the Los Angeles basin to explain geographic and temporal variation in aldehyde concentrations.

*Source*: Cartography by Ashley Marshall, based on data in Morris Neiburger and James Edinger, "Meteorological Aspects of Air Pollution in the Los Angeles Area," October 1947, 4, Box 20-05214-411 (3260 APBP0001), unlabeled folder, Kenneth Hahn Hall of Administration (Los Angeles County), Los Angeles.

the weather. "Prolonged combination of inversion and atmospheric stagnation," they wrote, could lead to "build-up of atmospheric pollutants to toxic levels."[50]

Roth and Swenson modeled their study design after the work of Harvard industrial hygienist Leslie Silverman, whose research team exposed research subjects to industrial vapors for eight-hour periods while documenting physical reactions, such as nasal irritation. The purpose was to identify a "sensory limit," a threshold before a subject experienced serious discomfort.[51] Silverman's research, however, had been geared entirely toward an occupational context, with study samples consisting entirely of "young, healthy" individuals most likely doing industrial work.

By contrast, the USC study broadened the sample. It included people of "all ages and conditions of health" so as to approximate the entire general population affected by the new air pollution. Its researchers built two arms: one of people aged twenty to forty, drawn from the USC student body, scientific laboratories, and APCD staff, and a second of volunteers, aged fifty to eighty-four, recruited by a local suburban newspaper, the *Pasadena Star-News*. Participants put on helmets with valves that allowed formaldehyde to enter enclosed space around their heads, and they were asked to rate, on a four-point scale, "odor," "irritation of nose," "secretion in nose," "irritation of eyes," "lacrimation (tears)," and "increased desire to blink" at various levels of concentration. Subjects in both arms reported irritation, and the elderly reported higher levels of irritation, suggesting they were most vulnerable to pollution. Irrespective of age, though, the threshold for irritation varied widely across subjects, with some responding to extremely low-level exposures and others not. It compounded the problem of smog, which now, it turned out, wasn't just a matter of getting rid of sources emitting higher concentrations of pollutants. Many in Los Angeles might be susceptible to even low levels of whatever smog turned out to be.[52]

Neither the UCLA nor the USC study offered much, however, on the persistent mystery of what smog *was*. Each had used aldehydes and formaldehydes, respectively, as proxies for smog, with Roth and Swensen noting that they were likely not the only "'guilty culprit' which is responsible for all or even most of the irritation caused by smog."[53] More inquiry on smog composition fell to H. F. Johnstone, a professor of chemical engineering from the University of Illinois. In early 1948, the APCD hired Johnstone and asked him to focus on sulfur compounds, which the agency suspected might be a chief reason for low visibility. Like the others, Johnstone emphasized local uniqueness: the role Los Angeles's particular mountain range and wind patterns played in trapping and recirculating polluted air during temperature inversion. The heart of his study, however, centered on adding new layers of detail to what had heretofore been generally described as "fumes," "smoke," "fog," and other generic terms. A key goal for future researchers, he argued, should be to identify the precise particle sizes associated with lower visibility or "maximum obscuration," along with their chemical composition.[54] This would allow researchers to pinpoint the exact concentrations of specific compounds needed to form smog.[55]

Johnstone zeroed in on sulfur dioxide ($SO_2$), which he noted had become a "a good measure of the total degree of industrial pollution."[56] In other locales, its concentration was directly related to distance from industrial sources: smelters, power plants, refineries, waste facilities, foundries, and the like.[57] It also had a tendency to oxidate—that is, bind to oxygen. When that happened, it formed other sulfuric compounds in aerosols—especially sulfuric acid and sulfur trioxide ($SO_3$)—that contributed to the thick mists plaguing other regions with reduced visibility. The remainder of Johnstone's sulfur discussion focused on promising, if still rudimentary, methods for controlling emissions. These techniques included filtration of sulfur compounds and the addition of other substances, such as ammonium or zinc oxide, which could convert $SO_2$ to less harmful sulfates.[58] If $SO_2$ was as central as Johnstone's analysis indicated, Los Angeles County had reason to worry. Despite progress, its own data showed that $SO_2$ concentrations were still eight times the recently imposed limits, with peaks in the morning at around 9:00 A.M., and once again in the late afternoon at around 3:00 P.M.[59]

On its own terms, the science was interesting enough, but it came with real political stakes. By linking $SO_2$ squarely with Los Angeles's industrial base, particularly large facilities, Johnstone issued a de facto indictment as he spotlighted industrial sources repeatedly. On visible emissions, he wrote that "the number of industrial stacks with visible plumes that carry for long distances is impressive."[60] And when discussing "sulfur balance"—a means of assessing sulfuric contribution from a source, then controlling it—Johnstone focused on the oil industry alone.[61] In Johnstone's estimation, smaller facilities, dumps, and automobiles didn't account for the bulk of the problem. Capping vehicle emissions, he hypothesized, wasn't the main answer given the lack of smog attacks in other cities with comparable traffic levels. Johnstone's suppositions were supported by the APCD's own estimates, which showed a considerable, but hardly majority, $SO_2$ contribution from automobiles.[62]

But although industrial firms were to blame for the immediate smog problem, the firms themselves would also be a major part of the solution. Once again, like many of his contemporaries, Johnstone played conciliatory chords alongside critical ones. Johnstone aimed his sharpest criticism not at industries but at the APCD, charging that its $SO_2$ limit was far less strict than England's. But even as he called for a more aggressive APCD, he maintained that it was "especially important to develop a feeling of cooperation and, whenever possible, to seek improvements through a spirit of civic pride, rather than by resorting to the law."[63] Johnstone assumed that Los Angeles's midcentury boom would continue unimpeded; his prescriptions were of a technical nature, anchored around limitation and amelioration of emissions. They were, in other words, the language of the industrial-ecological accord.

## Decision-Making amid Uncertainty

Despite the uncertainties about smog, the APCD began moving on regulation anyway, even as many others, including the federal government, had shrugged and rebuffed Los Angeles's attempts to involve them in local matters.[64] How far would the APCD now go? In late 1948, APCD director Louis McCabe issued a forceful statement to the board of supervisors, promising a slate of additional emissions standards and regulations, citing the recent research. McCabe's appearance came a couple weeks after a series of low-level tempera- ture inversions had resulted in such heavy overcast that more than half of the region's refineries closed down for a day on September 3, 1948. The results of the unplanned industrial strike were remarkable and revealing, amounting to a natural experiment. As McCabe put it: "The visibility has been much better and the pollution has been less intense. The clarity of the atmosphere on the leeward side of the idle refineries is in striking contrast to that of the operating plants."[65] He ended by discussing industrial sources of sulfur, but unlike scientists such as Johnstone who'd done the same, McCabe made the statement before a promi- nent public body.

As the district prepared for the next stage, residents continued to express frustration and impatience with the pace of affairs. A particularly charged pair of letters came from Pasadena mechanical engineer George Schuler, who argued that the new sulfur standards were far too low and still increased risk to vegeta- tion by "4000 times." More important than plant life was the ongoing and future human toll. Schuler was apoplectic, and in a list of two dozen "further facts and figures," he listed declining life expectancy, higher than average mortality rates, heart disease, suicides and homicides, population loss, multiple fainting spells by area entertainers, and a host of less grave (and by now familiar) symptoms, including irritated nasal and throat passages and lacrimation. It was all, in short, a "deadly menace," and it had one fundamental cause: the county's oil refineries, which were "the only source of smoke and fumes large enough to fill this entire valley." They were injuring and killing residents, Schuler charged, because of a weak-kneed regulatory agency staffed by those who "refuse[d] to do their duty" by closing refineries.[66]

Schuler wrote passionately and may have overreached a bit. Much of the work on health effects, in fact, was still unfolding, and studies performed thus far were small in size and cross-sectional, meaning that they didn't track sub- jects over time to see precisely how people fared after exposure. It thus wasn't possible to make authoritative statements about whether exposure to smog in the past caused an ailment in the future. Still, Schuler was no oddity, and he captured the mood of many residents who questioned the industrial-ecological accord and the path of civic consensus that it entailed and that the APCD pur- sued. In one missive, one resident identified only as the "wife of J. G. Schutte" singled out the current APCD executive secretary, Amos Thomas, as a pawn of oil companies who'd rebuffed her after she had written him. She wrote: "This is too serious a matter to neglect. If we have a man on the Control Board who is influenced by the big industries and oil companies and siding in with them against Dr. McCabe's courageous effort to abate this danger to our city, we should get rid of him at once so as to give Dr. McCabe full support in every way."[67] But her portrayal of APCD officials as lapdogs wasn't accurate. At the same time as Schutte's letter arrived, McCabe and the board of supervisors were working to rid the APCD of Thomas, calling him a "worthless appendage" in one internal memo that suggested Thomas was unsupportive of the APCD's efforts.[68] But McCabe sympathized with constituents' impatience. Persistently claiming the need for more science could amount to a "dangerous sedative," McCabe acknowledged, and he cautioned against dithering and "ephemeral research designed to divert or postpone enforcement activities against the many known sources of air pollution which are apparent to any unbiased observer."[69] But elsewhere, Supervisor Ford, in a note to another accusatory constituent, defended the APCD by emphasizing that the problem of smog in Los Angeles was distinctly challenging and that the underlying scientific questions required thorough answers, especially if regulatory actions faced legal challenges and attacks on its evidentiary base.[70]

And so, over the next few years, the APCD expanded its scope. The inspection and permit program grew, with the number of site inspections increasing by 1950 to 17,974, up from 1,474 in the agency's first year of operation. The number of hearings during the same period jumped from 317 to 1,228. Permits for control devices inspected and approved by the APCD increased from 24 in 1948, the first year of the permit program, to 899 two years later.[71] District officials developed a clearer picture of common sources. They were assisted by new technology—including mechanical filters and electrical precipitators collecting air samples—that could calculate the volume of specific emissions.[72]

The debate about sources and relative contributions to pollution now proceeded more concretely. Data from a 1951 "Preliminary Total Pollution Survey" provided figures for daily emitted aerosols—suspended particles—that were measured in tons, along with estimates of their decline since 1948. Some figures were striking. "Metals industry" facilities emitted 4,331 tons daily but reported a 22 percent reduction over the period. Likewise, "minerals and earth processing" plants emitted 3,994 tons but with a 27 percent decrease from 1948. Sulfur dioxide, the most studied compound, remained a problem, with 6,683 total tons emitted, 2,688 from fuel oil sources that reported no substantial reduction in emissions. Still, by the end of 1950, the district reported a 50 percent overall reduction in sulfur emissions since it had passed rule 53a, one of its biggest accomplishments to date.[73] And it could boast a staggering 77 percent reduction from non-fuel-oil sources.[74] Outside of specific sources, the district was also starting to produce tables showing associations between concentrations of various compounds and their effect on visibility, something that H. F. Johnstone had urged a few years earlier.[75]

Still, the pollution picture remained hazy. The identification of $SO_2$ had been an undoubtable leap from simply discussing pollution in such generic terms as "smoke and fumes." But emerging evidence was confirming that many more compounds might be at play. Sulfur control, while the most immediate success of early APCD actions, might in fact only be a small component of the problem. Crop damage had become "increasingly prominent" despite these $SO_2$ reductions, often occurring in areas with lower sulfur concentrations. Something other than sulfur seemed to be causing unique internal leaf hydration that resulted in "scarred areas on the backs of the leaves" and discoloration to "brown or yellowish white."[76] Officials asked similar questions about aldehydes, wondering if other compounds might contribute to unwanted ophthalmological and respiratory reactions.[77] One new corner APCD scientists turned toward was hydrocarbons. Their presence in automobile exhaust soon increased attention on booming Los Angeles traffic, which had previously remained a secondary concern. Household backyard incinerators were now subject to scrutiny, too.[78]

These scientific developments brushed up uneasily against politics. If it expanded the dragnet of potential pollutants, the county would test the cooperative accord with industry it had cautiously nurtured. Comprehensive as it was becoming, the pollution control program still depended mostly on voluntary compliance from industrial firms themselves. The county rarely took people to court except for the most egregious violations. As late as 1952, new district director Gordon Larson, in a presentation to the board of supervisors, still spoke of pollution control as a "community effort," one that required "cooperation and application of technical knowledge."[79]

But as more knowledge about pollution accumulated, however fragmented, a consensus approach to regulation came under scrutiny, much of it from residents. An illustrative conflict occurred around Bethlehem Pacific Coast Steel's mill in Vernon, an area with elevated levels of pollution. In 1951, a group of neighboring Maywood and Huntington Park residents petitioned the county about the plant. Even after a few years of regulation, the "smoke, gases, fumes, odors and fine air-borne deposits of unknown corrosive substances," they wrote, remained "almost insufferable and injurious to our health and comfort."[80] In fact, the mill had been on the APCD's radar for a number of years. It had been granted a number of "variances"—exceptions to emissions rules—with the APCD holding out hope that Bethlehem would be able to install control equipment and bring itself into compliance. At one point, the county initiated court proceedings against the firm and asked for an injunction, alleging that the plant's operation, particularly three open-hearth furnaces, violated a slate of rules. In response, the firm simply shut down the furnaces in question, pledging to switch to electric furnaces and other filtration equipment recommended by the county.[81] After Bethlehem's agreement, the county praised its "cooperation" and filed a motion to dismiss the case.[82] But even a year later, officials wondered whether Bethlehem would self-correct as promised. A year later, the APCD was questioned along such lines by Kenneth Hahn, a thirty-two-year-old newly elected county supervisor about to play major roles in air pollution control and South Central Los Angeles around health care.[83] Hahn wasn't alone. Supervisor Ford wondered whether Larson was hesitant to push for faster action from what he called "big industry."[84]

At the same time, the APCD faced parallel pressure from those more sympathetic to industrial firms. California Institute of Technology (Caltech) professor of mechanical engineering R. L. Daugherty, who also chaired the county supervisors' advisory committee to the APCD, questioned the aggressiveness of the APCD's action against Bethlehem Steel and industry at large. Daugherty's reaction shouldn't have been surprising. Since its conversion to a research university in the 1920s, Caltech had become a "dynamic nucleus" in the Southern California industrial boom, and Daugherty proceeded as one might expect.[85] He admonished Supervisor Hahn for his vocal questioning about the Bethlehem Steel incident, stating that "all the information that I have . . . indicates that the various steel companies in this area are making a serious attempt to minimize, if not eliminate, the air pollution which they produce." A pithy remark of Daugherty's captured postwar Los Angeles's fundamental conundrum of reconciling ecology with economy. "The only alternative" to allowing the steel mills more time to adapt "would be to close down these plants entirely, which would throw a great many people out of work and cause a financial loss to the community which I do not believe the community is ready to accept yet."[86]

## Science Solves Smog

In 1952, major new research on Los Angeles air pollution pushed scientific debate beyond an emphasis on sulfur dioxide and aldehydes. Notably, it emerged from Caltech, otherwise home to people who had downplayed pollution risk, and it came from the chemist Arie Haagen-Smit, who clarified much of the mystery surrounding what constituted smog. In a series of experiments, Haagen-Smit's research team explored what exact processes in the atmosphere created the chemical byproducts everyone had been calling smog. Then it turned to consequences. What kind of damage—and how much—did these byproducts do to plant and human life?

The APCD and Haagen-Smit had worked backward after noticing damage on plants in areas with lower concentrations of sulfur. This suggested that some other compound might be causing the crop injury.[87] But if not sulfates, then what? The cracking of rubber was suggestive. Tire manufacturers had noticed that their products deteriorated far more rapidly in Los Angeles and, further, that the time elapsing before rubber cracking was much shorter on smoggy days by margins of twenty-three to fifty-three minutes.[88] Even more curious: cracking resembled reactions to ozone, but how ozone might be forming in Los Angeles remained a mystery.

The Haagen-Smit team simulated the Los Angeles air basin using fumigation rooms where they exposed plants and humans to compounds that they'd found were capable of producing what they had observed in plants and rubber—that is, things other than the usual suspects of "sulfur dioxide, chlorine, hydrogen sulfide, or hydrogen fluoride." They substituted ozone ($O_3$) and "vapors of a cracked gasoline containing 20% [unsaturated hydrocarbons]," which were regularly emitted from various sources the APCD had identified. This addition of hydrocarbons resulted in "further development of the symptoms on all five indicator plants," just as had happened to vegetation all over Los Angeles.[89] The team delved further by redoing the fumigation and identifying effects of varying hydrocarbon concentration and structures.[90]

Hydrocarbons, however, weren't the full story. Nitrogen dioxide ($NO_2$), which had previously merited little attention, now assumed a more central role. In earlier research, conducted in the late 1940s, Haagen-Smit found that $NO_2$ could act as an oxidizing agent to hydrocarbons in the presence of sufficient sunlight.[91] That provided a pathway to *intermediate* byproducts (peroxides) and *final* byproducts (aldehydes and acids). By measuring concentrations of these newly produced compounds at various levels, Haagen-Smit determined that final byproducts had little effect on plants; the bulk of the problems stemmed from contact with the intermediate products of oxidation: peroxides. Examining nitrogen dioxide and hydrocarbon oxidation also yielded another finding: ozone was another byproduct of oxidation, and it resulted in the observed rubber cracking.[92] This ozone, in turn, could serve as another possible oxidizing agent for hydrocarbons, producing more unwanted products in an ongoing cyclical process.[93]

The experiments led to other important related findings on how the worst aspects of smog were created. It was the oxidation of hydrocarbons, the researchers found, that resulted in smog's trademark visibility-obscuring haze. Within only a few minutes, visibility was reduced to eight feet in one experiment, a consequence of aerosol formation during the process. Haagen-Smit, as the USC researchers had a few years before, also subjected human research subjects to the simulated smog environment, asking each person to record irritation with

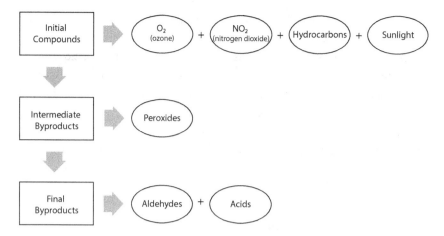

**Simplified rendition of Arie Haagen-Smit's schematic of smog formation, 1951.**
Among others, Haagen-Smit's experiments clearly identified the central role of
hydrocarbons and nitrogen dioxide ($NO_2$) in smog formation, while moving
attention away from the previous focus of air pollution control efforts, sulfur
dioxide ($SO_2$).

*Source*: "Second Technical and Administrative Report on Air Pollution Control in
Los Angeles County, 1950–1951," Box 20-05015-211 (APBP0012) (no folder), Kenneth
Hahn Hall of Administration (Los Angeles County), Los Angeles.

changes in hydrocarbon size and structure. As with plants, the intermediate
byproducts of oxidation were what triggered the adverse reactions, not the
hydrocarbons or nitrogen dioxide by themselves.[94]

Haagen-Smit's research carried several implications. Scientifically, the early
inquiries captured only part of smog formation: the focus on sulfur dioxide
had been somewhat misplaced. Sulfur dioxide and byproducts of its oxidation
could obscure visibility. But sulfur dioxide didn't react with hydrocarbons in
the same way—and result in similar consequences—as nitrogen dioxide. Likewise, the earlier focus on aldehydes had focused on *effects* (principally, eye irritation) but not on how they formed in the first place. Prior research had failed,
in Haagen-Smit's words, to look at emissions' "fate in the air."[95] "Pollutants from
the moments of their release are subjected to the action of natural components
of the air as well as that of other pollutants," he concluded.[96] Through three
experiments using plants, human research subjects, and rubber, Haagen-Smith
had identified *peroxides* as the chief culprit for the worst smog symptoms. He'd
learned how they formed. And he'd identified the sort of damage they did and
in what amount.

Haagen-Smit didn't touch politics, but his work's implications for industry
were unmistakable. "Estimates, as well as actual measurements," Haagen-Smit
summarized, "have shown that from 1000 to 2000 tons of hydrocarbons are

released daily into the Los Angeles atmosphere through evaporation losses in the manufacture and distribution of petroleum products and through incomplete combustion, chiefly from automobiles," the last previously an afterthought.[97] It wasn't that different from what countless APCD dispatches had said. But now smog had an identifiable life cycle that was not only more comprehensive and detailed but appeared in two prominent scientific journals. By moving scientific inquiry on smog from outside the walls of internal agencies and into the pages of *Industry and Engineering Chemistry* and *Plant Physiology*, research on the roots of smog and its effects gained new prominence.

## The Ambiguous Policy Role of Science

Haagen-Smit's findings were a watershed, but science had a more complicated role in Air Pollution Control District activities than one would think. Staring squarely in the face of scientific uncertainty, the APCD had in fact acted aggressively on smog way before the hydrocarbon discoveries. It'd long taken a multipronged approach toward smog, and it would continue doing so. In 1950, the same year as Haagen-Smit's discovery, the district declared: "Since each pollutant plays a different role in the formation of smog, a percentage change in any one pollutant does not necessarily reflect a corresponding change in the total smog problem."[98] Casting a wide net was paying off. From 1948 to 1951, declines were reported for aerosols (350 to 225), oxides of nitrogen (260 to 255), organic acids (140 to 90), and aldehydes (35 to 25). And sulfur dioxide continued to drop sharply, from 595 to 300 tons per day. But emissions of all types of hydrocarbons, the critical factor in Haagen-Smit's model, increased slightly, from 2,090 to 2,130 tons.[99]

Haagen-Smit's findings turned regulatory attention more squarely to hydrocarbon reduction. And it drew state-level attention to a local issue. In 1953, California governor Goodwin Knight convened a conference and appointed a Special Committee on Air Pollution consisting of not just Haagen-Smit but also Joseph Kaplan, UCLA's head of meteorology, Reed Brantley, Occidental College's head of chemistry, and John Poole, head of the science and mathematics department at John Muir College. The committee chair was Arnold O. Beckman, another Caltech connection. A former academic, Beckman had branched out into the private sector, forming Beckman Instruments, a firm that over the decades made him a millionaire via sales of meteorological devices.[100]

The most important sections of the Knight Committee's report dealt with culpability. As had previous public officials, the committee vacillated between consensus and conflict. Communitarian language infused the report's appraisal, with offending industries treated as both disruptors of the collective whole but also vital partners in taming that disruption. Its comments on automobiles were revealing. Knight Committee members wrote that "effective steps to control pollution from automobile exhausts appear to be among the most serious problems."[101] The solution, however, was to "secure aid from industry through improvements in engine design, better fuels, and development of corrective devices."[102] The optimal solutions were thus technical and achieved via consensus with auto manufacturers. It was a continuation of an ideal that animated the APCD from its early days.

Yet there were signs of cracks in the industrial-ecological accord. They came to the fore when the Knight Committee tackled the petroleum industry, which it identified as a primary target because of its heavy hydrocarbon contribution. The committee applauded the voluntary efforts of petroleum firms heretofore, remarking that in the future "the complete cooperation of the industry will be needed to reduce air pollution to an acceptable level."[103] But the optimistic tone of previous regulators was absent. If the current system failed, it would "lead inevitably to curtailment of industry or the imposition of onerous restrictions upon operations."[104] A battery of new restrictions suggested a more forceful stance toward the petroleum industry than the current one, which prioritized voluntarism. The committee proposed new rules banning "open" vapor-technique forms of petroleum extraction, such as "skimming ponds, separators, sumps and sewers." It argued for additional fume control regulations at filling stations and during transportation of gasoline, as well as limits on exhaust in vehicles themselves, either through the use of certain varieties of petroleum or through technical alterations to automobiles. Most ominously for the industry, though, was the committee's declaration that "the feasibility of reducing or relocating existing facilities and curtailing future expansion of air-polluting industries, such as petroleum refining, shall be actively investigated."[105] This meant, too, that the solutions offered by the Knight Committee, composed entirely of experts in the chemical and engineering sciences, were no longer just technical.

The prospect of restraining what'd become a core part of the Los Angeles County regional economy was now at least raised as an option, if not exactly highlighted. Though cooperation still ruled, conflict—if need be—was now more openly discussed than ever.

## Smog and the Boundaries of Health

Constituent complaints, the original impetus to regulatory intervention, had always starkly framed smog in health terms. So did the utterances of some public officials, such as Supervisor Ford, who'd early on characterized smog as a "grave menace to the well being and health of millions."[106] Framing smog as a health problem seemed self-evident enough. It was a surprise, then, when the Knight Committee deemphasized smog's health dimension. The committee called instead for "an all-out effort to get rid of smog," urging that officials not allocate resources "into channels which, however interesting"—read: medical research—"will not assist in reducing air pollution." Consequently, health barely came up in the committee's report except for quick references to eye irritation. When the committee characterized medical research as an unnecessary detour, it reaffirmed a central guiding tenet of Los Angeles County, which had moved preemptively, without worry about the need to wait for all evidence on human health effects to accumulate. The Knight Committee pushed that approach still further, writing that comprehensive smog abatement resulted in downstream effects and the elimination of all types of deleterious consequences (health or otherwise). "With the elimination of pollution, associated health hazards automatically vanish," the authors wrote.[107]

Deliberations in a Sacramento chamber were one thing. Elsewhere, residents continued to center, not sideline, the language of health whenever they talked about smog. In late 1954, Santa Monica resident Frederick Hehr warned that "even now too many deaths are caused by it, disguised as pneumonia, brain stroke and a few others. People even slightly sensitized will acquire a deadly sensitization if exposed to smog for weeks and months."[108] A year later, an ad hoc citizens' group issued a flyer titled "Warning: The Death Fog Is Coming." It spoke of refinery emissions "which are slowly embalming your living bodies from the lungs on out" and urged residents to write the board of supervisors "before you develop lung cancer and while you can still see to write."[109] And it intimated that the APCD was in the pockets of industry and withholding information about what was in pollutants, writing that to the district, "a refinery is a client, not a culprit."[110]

These residents remained apprehensive about the world around them. Despite regulatory progress, a prolonged smog attack on the city in 1954 demonstrated that the problem was hardly eradicated. And health professionals were concerned, too. From firsthand experience, physicians such as S. C. Glassman wrote to officials about "this unhealthful, dangerous condition." The results, Dr. Glassman said, were "more noticeable in the health of the people who have resided here during this time."[111] Robert Hope noted that he was "seeing more and more the effect upon my patients of smog," but that "one does not have to be a physician to postulate the fact that the air pollution . . . is very detrimental to our citizens' health in general."[112] Ophthalmologist S. S. Brown worried that eye irritation might cause "permanent damage," for which "the only sure relief is the removal of the cause—smog."[113] Paul Reed wondered "if the smog is capable of

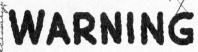

**Pamphlet with explicit health framing of air pollution, 1955.**
*Source*: "Warning: The Death Fog Is Coming," November 19, 1955, Box 25, Folder B III 5a ee, John Anson Ford Papers, Manuscripts Collection, Huntington Library, San Marino, Calif.

eating microscopic holes in the clothes, which people wear, what damage must it be doing to our eyes, the delicate membranes of the nose, throat, bronchial tubes and lungs."[114] Harold Lincoln Thompson, who'd practiced medicine for twenty-three years, stated that smog was a "serious hazard to the health of residents" and that, apart from irritation, more serious "lung and heart afflictions" might result.[115]

Individual residents and physicians weren't the only people keeping health alive in public discussion. Physicians' chief local lobbying organization, the Los Angeles County Medical Association (LACMA), took up the smog-health issue as well. The organization's involvement reflected air pollution control's broad political appeal and the unlikely allies it could draw. The association was typically opposed to large-scale state intervention on matters of health and was simultaneously engaging in fierce campaigns against national health insurance, just like its federal counterpart, the American Medical Association.[116] But on smog, LACMA not only supported the *expansion* of APCD efforts but criticized the officials for not focusing on health enough. It argued that the scientific research that the county had conducted so far on the chemical properties of smog required parallel attention to health effects. In 1951, LACMA had commissioned a survey of its membership soliciting physicians' impressions on smog and physiology. The 2,803 respondents echoed the physicians writing to Los Angeles County. Of them, 91 percent reported patients with eye problems they thought were attributable to smog, while 57 percent and 43 percent, respectively, observed lung and "psychoneurological" issues.[117] Three years later, in a statement issued in conjunction with Los Angeles medical schools, LACMA criticized the Knight Committee's argument that simply placing priority on elimination of all smog emissions would take care of its epiphenomenal problems, such as health effects. It was, in fact, "essential" to identify more precisely which compounds resulted in simple irritation and which had long-term health impacts. This required support for a research program that investigated "biological responses to smog," "metabolic research concerning absorption, fate and methods of excretion of smog constituents," "determination of systemic effects following absorption," and how "various intensity levels" resulted in "chronic and cumulative effects."[118] In private, LACMA was even more vigilant, internally debating the possibility of emergency oil refinery and traffic shutdowns, before deciding against them because of their "economic effect on the working people of this community." The association passed, however, a resolution chiding the board of supervisors for what it perceived as inattention to health.[119]

Los Angeles County Medical Association agitation escalated the Air Pollution Control District's interest in health. Largely due to pressure from LACMA, the agency drew on scientists from area medical schools and formed a Medical Commission on Environmental Contaminants to investigate the health effects of smog. It promised that such research, conducted at USC, was forthcoming. Lest the Knight Committee had left any other impression, in 1954, the APCD issued a public letter to county residents that reaffirmed, at least rhetorically, the agency's commitment to protecting human health. "No person and no industry, large or small, has the right to endanger the health of our people," the letter read.[120]

## APCD Restructuring and the Automobile Problem

Health focus or not, the Knight Committee catalyzed more expansion of Air Pollution Control District infrastructure. The agency increased its personnel from 117 in mid-1953 to 196 in mid-1955, with a maximum allowable number of 356 through 1956. It switched to a twenty-four-hour system of surveillance, which eliminated ad hoc enforcement driven primarily by response to impromptu complaints. And it looked into working with the county's regional planning commission, which proposed creating additional industrial zoning categories that would spatially isolate newly constructed facilities.[121] The agency pledged to follow through with all the Knight Committee's recommendations for controlling vapors from refineries and exhaust from automobiles.[122]

The most important ordinance since the APCD's caps on sulfur dioxide was rule 56, which required the installation of vapor-control equipment on petroleum storage tanks, a major source of hydrocarbons. In February 1954, the agency portrayed the initial implementation of the rule as a success, noting that an overwhelming majority of tanks slated for vapor control (103 out of 139) had properly adhered to its guidelines. Beyond the storage tanks, refineries themselves were subject to on-site inspections for excess hydrocarbon releases. An expanded permit system—from 50 to 700 in just three years—enabled such regularized oversight.[123] By mid-decade, the APCD boasted 340 fewer tons of hydrocarbons emitted daily. It was an important achievement. By the APCD's estimate, hydrocarbons—the critical compound in Haagen-Smit's smog model—accounted for more emissions than either sulfur dioxide or visible "dust and fumes" combined.

Los Angeles County zeroed in on oil extraction and automobiles as its two chief sources of interest for future air pollution control. The focus on them unleashed arguments over which was the greatest contributor and whether one deserved to be as scrutinized as the other. Cars hadn't been a major point of discussion in the first decade or so of Los Angeles air pollution control, but by 1955, this was no longer the case. Auto exhaust was rising due to federal highway infrastructure, along with skyrocketing vehicle usage stemming from Los Angeles's midcentury growth. Between 1939 and 1957, vehicle registrations had almost tripled, from 1.1 million to 2.9 million.[124]

Emerging scientific investigation on the automobile combustion process was showing that cars emitted more pollutants than previously thought. Caltech engineer Daugherty—who in the past tended to be a more conservative force within the APCD when it came to risk assessment—bluntly laid out several findings in a brief to the agency. Most automobile engines, in his experience, underwent "incomplete combustion" due to lack of sufficient air supply and time for compounds to react with one another. In an ideal combustion cycle, only carbon dioxide ($CO_2$), water ($H_2O$), and sulfur dioxide ($SO_2$) formed. More typically, though, an automobile emitted all the key components of smog: hydrocarbons, aldehydes, free hydrogen, and, previously unmentioned, carbon monoxide ($CO$), which Daugherty quickly mentioned might pose a danger in enclosed spaces.[125] Cars were, in other words, moving incubators of smog, and more than a million of them were rolling on the county's streets every day.[126]

Yet when it came to policy, Daugherty was characteristically more circumspect. More science didn't necessarily require more vigilance. "Until facts are obtained," Daugherty cautioned, "it would be premature to take certain drastic actions that mere uninformed people are advocating." And elsewhere, he tempered the ominous tone of his automobile exhaust brief by stating that he was unsure "whether it is the biggest factor or not" for smog, and he urged county officials to "appreciate the great difficulties that the automobile industry faces in alleviating this objectionable feature."[127] Similar sentiments came from such figures as Herbert Legg, another Los Angeles County supervisor, who regularly criticized the APCD not for lack of action but for too much activity. In the wake of the Knight Committee, he declared that the agency's rules had "involved the expenditure of many millions of dollars" by industrial firms to comply but that its rules were "found to be based on guesswork rather than upon proven scientific facts." Legg concluded, "There should be no more guesswork, whether it affects industry, the backyard incinerator, the automobile or any other prospective violator."[128]

These more cautious voices, whether scientists or politicians, pointed to a bigger issue: How much evidence was enough to justify another round of fresh regulations? A public meeting convened by the Citizens Committee on Air Pollution, formed by the county a couple years before, examined recurrent issues: what was "knowable" in smog science to that point; the future of the regulator-industrial relationship; and the relative smog contributions of suspected emissions sources. It brought together representatives from the Western Oil and Gas Association, the Southern California Air Pollution Foundation (a private group funded heavily by industry), the Pure Air Committee (another residents' group but unsanctioned by the county), and the APCD itself.[129] At the meeting's outset, P. S. Magruder, a longtime oil executive, spoke for the oil and gas association. He surprised the audience by publicly accepting Haagen-Smit's scientific finding pointing to the centrality of hydrocarbons.[130] The association's position, Magruder elaborated, stemmed not just from the science but also resignation over the lack of an alternative explanation. "We recognize," he said "that until we have something to refute the statement (if that is ever to be had) that hydrocarbons are the source of our trouble, we must put our house in order and we must recover as nearly 100 per cent of any emission of hydrocarbons as we can."[131] Magruder portrayed the county's petroleum firms as key participants in an antismog coalition and a larger community interest, not as antagonists. "We are citizens of this community just like you are.... We have stakes of a financial nature in this country just as you have. We expect that this country will grow, but it certainly is not going to improve in its growth if we have an undesirable and uncomfortable situation that is caused by smog," he continued.[132]

Magruder was still singing the industrial-ecological accord. Subsequent discussions between Magruder and the participants consisted of technical overviews of how to control vapor loss in refineries, which all the participants characterized as a fusion of effective self-policing with county oversight. When there was conflict, it centered on which exact phases of petroleum production deserved the most blame for emissions that remained hard to reduce. In two phases—oil field extraction and refining—Magruder claimed that vapor control systems could account for significant improvements. Where one couldn't report improvements, he continued, was in the third phase: "marketing," or transportation of the goods from refineries to the actual tanks of vehicles. There, hydrocarbon losses had risen in the past year, from 29 tons in 1953 to 37 tons presently.[133] Nearly all of it, he argued, came from the 8,500 independent filling stations (not overseen by oil producers), which had yet to install similar protective equipment to trap vapors. More important than filling stations, though, was what happened after vehicles left. Ultimately, both filling stations and auto exhaust were tied to the county's population growth, and it showed no sign of declining. From 1940 to 1950, it'd increased from 2.7 million to 4.1 million people. By 1960, the figure would reach 6 million.[134]

If filling stations were a problem, how was the county to address it? One possible solution was to pass an indirect tax onto the consumer, via price increases, which could then provide revenue for independent station owners and automobile manufacturers to install vapor covers and develop new carburetors and afterburners that emitted less exhaust. To Magruder, consumers would accept any hike if presented as a collectively mounted solution: "If we had the answer, and could say, Joe Dokes, we can assure you that if you will all come out here and do this, that and the other, there will be no more smog, or it will be very mild—I believe they'd go for it."[135] John Rice, speaking for the county's Citizens Committee on Air Pollution, echoed these sentiments and added that smog controls might even be marketable, a way to signal a business's commitment to a civic mission. He added that "it would be very thrilling ... to the whole public of this county if they could see at each filling station something being done affirmatively in connection with the air pollution problem."[136] Magruder and Rice weren't the only ones sounding a communitarian tone. Joseph Sternbach of the Pure Air Committee—typically a more critical organization—praised the industry as well, starting with its acceptance of the hydrocarbon research.

"We're sitting across the table from someone whom I have regarded as a dragon," he said. "The oil industry has represented to me a bogey-man, a dragon, something you couldn't approach and talk to."[137]

Though a commitment to cooperation and community spirit infused the meeting, there was uncertainty over what should come next. Part of that flowed from the nature of environmental science, which could be maddeningly imprecise on a number of counts. Although air pollution control officials could estimate how many tons were emitted from various sources, the figures were calculated by obtaining samples and making statistical projections for a total. And even with those projections, it wasn't always easy to gauge how much of a particular compound actually contributed to smog and thus what the right emissions cap might be. For instance, hydrocarbons emitted outside certain time periods (daytime) and meteorological conditions (certain wind speeds) wouldn't undergo the oxidation process Haagen-Smit had identified. It also wasn't easy to connect specific sources to emissions. Auto exhaust from *transportation* of gasoline, for instance, was often classified as coming from gasoline *production*.[138] In the end, science was important, but less so than it seemed at first glance. All its ambiguities resulted in an implicit commitment to just continue as the APCD always had, even when gaps in scientific knowledge still existed. Just "attack every known source," as the Pure Air Committee's John Rice put it.[139] A year would make a big difference.

## Recentering Health

Like the Knight Committee, the 1954 roundtable didn't make health a central point of emphasis. But it also didn't relegate it. Health only came up once, but it did so during a discussion over whether costly air pollution equipment would be justifiable "aside from the health terms."[140] The health benefits of air pollution control, in other words, were taken for granted. The initial decentering of health by public officials, then its reemergence, wasn't unique to Los Angeles. It paralleled smog discourse in other areas. The initial response to a weeklong December 1952 smog attack in London, historian Peter Thorsheim notes, wasn't healthcentric, and the press "said virtually nothing about its possible health effect." Only when officials later suspected a connection to elevated mortality during that week—and investigated it—did the interpretation of London smog became more explicitly oriented around its health effects.[141]

That was the case in Los Angeles, too, as preliminary results of health research on smog started to appear. In December 1954, the board of supervisors convened a "Special Advisory Committee on Smog."[142] It arrived as John Goldsmith and Lester Breslow, of California's Bureau of Chronic Diseases, initiated studies of smog and health effects.[143] The real splash came, though, from Paul Kotin, a USC professor of medicine, who published several articles examining the potential relationship between exposure to hydrocarbons and lung cancer. Writing in the *Public Health Reports*, Kotin surveyed an emerging body of work on potential carcinogens found in a number of products, including arsenic, selenium, and hydrocarbons. He discussed their emergence alongside a more disturbing trend, writing that "large-scale introduction of industrial pollutants into the atmosphere is entirely compatible with the latent period now generally accepted for the development of lung cancer, which ranges from 10 to 40 years."[144]

Kotin based his provocative pronouncement on research he'd conducted with the Air Pollution Control District during the past few years on carcinogenicity of auto exhaust. In 1952, Kotin's researchers collected air samples for a little more than a month. They were obtained at two sites, one located in the industrial town of Vernon, the other in Los Angeles, near a busy freeway intersection. The samples were then used to create a liquid solution designed to approximate smoggy Los Angeles County air, which researchers then rubbed on lab mice. After fifteen months, more than a dozen mice exhibited tumors. It was an incidence of 42 percent, which the researchers suggested might actually be low, given that tumors could still form in remaining mice.[145] Even more striking: none of the unexposed control mice had died, and none developed tumors.[146] The results were similar in two other groups of mice, one exposed to a solution derived from air samples of gasoline exhaust, the other to diesel, which contained even higher concentrations of hydrocarbons. In the first (gasoline exhaust), 44 percent of the experimental group exhibited tumors, while in the second (diesel exhaust), that figure jumped to 85 percent.[147]

Still, the findings came with caveats when it came to lung cancer. Although the experiments demonstrated carcinogenic properties of hydrocarbons, they had manifested as *skin* tumors. In Kotin's view, however, that already was sufficient for action from a "preventive-medicine and public-health point of view." That there was still uncertainty about the exact connection between hydrocarbons and lung cancer "in no way militates against regarding their atmospheric presence as anything but a potential hazard."[148] A year later, at the Third National Symposium on Air Pollution Research, Kotin discussed a subsequent experiment that produced lung tumors in mice. But the presentation lacked more precise details, including the exact biological mechanisms at play and the level of smog required.[149] There were other mysteries. In each of the experiments, after collecting air samples, Kotin decomposed them to identify a number of hydrocarbons present, most importantly benzopyrenes, which were known carcinogens. Less clear was what exactly happened to them *after* emissions from a source. Kotin hypothesized that the presence of an "external eluting agent"—capable of separating hydrocarbons from soots so that they could enter human bodies—might be necessary for "cancer initiation."[150]

Limits notwithstanding, Kotin's findings caused a stir, generating headlines not just in Los Angeles County but across the country. Yet the challenges of pinpointing smog's exact health ramifications persisted. In 1955, the California State Department of Health issued *Clean Air for California*, which underscored the provisional nature of health inquiries. A year later, officials from the APCD, the Los Angeles County Medical Association, and the private Stanford Research Institute gathered in front of the press to debate the difficulties of health research. Carl Miller, a *Wall Street Journal* reporter, opened the event by declaring that "probably no other aspect of smog quite concerns all of us as much as its possible effect on our health," before going on to state that much "confusion" existed around the issue.[151]

One conundrum was conceptual. If one viewed health as the World Health Organization did—as not merely "absence of disease" but "complete physical, mental, and social well-being"—there was little dispute that smog was associated with health, given the physiological irritation and feelings of unpleasantness well documented by both Los Angeles residents and laboratory experiments. But if one defined health more narrowly, as a series of physiological signs, it wasn't yet clear how smog damaged human bodies, if at all. And little was known about accumulated harmful effects that weren't immediately obvious. As the Stanford Research Institute's Dale Hutchinson put it: "We haven't any information, for example, on what is sometimes termed as the synergistic effect—what happens when you get several pollutants that a person is breathing, for example, for 16 hrs. a day; or what are the long-range effects of some of these things. What is going to happen to me when I am 84 as a result of having breathed smog for 40 years?"[152]

Laboratory work on mice existed, but studies conducted in the field among actual living humans were a whole other matter.[153] An obvious hurdle was simply the lack of sufficient time that had passed before one could design a study to investigate links between someone's past smog exposures and current ailments. "Even the most adequate of medical research programs will not produce the answers we require overnight," remarked the APCD's Leslie Chambers.[154] What existed were a crop of cross-sectional studies, which their authors claimed showed elevated mortality rates during heightened smog at a single point in time.[155] But this work, at best, was hypothesis generating, given the host of other variables that might explain such an outcome.[156] And it did little to identify precise pathways connecting smog to morbidity and mortality. Interest in health may have been growing again, but findings about exact effects and causes remained underdeveloped. For people such as Goldsmith and Breslow, who had conducted some of the first epidemiological studies of air pollution, it still wasn't a reason to dismiss the health dimension. Writing in 1958, a few years after their first studies had appeared, they admonished those who would "derogate study of the health effects in favor of control efforts alone."[157]

## Triumphs and Limits: Two Cheers for Air Pollution Control

Even without full scientific knowledge about smog and, later, its human health effects, the Air Pollution Control District proceeded at a furious pace for the better part of the 1950s. Uncertainties had always existed over the relative importance of different pollutants, and the agency had always cast a wide net. Since rule 53, which limited concentrations of sulfur dioxide, it had passed a slew of other similar measures. Amendments to rule 53 covered additional material lost in combustion during industrial processes, particularly carbon monoxide, and applied to all industrial sources. Rule 54 targeted "dust and fumes," capping emission at 40 pounds per hour for facilities processing more than 60,000 pounds of material in the same time span. In addition to rule 56, which required vapor-controlling equipment on tanks, rules 59 and 61 expanded the vapor controls to two phases identified by the APCD as points of concern beyond the original source: separation into liquid and the marketing phase, when gasoline was loaded into trucks and trailers.[158] Rules 57 and 58 outright banned open fires and backyard incinerators, both typically used for waste disposal. This enraged a faction of homeowners and real estate interests who saw the measure as overly aggressive, an affront to property rights, or a red herring away from more substantial sources of industrial pollution.[159] The APCD didn't care.

Toward the end of the 1950s, the agency turned its eye to the automobile. But it deviated from the industrial-ecological accord that Los Angeles County had embraced since the end of the war. The shift resulted in protracted conflict that extended into the next decade. Automobiles were difficult to control. They were nonstationary and lacked equipment for controlling exhaust. But the technological limits, in the eyes of some county officials, were caused as much by automobile firms' foot-dragging as by an engineering lag. As it had with other industry groups, the county had reached out to automobile manufacturers, sending representatives to meet executives for a week in Detroit. At a 1955 meeting, county officials were briefed on prototype devices designed to reduce emissions by limiting air flow, particularly during deceleration, which accounted for a majority of hydrocarbon loss. Working together as a "non-competitive and non-profit basis," automotive firms overseen by the Automobile Manufacturers Association planned for the release of an initial device for 1958, which the county planned to mandate on all vehicles as a rule. The meeting ended on an optimistic note, with the manufacturers praising the county for its strong public stances on incinerators, which they interpreted as a sign of across-the-board enforcement and lack of favoritism toward one or another polluter.[160]

But within a year, Smith Griswold, fresh into his first year as APCD director, questioned the manufacturers' commitment, leading to a testy private rebuke from manufacturers themselves. Supervisor Kenneth Hahn was even more aggressive, hounding individual executives about their sluggish pace. Although manufacturers had sent some pilot contraptions to the APCD, it looked doubtful that they'd meet the 1958 date for a completed device. Whether that was due to lack of collective commitment or genuine engineering challenge was beside the point. It left a large hole in the county's air pollution strategy, which had yet to address the most rapidly growing source of emissions in the region via a rule.

The foot-dragging by car companies wasn't the only problem. Even if the ideal device did emerge, Griswold wondered whether the emergence of such a device would result in as substantial a net benefit as hoped, given the consistently rising number of automobiles in the region. According to one estimate, even if the hypothetical device could reduce hydrocarbon loss by 25 percent, "partial control," Griswold noted, might in the end be "marginal in terms of the triennial increase in the County automobile population."[161] Griswold was onto something. Between 1945 and 1955, the car population had doubled, from a little more than 1 million to about 2.5 million. It was projected to continue to 3.5 million by the next decade, more than enough to offset a device that reduced an individual vehicle's emissions.[162]

If the dividends from a device limiting hydrocarbon losses—were it to ever appear—wouldn't be as consequential as hoped, were automobiles themselves a diversion, and might a more productive focus be petroleum itself? Environmental scientists had started investigating whether the specific hydrocarbon composition in fuels increased the likelihood of oxidation, in turn critical to creating smog. The APCD's own Paul Mader and Leslie Chambers were looking into an association between fuel composition of commonly used automobiles and volume of oxidation products (in this case, aldehydes).[163] In one experiment, researchers compared the effects of premium fuels with a special laboratory-modified one containing no hydrocarbons. After running both in the same motor, they found that the modified fuel yielded a lower volume of oxidation products: 1.60 parts per million (ppm) versus 3.46 ppm for total aldehyde concentration after an hour of combustion.[164] The findings set the course for learning more about fuel composition itself, particularly olefins, a class of hydrocarbons that the researchers hypothesized might be more likely to result in smog. It also meant more ambiguity, not clarity.

The focus on automobiles and fuels pointed to another blind spot of the antismog campaign as it evolved: the centrality accorded to hydrocarbons. Hydrocarbons, of course, had captured everyone's attention because of their role in forming smog. But did the heavy focus on them come at the expense of other pollutants? Although rules limited sulfur and carbon monoxide emissions, as well as dust and fumes from such industrial sites as steel and textile mills, these other compounds ceased to be as strong a focus even if they played important roles in pollution that had nothing to do with Haagen-Smit's oxidation process. (This was to say nothing, too, of pollutants that were not "detectable by sight and sting," in Christopher Sellers's phrase.)[165] Health studies—already relegated to second position by Governor Knight's committee—came to center on hydrocarbons alone rather than on a larger array of compounds that might prove equally harmful to human health. Only toward the late 1960s did the health risks of other emissions return to prominence in both scientific research and regulation.[166] These included sulfur and nitrogen oxides, as well as particulate matter: tiny, barely visible (sometimes invisible) aerosols and solids that get lodged in people's lungs.

An additional reason for the sidelining of sulfur dioxide, plus other compounds, may have been Paul Kotin's claims about hydrocarbons and lung cancer, which years afterward looked monocausal and reductive. This was especially the case when one took into account Kotin's later assertions that air pollution, not smoking, was the leading cause of lung cancer, a proclamation he first made in a 1956 article published in *Cancer Research*. "There is at present no convincing evidence that tobacco possesses the necessary qualifications for the initiation and promotion of lung cancer," Kotin boldly wrote. Almost all of the *Cancer Research* article was devoted, however, to a literature review of studies such as those Kotin had conducted on hydrocarbons and carcinogenicity and offered nothing to support the statement about tobacco. Despite this, Kotin pressed the exclusivity of the connection between air pollution and lung cancer for years, beyond scientific journals and in the mainstream press. Left unmentioned in the media coverage was Kotin's simultaneous presence on the scientific advisory board of the Tobacco Industry Research Committee, an industry front group that downplayed the cigarette and lung cancer link for decades. As an influential air pollution researcher in Los Angeles County, Kotin's efforts diverted agency attention away from health outcomes other than lung cancer and compounds other than hydrocarbons.[167]

In this regard, the biggest omission from the program's purview was tetraethyl lead, common in gasoline. In a 1955 memo by Caltech's R. L. Daugherty outlining the hydrocarbon problem, tetraethyl lead received only a passing mention. A 1957 presentation by automobile executive J. M. Campbell in Los Angeles County entitled "What We Are Doing about Combustion?" similarly glossed over lead, mainly discussing a single 1927 Bureau of Mines study downplaying the health effects of leaded gasoline.[168] Even the APCD's own Smith Griswold referred to lead as not present "in sufficient quantity to constitute hazards in their initial form."[169] The position was consistent with that of the Lead Industries Association, a lobby for companies that made lead-based products. It'd long claimed that the human body could tolerate low levels of lead. The chief promulgater of this assertion was Robert Kehoe, a prominent industrial hygienist funded by the Ethyl Corporation, a top leaded gasoline manufacturer. The Kehoe position on lead was a consensus many public health practitioners accepted for decades. It would not be challenged prominently until the mid-1960s by Clair Patterson, a Caltech professor of geochemistry.[170] Until then, Kehoe and other Ethyl employees regularly wrote letters and gave speeches dismissing the dangers of lead. Writing to the APCD, as he did to many other agencies across the country, Kehoe cautioned in 1950 against "any very striking conclusions concerning the importance of minute quantities of lead in the atmosphere" and downplayed "the increment due to the use of leaded gasoline," arguing that it was "difficult to isolate."[171] A draft of a 1954 public statement from Ethyl, circulated among Kehoe and two Ethyl executives, referenced Los Angeles pollution but then claimed that "lead in small enough quantities is not poisonous. There is lead in all the food we eat and water we drink, as well as in all the air we breathe. The average city-dweller takes in daily about 30 times as much lead from his food and drink as from the air he breathes. He doesn't accumulate this lead permanently in his body, but excretes it and so keeps in balance."[172]

Still, in the years immediately preceding the challenge to these ideas on lead, some environmental health scientists had already begun investigating the health effects of airborne lead exposures from gasoline. Although their analyses operated squarely within preexisting assumptions on lead and health, they occasionally scratched the edges of the consensus. A national 1960 conference on air pollution and health, for instance, featured a symposium on lead and carbon monoxide exposures. One paper by Joseph Aub, who'd spent most of his career at Harvard Medical School and Massachusetts General Hospital, compared organic lead and inorganic lead intoxication. Organic lead poisoning occurred through skin absorption and eventual passage to the intestinal tract and had drawn the bulk of researchers' attention. Inorganic lead intoxication, which could result after organic lead was burned in tetraethyl gasoline, occurred through inhalation and passage through lungs. The latter pathway, he suggested, resulted in much more absorption of lead than occurred via the gastrointestinal tract. Elaborating further in a panel discussion, Aub remarked: "My point of view is that the only important thing is the total amount of lead that is taken in per day, regardless of where you get it. However, the amount taken in by lung is more toxic than that taken in through the stomach." The remarks were notable coming from Aub, who was one of the most high-profile defenders of the Kehoe consensus and himself also a recipient of lead industry funds. Although he didn't budge from the position that only high levels of lead exposures were toxic, Aub allowed, in however qualified a manner, that lead exposures from automobile exposures might pose more of a threat than other pathways. This made the APCD's sidelining of the leaded gasoline threat all the more lamentable, even if it was in keeping with prevailing views toward lead at the time.[173]

Airborne lead exposure eventually shaped up to be one of the central tragedies in public health regulation, persisting into the 1970s all while remaining marginalized in lead debates, anchored as they were around housing stock and lead paint. It was not until 1970 that California adopted a lead threshold of 1.5 micrograms per cubic meter, which became the federal standard in 1978. By then, manufacturers were phasing out lead anyway because of the damage it caused to new catalytic converters.[174] The standard would not be lowered again until three decades later, when a growing counterconsensus finally emerged around the dangers of low-level lead exposures.[175] Public awareness of airborne lead, however, had grown throughout the 1960s. In 1969, a year before the California standard, a new advocacy group called the People's Lobby had condemned "existing laws and devices" that "do not in any manner control the pollution of our bodies with lead."[176] The group—hatched in the wake of a failed attempt to recall Governor Ronald Reagan—was setting its sights actively on environmental regulation and what it perceived as insufficient aggressiveness.[177]

Another major constraint on the APCD was its unfolding in concert with regulated industries. Although the agency was no pushover, it often accepted the industry's terms of debate. The voluntarist approach rested on industrial firms' wish to abide by rules that were ultimately ameliorative, such as using vapor covers and hydrocarbon reducing equipment. Writing on the Los Angeles Chamber of Commerce's influence on what I have called here the industrial-ecological accord, historian Sarah Elkind has written that the organization "protected the Los Angeles business and industrial community from more stringent regulations and ensured that air pollution policy met its own institution goals."[178] Many other regulatory proposals never received significant follow-through: implementing aggressive zoning, limiting construction of new industrial sites, or relocating existing ones. This inaction left open the question of whether Los Angeles County's commitment to perpetual industrial growth and boosterism would ultimately triumph over human health and livability.

Then there was the question of environmental health inequality. One of the areas almost directly in the path of the wind patterns that Morris Neiburger had identified in the mid-1940s was Watts, where almost all of Los Angeles's Black residents lived, squeezed between Inglewood and the industrial suburb of Vernon, an early source of interest during the nascent days of the APCD. After a 1965 riot, Watts was about to become the site of a huge wave of infrastructural investment designed to address severe medical neglect of the area. But the very world where patients lived and the air they breathed outside of the new medical facilities was a whole other matter. Not far away were waste sites, airports, and the burgeoning ports of Los Angeles and Long Beach, part of an overall pattern of zoning that concentrated industrial sites in certain areas and made environmental health burdens most felt by residents of low-income, often racially segregated neighborhoods.[179] Things weren't helped by what historian Eric Avila has characterized as "the age of the freeway." Beginning in the 1940s, Los Angeles County—spurred by soaring population growth, a doubling of automobile registrations in a two-decade period, and street crowding—embarked on a highway construction boom fueled by generous state subsidies. It ultimately resulted in a Los Angeles system that increased "four and a half times" in size between 1950 and 1955, doing so at the expense of a number of working-class Latino and minority neighborhoods, where buildings were bulldozed and cleared to make way for highways.[180]

In an era of robust growth, freeways were a paradox, and they captured the fundamental weaknesses and strengths of even the most robust of local air pollution programs. In seeking to provide relief from congestion, the new roadways instead opened the gates to even more of it but on a larger scale, bolstered by the "national, state or intercommunity" automotive connections that a 1943 regional plan had called for. It was a version of a persistent conundrum: how to accommodate economic growth and boom while curtailing its ecological excesses, and freeways made it a problem bigger than any local agency could handle. That's because Los Angeles County's air pollution problems had now become those of neighboring San Bernardino, Ventura, and Orange Counties, too. Recognizing the illusory nature of local county boundaries when it came to air pollution whose sources crisscrossed multiple regions per day, California created a locale-transcending agency called the Air Resources Board (CARB) in 1967 to oversee the entire state. It made the dean of smog research, Arie Haagen-Smit, its first chair.[181] The need to scale pollution control efforts up still further came in 1970, when the federal government created the Environmental Protection Agency and passed the Clean Air Act to oversee emissions across the country.

Yet local air pollution strategies still persisted in these new forms. The Air Resources Board borrowed most of its regulations straight from the APCD (down to the exact enumeration of rules), and the tactic of preemptively targeting both sources and particular substances, whether oxides or hydrocarbons or whatever else, with strong emissions caps had first been perfected in the smoggiest of Los Angeles days. And in something of a full circle, the Environmental Protection Agency listed as one of six so-called criteria air pollutants sulfur dioxide, the first compound targeted by the APCD.[182] Further, it allowed CARB to set state-level standards more stringent than federal ones, while CARB allowed the same for county-level agencies below it: the idea being that local conditions might deviate from overall national or state ones and thus require tailored and specific regulations. In 1955, President Dwight Eisenhower had remarked that pollution was "a uniquely local" dilemma. He'd been both wrong yet also quite right.[183]

The Los Angeles air pollution story was one of striking efficacy, however imperfect, and unlikely unity, however fraught. Its medical care story was something else. A decade after the heyday of local air pollution control, the Watts riots of 1965 forced Los Angeles to confront who'd really gotten to participate in two decades of Los Angeles growth and who'd been excluded from it. Civic tranquility, with the occasional hints of fracture, now turned into explosive conflict, and medicine was not insulated from it. The Los Angeles medical world wrestled with how to reverse racial marginalization, who exactly would get to shape solutions, and how whatever they devised would survive an emerging era of fiscal stringency.

# 3

# Los Angeles

## Health Politics and the Fire Next Time

Los Angeles's air pollution control program had occasionally conceded to industry; contained more than its share of regulatory opportunities not grasped; and never quite—to this day—harmonized the contradiction between capping emissions amid runaway industrial growth. Nevertheless, its creators had reasons to boast. Even before the science of smog was settled, they had created a robust countywide edifice with buy-in from varied municipalities and constituencies throughout a vast and growing metropolis.

But the civic unity that characterized smog abatement belied pervasive inequalities underneath. It'd be in another domain of health politics—medical care—where long-simmering fractures within the city would come to a boil. Those who brought attention to it were the mix of the expected and the unexpected.

One of the unexpected turned up before the Los Angeles County Board of Supervisors in 1966. A few years removed from the Bay of Pigs Invasion and the Cuban Missile Crisis, Central Intelligence Agency (CIA) personnel were probably among the people you'd least imagine opining perceptively on racism. And when they did, it was usually in the name of funding counterinsurgencies to stamp out civil rights activism.[1] Former agency director John McCone's words were all the more striking, then, when he remarked: "We concluded that the sickness in the center of our city caused an explosion, a formless, quite senseless, but almost hopeless and violent protest engaged in by a few, but bringing distress to all. The health problems in South Central Los Angeles did, in our opinion, contribute materially to the crisis in our city."[2]

McCone was talking about the 1965 riots in the Watts neighborhood of Los Angeles, just under a year earlier. And while his remarks flung some aspersions on the rioters' tactics and virtuousness, they contained an admission that there were real grievances behind the rioters' actions. This admission was one many people in his professional strata were forced to make during the long, hot summers of the 1960s when waves of cities in the United States, from Plainfield and Newark, New Jersey, to Cleveland and Detroit were wracked by what observers euphemistically called "civil disorders."[3] Watts drew more attention than almost any of them, and in a single week, it dispelled the idyllic image California's boomtown wanted to project. Kitschy Spanish Art Deco, palm trees, classic Hollywood, and beachfronts gave way to reckoning with police brutality, residential segregation, material deprivation, and widespread racism too long ignored.

McCone's remarks came not just at any hearing but one specifically about medical maldistribution. His remarks mentioned "health problems in South Central Los Angeles," where Watts was located, and they were part of a larger discussion about the need to deliver to the area much-needed medical infrastructure that'd been absent for decades. As the chair of the commission assessing the reasons behind the rioting, McCone had overseen a report that concluded that Watts was nothing less than a medical desert and that'd recommended the construction of a full-service public hospital as a solution. Now, the CIA man was impatient and was returning to Los Angeles County with a message: get on with it.

Until the riots, Los Angeles County's health care system hadn't experienced any of the sustainability problems that wracked New York City's in the immediate years after World War II. But maldistribution was another story. And so, heeding McCone's call to action, get on with it government officials did. They didn't anticipate demands for community control that'd soon follow and a radically different fiscal climate that'd soon threaten the sustainability of the new infrastructure they'd offer for the problem of medical maldistribution in Los Angeles.

### County Growth, Hospital Boom

In the few decades preceding Watts, nobody would've predicted that health would be key to analyses of the riot and solutions proposed in the wake of it. Before World War II, the system was modest and sleepy. After the war, it underwent remarkable growth, in tandem with the region in which it sat.

The largest and oldest of the county hospitals, Los Angeles County General, served as the teaching facility for several medical schools, with a particularly strong tie to the University of Southern California (USC) School of Medicine. In the early twentieth century, university affiliation proceeded on a largely casual and improvised course for decades. The postwar period saw more formalization of the relationship, with a $419,000 contract signed in 1953 between USC and the county, which compensated the school for personnel and supervision of County General's training programs.[4]

The Los Angeles County system had added only one minor facility during the interwar years, Olive View Hospital, in 1920. But after World War II, it needed to expand rapidly. Officials estimated a total shortage of 1,686 acute general care beds in Los Angeles across both voluntary and public sectors that the hospital could help alleviate. To ease the shortage, the county acquired a military hospital in 1946 and converted it into a 700-bed facility, Harbor General Hospital, aimed at southwestern Los Angeles. In contrast to a New York system facing infrastructural limits and personnel flight by the late 1950s, the Los Angeles counterpart experienced robust postwar growth. Five years after its creation, Harbor General entered an agreement with the UCLA School of Medicine, modeled after the County General–USC affiliation, thus providing the county with two academically affiliated hospitals.[5] County oversight, like air pollution regulation, became further enforced with a county-city merger of health services departments in 1964.[6]

Los Angeles affiliations weren't just free of sustainability crises. They also didn't run into political discord over governance, as happened in New York in the early days of public hospital affiliation. One reason for that was simple tradition. From County General's inception, medical schools had been involved in its operations but had never assumed administrative control over institutions' individual governance. Most staff at public hospitals thus saw affiliation as a necessity, not an outside incursion by private medical centers. In 1958, for example, when UCLA officials announced that they might end the Harbor General affiliation, several members of Harbor General's attending staff responded that they wouldn't want to work at a public hospital unconnected to an academic medical center. The character of Los Angeles County further blunted any hostility to affiliation. The small number of public hospitals, amid geographic sprawl, discouraged development of the strong localist ties to hospitals that existed in New York.[7] "Every neighborhood its own hospital" was hardly the mantra of Los Angeles County in the 1940s.

Unburdened by New York–level sustainability crises, Los Angeles County health officials could focus on expansion. Following the Harbor General facility acquisition, Wayne Allen, the county's chief administrative officer, remarked that "this unit alone is not enough," given the region's expected population boom.[8] Officials commissioned studies on medical needs, and the results showed that current infrastructure was inadequate to the task. Far from the 1,688 figure predicted during wartime, two needs assessments argued that the county required slightly more than 8,000 beds, about one-third of which should be in public facilities. The county saw the problem not just in the numerical aggregate but also in spatial terms. It divided the county up into twenty-one hypothetical health districts, calculating ideal bed needs for each one based on population counts. The conclusion: future health facilities ought not be built indiscriminately but planned and sited carefully according to patient demand and where it did and didn't exist. In the words of Arthur J. Will, the county's superintendent of charities, the county would be "best served by a decentralized and appropriate distribution of hospitals throughout the entire County area."[9]

And so, infrastructural growth continued. In 1955, the county leased the 200-bed private Methodist Hospital in southwest Los Angeles for ten years, renaming it the John Wesley County Hospital. It purchased the facility to ease ongoing burdens at the other two main county hospitals and to provide more care for the area. The county rebuffed repeated attempts by a physicians' group to sublease the facility for private use, with its lead attorney arguing that county medical needs were still too great to give up any more beds. It was all a sign of the county's commitment to providing more public facilities for the medically indigent, and a decade later, the city purchased the Wesley hospital outright.[10] Advocates pitched expansion as integral to Los Angeles County's civic consciousness and economic growth. For James Hamilton, the consultant who'd conducted one of the citywide hospital surveys, the county, via the addition of more hospital beds, needed to cultivate a widespread appreciation of general hospitals as "a fundamental community service institution which forms part of the bulwark of community life, which must be preserved and developed to gain the health and happiness so constantly sought by its citizens." Los Angeles County's "expanded economic development," he argued, "requires a balanced expanded health program to maintain its pace."[11]

If Los Angeles was the exemplar midcentury booming metropolis, health care was going to be an integral part of it. But the robust growth of Los Angeles County hospitals in the 1950s hardly proceeded without problems. Into the 1960s, personnel shortages wracked the system, though they took on a different form than those in New York City. On the East Coast, employees at all levels fled or avoided the public system entirely. In Los Angeles County, by contrast, the problem wasn't exodus but perpetual shortage caused by rapid population growth and heightened patient demand, especially for outpatient care. County facilities had trouble keeping up. Speaking in 1957 before the board of supervisors, one County General executive estimated that admissions had spiked by 54 percent in the past decade, with outpatient clinic volume up by 78 percent. The result, he recounted, was "as many as 2,750 outpatients . . . in our clinics every day," and regular "overcrowd[ing]" from facilities ill-equipped to deal with the pressure.[12] Residents complained, too. Albert Gilpin asked county supervisors to "relieve the suffering and hardship imposed on county hospital outpatients." He recounted three and a half hours "spent sitting on a hard bench with dozens of men, women, and children all sick seeking medical aid" and feeling that "the employees of the outpatient dept . . . make no effort to get these cases attended to."[13]

Patients weren't the only ones upset. So were hospital personnel. In 1957, Local 347, the union that represented city, county, and state employees, studied the stresses on labor created by heightened patient demand. It pointed out that the "average hours of bedside nursing care per patient" were below the hospital management minimums of the time. They stacked up poorly, too, against private hospitals in the area. Compared to Cedars of Lebanon Hospital, for example, County General recorded average nursing care hours of 2.83 compared to Cedars' 6.285.[14] It was a staff, in other words, spread dreadfully thin. County hospital administrators had begun hiring licensed vocational nurses to fulfill the functions of increasingly scarce registered nurses, and everyone was often "doubling up and work[ing] double shifts and working on their days' off," in the words of Alfred Charlton, Local 347's business manager.[15] The union's diagnosis matched the county's. That same year, Roger Egeberg, County General's medical director, estimated a countywide shortage of 800 nurses.[16]

The mounting attention given to these problems generated a swift policy response. Board of supervisors chairman John Anson Ford wrote that there was no excuse for "the kinds of human neglect" that he was "satisfied is taking place in our great institution," pledging county action and portraying the facilities' faults as an opportunity to be seized.[17] The county followed by placing three bond measures on the ballot to raise funds for alterations to County General. All three measures received majority votes, with 62.9 percent voting in favor of a dedicated outpatient wing, 54.9 percent for a rebuilt nurses' residence, and 53.2 percent for a new interns and residents building, but they failed to overcome the county's two-thirds majority requirement. Still, although not overwhelming, the majority results indicated the existence of a substantial public constituency for the hospitals, confirmed two years later when the county floated another $19.9 billion hospital bond that did pass.[18] It allowed the county to proceed with the County General upgrades, which freed up space usable for at least 200 additional outpatient beds. Beyond that, the hospital reported steady rises in internship and residency placements, a sharp contrast to declines faced by New York City at around the same time. The nursing shortage remained a challenge, but by mid-1959, rates of new hospital staff outpaced rates of new patients, 10 percent to 9 percent.[19]

## The Underside of Medical Boom: Maldistribution in Watts

In 1946, James Hamilton had argued that economic growth and medical care expansion ought to proceed in tandem. And the county had obliged, acquiring three new facilities and cementing ties to prestigious medical schools. This development occurred alongside a huge national investment boom in hospital construction, best exemplified by the Hill-Burton Hospital Survey and Construction Act that same year, which appropriated $75 million for building hospitals. Almost all of it (93 percent) went to Jim Crow states, however, which meant segregated wards and subpar care for African Americans in the South.[20]

That's not exactly what happened in Los Angeles County. Instead, during Los Angeles County's public hospital boom, large areas—and the people in them—were entirely passed over. Hamilton had warned of it, interrupting his rousing call by reminding officials that "we must also face the problems of the racial and so-called minority groups for which the hospital facilities easily obtainable by them in this County is pitifully small."[21] His admonition went unheeded. And in the mid-1960s Los Angeles would soon see what happened when officials didn't "face the problems" of which Hamilton spoke.

Throughout the decade and a half following Hamilton's statement, Los Angeles had become home to a steady influx of westward-bound African Americans. Though less remembered in the popular imagination, it was a stream no less consequential to the Great Migration than others from the South to the Midwest and Northeast, and it resulted in rapid demographic change. In 1940, 75,209 African Americans lived in the county. By 1960, that number grew to 451,546. The conditions African American arrivals confronted were just as arduous as those faced by their counterparts elsewhere.[22] Virulent racism in the housing market severely limited their residential options, and on top of that was white flight from neighborhoods when Black residents arrived. The cumulative result was a Los Angeles riven with residential segregation, where most of the city's Black population was funneled, marginalized, and spatially concentrated into South Central Los Angeles. Two of its most well-known areas were the adjacent neighborhoods of Watts and Willowbrook, 95 and 80 percent Black, respectively. There, in the words of historian Josh Sides, residents "increasingly found that the neighborhoods in which they had invested much of their time and energy were deteriorating rapidly." In 1962, the Los Angeles County Welfare Planning Council described the area as one dotted "with unpaved roads and old houses" alongside the "low rental and low dwelling unit values" that "predominate[d] in such sections." In it, there were "no large shopping centers to focus community activity or traffic." It was a place that "[gave] the impression of being largely unplanned," with "marked over-crowding" in some parts next to "large patches of land with relatively low population density." And despite the achievements of air pollution control countywide, other environmental health hazards were everywhere. Industrial expansion from neighboring Vernon meant that parts of South Central were "littered with industrial debris and saturated by industrial liquid runoff." The unpleasantness was compounded by lack of

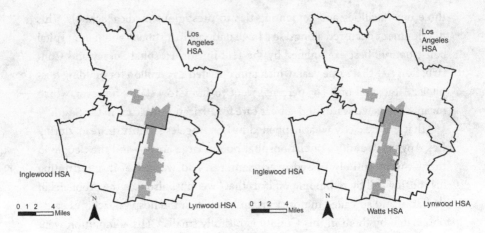

**1960 census tracts with 75%+ Black populations before/after new Watts Hospital Service Area.** The first map shows boundaries of three contiguous existing Hospital Service Areas at the time. The second shows the new boundaries proposed by White for the Watts HSA (eventually adopted by Los Angeles County) and how it foregrounds the particular social geography of the area. (Its boundaries are carved from the previous HSAs.)

*Source:* Author's calculations and cartography based on 1960 U.S. Census (National Historical Geographical Information Systems database, Minnesota Population Center, University of Minnesota. Note: These diagrams were created by identifying the census tracts that comprised each HSA. Tracts for the Watts HSA are found in "Appendix C: State Advisory Hospital Council Meeting," March 7, 1966, Box-Folder 1.24.2.6.5.8, Papers of Kenneth Hahn, Manuscripts Collection, Huntington Library, San Marino, Calif., which also indicates which of the contiguous HSAs each tract was used to form. I could not find a systematic tract-to-HSA directory for those unlisted in this document despite a thorough canvas of the annual *California State Plan for Hospitals*, which provided boundaries but not tracts. I estimated the tracts by georeferencing a map of the boundaries and HSA boundaries to census tract boundaries. I believe this estimate is mostly reliable, though not perfect, with an unavoidable drop-off or addition of a few tracts per HSA. For tracts partially within HSA boundaries, I chose to exclude rather than include. The HSA map is in Arthur Viseltear, Arnold I. Kisch, and Milton Roemer, *The Watts Hospital: A Health Facility Is Planned for a Metropolitan Slum Area* (Arlington, Va.: U.S. Department of Health, Education, and Welfare, 1967), 60.

effective public transportation in the region, especially when the Pacific Electric railway system ceased operation in 1961 and was replaced by "notoriously unreliable and inconvenient" bus service, most of it subcontracted to independent firms.[23]

The county hadn't entirely ignored the area's health needs and had acknowledged geographic barriers to hospital access for those isolated in South Central Los Angeles. Discussing their efforts, county officials described a growing population in the area "seriously in need of public health services." But it combined the statement with thinly veiled antipathy for those who lived there. The

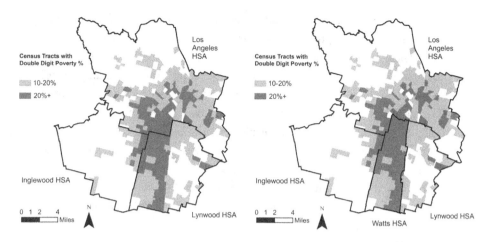

**1970 census tracts with double-digit poverty percentage before/after new Watts Health Service Area.** The first map shows boundaries of three contiguous existing Hospital Service Areas at the time. The second shows the new boundaries proposed by Sol White for the Watts HSA (eventually adopted by Los Angeles County) and how it foregrounds the particular social geography of the area. I used the 1970 census because it was the first to incorporate a poverty rate measure. I relied on the Social Explorer database's "Poverty Status for Families" variable, recalculated from the original manuscript census. Though imperfect in many ways, it provides a sense of the spatial distribution of poverty.

*Source*: Author's calculations and cartography based on 1970 U.S. Census (Social Explorer database and National Historical Geographical Information Systems database, Minnesota Population Center, University of Minnesota).

county's health officer, Roy Gilbert, wrote that the population's "low income combined with high birth rate and relatively low levels of hygienic standards serve to develop public health problems" that a health center could alleviate. Such a facility would "bring our indolent and indifferent segment of the population under official public health influence to a significant degree."[24] This wasn't exactly a testament to a county health system that showed much regard toward Black residents. Still, under pressure from the Los Angeles Urban League, the county constructed a health center in South Central Los Angeles.

Overall, the county's efforts were indeed modest and existed alongside independent initiatives elsewhere. In 1946, a group of left-leaning physicians and activists had founded the Community Medical Foundation (CMF), which operated an outpatient facility in the Watts area. From its inception, the foundation saw the center as a way to demonstrate an alternative mode of health care delivery grounded in prepaid group practice, where everyone paid flat fees and got access to everything in an operation. And it was a political instrument, too, one that catered to low-income and minority patients and foregrounded its nondiscriminatory policy in various printed materials. Like Gouverneur in New

York, the CMF also worked to cultivate close ties between neighborhood and facility and patient and provider. Administrators regularly discussed how a "consumer voice" could play an integral role in the center's operation. Educational programs included lectures on "social factors affecting health," including one on the role of housing, while operations attempted to reduce hierarchy, with physicians regularly instructed on how to handle patient complaints and effectively communicate without jargon. By the mid-1950s, however, the CMF floundered. One problem was simply scale. Financial self-sufficiency proved hard to achieve, and in 1954, the organization found itself $14,000 in debt.

The biggest barrier, though, came from outside the center itself. Stephen H. Fritchman, the CMF's president and a reverend at the First Unitarian Church, had drawn attention from the House Un-American Activities Committee, stigmatizing the entire operation at a time when the Los Angeles County Medical Association was waging a vigorous campaign against prepaid group practice and other deviations from traditional fee-for-service models. Soon, the organization was defunct. Even before then, the relationship between the facility and its original clientele was fraying, for it had moved, four years earlier, northward from Watts due to declining public transportation in the area. While the move rendered the center more accessible to some, it left another unmet need in the South Central Los Angeles medical landscape.[25]

The early 1960s saw other small-scale endeavors, with mixed success. In 1964, working by himself, a Black pediatrician in Watts, Sol White, proposed a 150-bed "nonprofit community hospital." White failed to attract much funding. A more successful simultaneous initiative of his came, however, when he lobbied for the creation of a new Hospital Service Area (HSA) that would be carved out of two existing ones. To White, existing administrative cartography obscured patterns of hardship, and his proposed HSA would draw it out.

White was right. As currently constituted, the heavy racial segregation and economic deprivation of Watts disappeared into contiguous HSAs: Inglewood, Lynwood, and Los Angeles. He carved the new Watts HSA by extracting the most racially and economically segregated areas from the neighboring Lynwood HSAs and Los Angeles HSAs to the north and east. The Black isolation index—a standard metric for measuring segregation, with 1.0 the maximum—for White's new Watts HSA was 0.83, compared to 0.79 for Lynwood and 0.71 for Los Angeles as those HSAs existed in their current state.[26]

In turn, White hoped that carving out a new area for Watts would "create, stimulate and promote the growth of health and allied facilities in an area of tremendous need."[27] The proposal piqued the interest of Supervisor Kenneth Hahn, whose district included Watts, and he initiated an inquiry with the county's Hospital Advisory Commission.[28] It wasn't an insignificant development. As was the case with air pollution, true power in Los Angeles over a host of issues, including health services, rested with the county board of supervisors. For any idea to get off the ground, its commitment was the necessary first step.

## Maldistribution Assumes Center Stage

Supervisor Hahn and the county ended up doing more than just redrawing administrative boundaries. Because in August 1965, Los Angeles boom turned to burn and Watts erupted in riots that lasted for 144 hours, or almost a week.

The events had begun when a Black motorist had been stopped by the California Highway Patrol (CHP) and a heated argument had ensued, escalating to physical blows with his mother (who had since arrived) and other members of a crowd that gathered. Rumors of CHP assaults—including on a woman who appeared pregnant—soon spread, igniting a response that targeted South Central stores for both robbery and, in some cases, arson. What came afterward was a melee that included the CHP, Los Angeles Police Department, and National Guard, some armed with machine guns. It left 34 people killed, most of them Black, and 1,000 injured.[29]

Nationwide, analysts would debate the causes of riots, culminating in the 1968 Report of the National Commission on Civil Disorders: the so-called Kerner Report. But Los Angeles's assessments came sooner. Its riot commission, chaired by former CIA director John McCone, focused heavily on two themes: police brutality and deprivation of basic social needs, including housing, trash pickup, and fairly priced food. The CHP encounter merely symbolized accumulated grievances: the small flame that made an already filled canister pop. Medical care was spotlighted, too, in an entire section dedicated to "welfare and health" that endorsed "serious consideration" of a "comprehensively-equipped hospital" in the area.[30]

The recommendations were based largely on the findings of Milton Roemer, a UCLA professor of public health who offered vivid details about the landscape of South Central Los Angeles health care in a supplementary study conducted for the commission. Roemer was unsparing. He depicted an area shut out of the postwar medical care boom, both nationally and at the county level. Watts, for one, simply didn't contain many personnel. The two county health districts within the region contained physician-to-population ratios of 38 per 100,000 and 45 per 100,000, far less than half the countywide ratio of 127 per 100,000. The absolute numbers made the point even more starkly: 106 doctors total for a population of 251,000. The numbers got worse as one probed. Only 17 (or 16 percent) were specialists, compared to 55 percent nationally, and of them, only 5 were board-certified. Further, even if the physicians were acting in the best of faith under trying circumstances, Roemer observed that "there are inherent limitations to the quality of medical care that can be rendered in an isolated medical office. . . . Laboratory and x-ray facilities, not to mention professional consultation, are usually unavailable in such a setting."[31]

For medical care, then, residents had few options. One was to see local physicians of uncertain quality. They could also visit small neighboring hospitals, some of which were propriety for-profits, some of them individual nonprofit voluntary institutions with no affiliations to universities or larger facilities. Of the eight for-profit hospitals in the area, Roemer noted that only two were accredited. The inspection reports for them were miserable. For one facility, a 1964 assessment had "ordered the kitchen to be cleaned, mice-droppings to be removed, infected dressings to be incinerated, a registered nurse to be on duty for the 11 P.M. to 7 A.M. shift, the doctors to sign medication orders, and several other actions reflecting serious deficiencies." And in another, inspectors "indicated cockroach infestation near the coffee urns, torn or missing screens, no written manual of maternity nursing procedures, [and] inoperative nurse-call signals."[32] Fortunately, the small number of physicians and the poor hospitals surrounding Watts weren't the most common source of medical care. That distinction belonged to County General, which was eight to ten miles from an area with poor public transportation and low rates of automobile ownership. Roemer estimated that 40 percent of Watts patients went to County General if they required hospitalization, all the more astonishing given its distance. It was an exhausting and arduous trip for anyone willing to make it. A one-way trip could take more than an hour if done by bus, and the burden, Roemer speculated, impaired continuity of care and the likelihood of making follow-up visits.[33]

The three county-run clinics in the area, geared toward maternal and child health services, were no better. They, too, suffered from a low personnel-to-patient ratio, with one public health nurse per 5,230 people, less than half the standard of one to 2,000 countywide. For expectant mothers, what resulted was a disjointed system of prenatal care, beginning with two-week to one-month wait times to attain an initial appointment, followed by rushed examinations when one finally saw a physician, often as late as the last trimester. The distance to the county hospitals, where most deliveries occurred, compounded the already elevated risks for complications. In Roemer's view, it was "small wonder" why vital statistics for the region looked the way they did. In one of the two health districts in the area, maternity mortality was 8.9 per 10,000 live births (compared with 3.5 at the countywide level), premature babies at 12.4 per 1,000 (compared to 7.5), fetal deaths at 17.8 per 1,000 (compared to 13.6), and infant mortality at 38.7 per 1,000 (compared to 23.2).[34]

Roemer's study depicted an entire world cut off from the fruits of the mid-century economic and medical boom. Like the official riot commission, Roemer recommended construction of a new hospital for the area. But he intertwined a parallel critique that suggested that his observations were symptomatic of something bigger than medical care itself, arguing that "the operations of the free enterprise market in medicine, which prevails in the United States, have yielded in the Riot Area the meagerest of resources."[35] For Roemer, many of the observed problems surfaced before patients had any contact with actual medical care, and he noted that "cockroaches and other vermin abound[ed]" in poorly maintained dwellings that flouted housing codes. Medical care ultimately only touched the surface of a bigger problem. "The basic fact is that the heath service problems of this Area—or almost any depressed locality in the United States—spring from social and economic causes with very wide and tortuous roots," he wrote. "The difficulties we see in the Riot Area, in health as in other fields, are only the final excrescence of malfunctions and failures in our whole society. Their correction, therefore, requires action on a very broad scale, including the State of California and the nation as a whole."[36]

These words weren't surprising coming from Roemer, who had been a victim of political red-baiting during the 1950s because he'd been involved with various leftist causes. At the lowest point, the federal government had revoked Roemer's passport and sent him fleeing to Saskatchewan, where he'd helped developed Canada's national health insurance system.[37] Now he had returned to the United States and brought his political acuity to bear on a political hotspot of the 1960s. It was a country different from the one from which he'd been exiled. Red-baiting and repression had given way to fury and rage over racism and deprivation.

## The Riot Response: Fixing Medical Maldistribution

The riot unleashed a torrent of policy responses. Sol White, whose own clinic had burned during the riots, revived his proposal for a "Watts Community Hospital," gaining a hearing before the State Advisory Hospital Council, which had the final word in approving construction. The council ultimately rejected White's plans, skeptical of whether the facility could really be funded by local neighborhood advocacy groups, as White proposed. But it was also likely uncomfortable with the ideological tilt of White's project. One of his supporters, a physician named Julius Hill, who was president of the Golden State Medical Society, a Black physicians group, had declared: "We are sick of the dole and the paternalistic attitude. We want to encourage self-esteem and self-sufficiency in the community and we feel that giving the community the responsibility of supporting its own hospital will install those qualities," while another, the Rev.

James Hargett, stated that "the community no longer wants things done for it—it wants to do things for itself."[38]

If unabashed Black nationalism was too much, another proposal came from county supervisor Kenneth Hahn, who suggested creating a nonprofit corporation to oversee a Watts facility funded via federal hospital construction dollars. The Hahn proposal gained traction. Support came from the Watts Health Advisory Committee, an ad hoc group formed by the State Advisory Hospital Council, and it included neighborhood activists, the president of the Watts Community Labor Action Committee (a local labor union consortium), two medical school deans from UCLA and USC, and a county health official. The Watts Health Advisory Committee argued that the new hospital would be a "center for community pride" and "for promoting interracial harmony."[39]

Others saw the hospital as a political buffer. The Compton chapter of the National Association for the Advancement of Colored People asserted that a "hospital facility would satisfy grievances of long standing."[40] And John McCone himself declared that deprivation of health services fomented fury.[41] In February 1966, the county board of supervisors endorsed the hospital's construction, with its precise location and funding mechanisms to be determined.[42] Its unanimous vote was undoubtedly a product of the moment and the new political pressures that emerged from the riots' ashes.

Fissures soon disrupted the consensus. On one side were hospital advocates who wanted to proceed with all deliberate speed. Supervisor Hahn, who'd originally advocated for the formation of a nonprofit corporation, had since decided that the county should float hospital bond measures in the upcoming June 1966 primary election for funding. They'd be similar to those used to fuel expansion in the immediate postwar period, including Los Angeles County General Hospital. (The key difference was that those bonds had gone toward mere improvements, not construction of an entire facility from the ground up.) In the middle were the other supervisors, who remained supportive of the hospital but felt that Hahn was proceeding too fast without cultivating a base of political support beyond the Watts area. If the bond measures themselves failed, they worried that the entire project itself might be jeopardized. These concerns were doubly serious given California's requirement that local ballot propositions pass by a two-thirds vote.[43]

But a third camp questioned the idea of a government-run hospital altogether. These critics coalesced after the county's Hospital Advisory Commission moved to delay construction pending further study on feasibility.[44] Critics didn't deny that infrastructural deficits existed, but as a long-term course, they questioned the wisdom of a government-funded facility with huge fixed costs. The proposal for the hospital had expanded, with calls now for a total bed count ranging from 438 to 1,000.[45] Moreover, the hospital itself wouldn't be a medium-sized specialty facility like John Wesley Hospital but a comprehensive "Class A" institution featuring a full slate of outpatient, inpatient, and emergency services—and it would include an affiliated medical school that would be built at the same time.[46] It represented, in other words, an enormous commitment.

There were other considerations beyond the financial risks. Given the perennial shortages in available staff at the other county hospitals, one member of the advisory commission wondered whether an adequate level of staff existed for a new hospital. The critics also asked whether "one central hospital" would be preferable to decentralized, small-scale centers catering to specific needs. They expressed concern that a full-scale institution might attract patients from outside Watts *to* the new facility and result in falling use at other hospitals. While beneficial for stressed facilities like County General, such a development could prove problematic for smaller hospitals that'd lose patients. Finally, impending Medicare and Medicaid had skeptics wondering if a new public facility was necessary; by supplying patients with insurance, the new programs had the theoretical ability to give patients more institutional choice beyond public hospitals.[47] That was certainly something observed in New York City and elsewhere in the nation.

Political subtext lay beneath these technocratic considerations. Although they chose their words carefully, some skeptics faulted the project for its concern with Watts. They did so with language that carried racial subtext. In remarks to the board of supervisors, Alex Rogers, the Hospital Advisory Commission's vice chairman, remarked: "I think that this type of hospital service area should be properly developed to take care of all citizens in an area, not one group who happens to be more vocal and more emotional than other citizens," he added. Many critics' remarks accentuated the racial demography of the area. Beulah Black, a longtime social worker in East Los Angeles, remarked: "I have been working with the colored people and I love them," before voicing skepticism over the fast pace at which hospital plans were moving.[48]

Hahn rejected the criticisms and the calls from his fellow county supervisors to slow down. Slamming those who might take refuge in more "investigations and commissions," he rebutted that "kindness and a few high ideals will not do what needs to be done." Instead, "by building a quality hospital, jobs will be created, services will be rendered, lives will be saved, and the health of the community will be improved."[49] At the same time, Hahn was keenly attuned to the racially tinged political minefield around the hospital, and he modified his pitch to cultivate the widest possible appeal. At one point, he emphasized that the area directly east of South Los Angeles, Florence-Firestone, contained substantial "Mexican American" and "Caucasian" populations that also stood to benefit from the hospital. These concerns mounted in the months leading up to the June election that'd decide the fate of the bond measure. Hahn deliberated on how to persuade Los Angeles newspaper publishers of the "over-all value of the project to the entire community" and underscored that the "hard sell of this issue must be on a County-wide basis."[50] In campaign materials, proponents of bond measures emphasized benefits beyond Watts. One pamphlet, entitled "Better Health for Everyone," claimed that the new hospital would provide relief from overcrowded hospitals elsewhere, while several others repeated that "disease knows no boundaries." It "plays no favorites. . . . It touches the young and the old, the rich and the poor. It strikes any neighborhood." The rhetoric tapped into the ideal of a universal Los Angeles community.[51] The motives behind this approach were understandable enough, given the nature of some Watts hospital doubts. Shortly before the election, the *Los Angeles Times*, for instance, characterized the Watts hospital "as a sop to the Negroes, as a reward or a pacifier following the racial disturbances in the area."[52]

The strategy worked, and the hospital attracted a swath of supporters, from the Los Angeles Chamber of Commerce and Property Owners Tax Association to the Los Angeles County Federation of Labor and assorted Watts neighborhood groups. But the majority vote (62.5 percent) fell just short of the two-thirds percentage required for passage of the bond measure.[53] Hardly deterred, Hahn resurrected an alternate proposal of his: forming a nonprofit corporation that could raise capital from public and private sources. Fellow supervisors were more split toward the plan, but it won with a three-to-two vote. The eventual resulting entity took the form of a county-city public authority that received funds from its bond sales and matching state and federal funds. It'd lease the facility to the county government itself and play no role in the hospital's administration.[54] By mid-1968, the city of Los Angeles and the county had approved and implemented the plan, with the Los Angeles County Southeast General Hospital Authority offering $22.5 million in construction bonds, amortized over twenty years.[55]

Hahn's actions reflected his commitment, even zeal, for the project after the bond vote had jeopardized it. But the creation of the public authority raised a number of questions going forward. Despite talk of the hospital as an anchor and symbol for Watts community pride, the eventual means by which it was created was strikingly undemocratic and came from Hahn's political strong-arming of Los Angeles elites, namely his fellow supervisors and bondholders. That these were the patrons—all from California's white political power structure—raised questions about who would call the eventual shots when the hospital came to fruition. Besides governance questions, one other detail had been conspicuously brushed over by all parties, no matter their position on the hospital. On the planned site stood the Palm Lane Housing Project, whose 301 households were given a few months' notice and told to relocate once hospital funding was assured in late 1966.[56] County politicos weren't the only ones who expressed little concern. So did many of the local Watts advocates. The obliviousness reflected just how much postriot aspirations were being projected onto the promise of a brand-new hospital for the area.

## A Community Health Experiment for Watts

During all the planning and political jockeying over the Watts Hospital and how to fund it, the University of Southern California was developing its own parallel medical care experiment. Like Gouverneur in New York, the eventual South-Central Multi-Purpose Service Health Center (Watts center) was one of a handful of pilot sites for the Office of Economic Opportunity's neighborhood health centers program. As with Gouverneur, the idea of this War on Poverty program was to bring medical care to areas where severe shortages of such services existed. Plans for the Watts OEO center had accelerated after the riot. Announcing a $2.4 million award, Sargent Shriver, OEO's director, remarked that the facility would be "crucial in view of the lack of health facilities immediately available to the residents of Watts."[57] It would house a comprehensive "medical unit" offering basic medical care, targeted initially at the 30,000 people living in the most economically hard-pressed section of Watts.

But as with Gouverneur, the program was about more than just filling enormous gaps in health services. It would realize a community health vision that bridged health services to the specific surroundings where delivery took place. To that end, an announcement in the *South End Bee*, a local Black newspaper, announced that "priority for employment will be given to applicants within the area in the following order: (1) unemployed; (2) under-employed; and (3) employed." Only after employment for people living within the center's catchment area was "exhausted" would listings be opened to those outside.[58] Employees would then join health teams and canvass Watts to inform potential patients of the center's services, plus help residents navigate other social service agencies in the neighborhood that dealt with job training, housing, and education, many of them also funded by OEO. At the same time, they'd inform the center's staff about surrounding conditions, helping them "view health as a totality, including psycho-social as well as physical elements." Local employment at the center served an additional function: on-the-job training, part of a national movement to nurture "para-professionals" in health careers.[59] The most important mechanism for blurring the boundaries between health care and surrounding social environs, though, was a lay council, like the one at Gouverneur, mandated by OEO's "maximum feasible participation" requirements.

How much power this lay council would have over day-to-day operations remained to be seen. It didn't take long for contests over governance to surface.

USC threw considerable institutional muscle behind the project, with its dean and associate dean, Roger Egeberg and Robert Tranquada, overseeing administration. Elsie Giorgi, an eminent UCLA and Cedars-Sinai physician, joined as the Watts center's medical director, while the city of Los Angeles donated an 86,000-square-foot plot of land.[60] Unsurprisingly, bringing in these doctors came with no small share of tension. Their professed commitment to breaking hierarchy and professional walls was nothing short of radical, especially in a sector like medicine so premised on them. But while they supported active lay involvement, the center's academic designers simultaneously saw the Watts constituents as subjects with capacities requiring development by professional outsiders. In one grant proposal, for example, they declared that the program would help test whether "maximal involvement of the community residents in solving their own problems decreases social dependency."[61] In another, they wrote that "community participation will be maximum and meaningful and aim at general improvement through self-help in every phase of the operation. . . . It can be very safely assumed that this type of participation will produce eventual self-esteem and self-sufficiency, by overcoming the powerless of the poor, and allowing them a greater control over their own lives and welfare."[62] How helpful or constricting a guiding hand would the USC outsiders prove to be?

The university's involvement made that question an uneasy one. It wasn't the same institution it had been in 1953, when it had affiliated with County General, but had since become a major player in Los Angeles—and not just in medicine but also in real estate. In the few years before the riot, it had lobbied the city council for permission to expand dramatically by fifty-eight acres, potentially displacing hundreds of mostly Black households. Although several miles north of Watts, the Hoover Redevelopment Project (named for a north-south street that ran throughout Los Angeles) drew the fury of critics who saw an overt USC land grab. The university's reputation had consequences for the Watts health project. For Jim Bates, the project's hired community organizer, the university's involvement aroused justifiable suspicion. A Black alumnus of USC, where he had played football, Bates knew the institution firsthand and was uniquely situated to write about its dynamics with neighbors. In a memo, Bates summarized the early months of the project and described how hard it was to get people to overlook USC's involvement. As he told it, Watts residents were pretty blunt: "We just don't want the University of Southern California in Watts under any circumstances." "Agency representatives that were approached appeared evasive and sometimes hostile," Bates noted. "It became very apparent in Watts that the community considered a common enemy; and the University fitted that description to the last detail."[63]

The university felt the suspicion. All three administrators for the Watts center—Egeberg, Tranquada, and Giorgi—were white physicians, with Tranquada and Giorgi assuming day-to-day supervisorial roles. Decades later, Tranquada reflected on these early years. Entering Watts somewhat reluctantly, Tranquada, then a young associate dean, knew little about the social history of the area, having been asked out of nowhere by Egeberg if he'd be interested in taking on the project. He recalled discovering "immediately that we were neither appreciated nor trusted," then realized that "there was no basis of experience that the residents of Watts had which would have encouraged, or even allowed, them to trust us." Summarizing the general sentiment, Tranquada wrote that many felt "the only reason USC would make such a move was because they somehow were to make a huge profit from the venture—why else would a Honkey university that had never before paid any attention to Watts and its people suddenly seem concerned?" Suspicions went beyond money. "It was said," Tranquada recalled, "that USC needed more guinea pigs with which to teach its medical students and that was the reason for moving into Watts."[64] Fear of incursion and exploitation from a university behemoth—right down to the image of human guinea pigs—wasn't exclusive to Los Angeles, and it bore huge similarities to the rhetoric opposing affiliation battles in New York City. But here, the language came with an additional racial subtext, born of decades of marginalization.

Besides suspicion surrounding the academic behemoth up north, there were immediate brass-tacks issues, too. Virtuous founding words—"the philosophy is that of doing 'with them' rather than 'for them' or 'to them'"—were one thing in a proposal and quite different in the mundane world of everyday practice.[65] As its community organizer, Bates had the thankless task of forming a Community Health Council (CHC) mandated by OEO's Community Action Program, similar to New York City's Lower East Side Neighborhood Health Council–South. He needed to devise a method of assuring legitimate community representation but wondered anxiously how exactly to do so.

Bates's initial steps demonstrated his keen understanding of heterogeneity within Watts. He first asked Watts social service agencies and advocacy groups to nominate two candidates for membership on the CHC. The candidates then responded to questions gauging their knowledge and views on four subjects: "health need" in Watts, "community awareness," "role of Health Council," and "future effects of the health center," with interviewees receiving scores that determined whether they would move on to the next stage. The questions themselves were less about testing factual knowledge so much as they were an open-ended means of ascertaining general proclivities. Bates remarked that "we did not want to infer that the applicants should have experience in policy-making because we would be omitting many of our capable indigenous leaders." For instance, questions on "health need" weren't "attempting to find out if the applicant could define comprehensive care or any other medical details" but, rather, were a way of seeing whether applicants were aware that resource deprivation

**Table 3.1. Watts Health Project: First Community Health Council's demographic composition**

| Sex | Age | Years in California | Years in Watts | High school graduate | Training after high school |
|---|---|---|---|---|---|
| Male | 21 | 20 | 11 | Yes | No |
| Male | 23 | 23 | 13 | No | No |
| Female | 23 | 23 | 20 | Yes | Yes |
| Male | 25 | 22 | 22 | No | No |
| Male | 31 | 31 | 31 | No | No |
| Male | 36 | 15 | 9 | Yes | No |
| Female | 37 | 23 | 19 | Yes | 2 years college |
| Male | 38 | 10 | 7 | No | No |
| Male | 39 | 39 | 32 | No | No |
| Female | 40 | 7 | 7 | No | No |
| Female | 40 | 23 | 10 | Yes | Yes |
| Male | 44 | 23 | 20 | Yes | 2 years college |
| Female | 46 | 31 | 31 | Yes | No |
| Female | 50 | 37 | 25 | Yes | Yes |
| Female | 53 | 29 | 20 | No | No |
| Female | 62 | 62 | 13 | Yes | Yes |
| Female | 64 | 27 | 27 | Yes | No |

*Source*: Rodney Powell, unpublished essay on the South Central Multipurpose Health Center, in private collection.

existed in the first place and if they had creative thoughts about how to address it. Many questions reflected the health center's birth in a time of political tumult. It wasn't the typical health center interview, after all, that asked: "What do you think about the Black Nationalists?" "How do you feel about the riot/revolt of August 1965?" and "What constitutes good leadership in the community and why?"[66]

Then there were more objective characteristics taken into account. Bates screened as well for rough geographic proportionality from different parts of Watts, then further whittled down by age. Bates aimed for a minimum of six council members in the twenty-one-to-thirty age bracket, five in thirty-one to forty, four in forty-one to fifty, and four in fifty and over. Age quotas, Bates remarked, were a "necessary evil" to achieve something approximating representativeness. At the same time, they allowed a mixing of political sensibilities, from radical to risk-adverse, that the Watts project administrators saw as roughly associated with age cohorts. The first CHC assembled was all-Black, containing seventeen members: nine women and eight men. Six possessed some level of higher education, and of those, all but one were women.

Assembling the CHC wasn't what created conflict. What caused problems was lack of clarity over what exactly the council was supposed to do and how much power it really held. A few months after the receipt of the OEO grant,

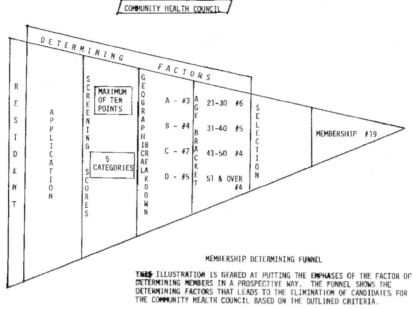

MEMBERSHIP DETERMINING FUNNEL

THIS ILLUSTRATION IS GEARED AT PUTTING THE EMPHASES OF THE FACTOR OF DETERMINING MEMBERS IN A PROSPECTIVE WAY.  THE FUNNEL SHOWS THE DETERMINING FACTORS THAT LEADS TO THE ELIMINATION OF CANDIDATES FOR THE COMMUNITY HEALTH COUNCIL BASED ON THE OUTLINED CRITERIA.

THIS PROCESS TENDS TO TAKE AWAY THE MANIPULATION FACTOR THAT IS USUALLY PREVALENT IN SUBJECTIVE ELIMINATION PROCESS -- ESPECIALLY IN THE FACTOR SUCH AS:  GEOGRAPHICAL BREAKDOWN AND AGE BRACKET.

Figure 2

"Membership Determining Funnel" for Community Health Council, ca. 1966.
*Source*: In private collection.

Augustus Hawkins, the Black Democratic congressman who had served the area for twenty years, wrote to USC. He inquired about why the council had been slow to meet and operate, emphasizing that further delays would "only add fuel to a flame of doubt and skepticism that plagues the opposers of your program."[67] Robert Tranquada replied that the problem arose because of inherent vagaries in "maximum feasible participation" and community administration.[68]

Four months before the inaugural CHC meeting—and two days after Congressman Hawkins's prodding letter—Tranquada and Elsie Giorgi debated how the CHC could really work. Interest in the center was growing, along with clamor from residents demanding clarification of the CHC's exact role and powers.[69] Adding to the frustration was how much time had elapsed since the ground breaking for construction. The facility wouldn't open until mid-1967, almost two years after its conception, fomenting frustration. But by the late summer of 1966, the CHC and other residents had issued demands about how the center should be run. One called for the $2.4 million OEO grant to be channeled to a local Black-owned business, out of USC's hands. Another pushed for limited hiring exclusively to Black applicants (in reality, achieved de facto by the center's geographically preferential hiring). A proposal that only Black firms receive future contract work—set-asides adopted around the country—clearly irritated university staffers, who characterized it as the "ignoring of normal prudent business practice," such as competitive bidding.[70]

The most substantial of the demands, though, centered squarely on governance. The CHC argued that its members ought to have the final word on hiring of professional and nonprofessional staff, superseding the authority of the project's academic directors. Uncertainty about the council's proper role grew to the point where USC planners reached out to OEO and discussed the logistics of implementing "maximum feasible participation." Writing on the difficulties of merging politics and medicine, Tranquada and Giorgi stated that one reason behind "not infrequent misunderstandings between grantee [USC] and poverty community is the vastly different order of priority of concerns which each holds." For medical providers, "the provision of good medical care" was "top priority." But for the "poverty community," there was a desire for more, including "concerns about transfer of authority from the power structure, economic security" and the "playing of a new role in society." In short, local people wanted community control.

Both Tranquada and Giorgi held firm that final authority needed to end with university supervisors, not the council, but they agreed that clearer delineation of authority could ease some of the tension. What resulted was a series of tradeoffs. On hiring personnel, the council would split duties with USC, with the CHC chiefly responsible for nonprofessionals while USC handled professionals. The university would have final say over the center's overall budget, but Tranquada and Giorgi proposed giving the council input over how it was allocated. Within the context of academic medicine, this affirmation of a role for a community council was novel and powerful, far more than just a gesture.[71]

## Mounting Medical Governance Battles

Yet the crises of governance were hardly over. A second source of conflict came from the roughly fifty Black fee-for-service physicians working in Watts, most of whom belonged to its Charles R. Drew Medical Society, named after the eminent African American physician who'd died young at forty-five after a car accident and who'd played a leading role in developing blood banking and later fought the Red Cross's decision's to segregate supply "by race."[72] The Drew Society's leadership, which had not been consulted and played no role in conceiving the Watts center, felt that it was in the best position to gauge the health needs of Watts residents and should control the facility's "policy making body," along with "responsible community organizations."[73] To these Black physicians, the new health center threatened "doctor-patient-community relations," and they declared that "self-help should be promoted rather than a free total replacement" like the USC-OEO project. Such "outside help," if it must exist, ought to be developed in concert with "physicians and people who work in the area so that a feeling of self-accomplishment is motivated to the establishment of total health needs in a presently indigent, hostile community."[74]

The Drew Society proposed an alternate course. It demanded that it hold veto power over personnel decisions (including ones that USC had already made); approval of all construction to ensure Black participation; oversight over OEO funds; and compensation for "overhead costs" it incurred fulfilling these duties. Other recommendations seemed designed to ensure the Drew Society physicians' economic hold on the Watts medical marketplace. One declared that "existing patient-physician relationship[s] must be scrupulously honored by all personnel" of the new facility, while another proposed that the clinic only accept "medically indigent patients," potentially ensuring a stable pool of more affluent, paying patients for the Watts physicians.[75]

This opposition from Black private physicians mounted. Profiled in *Time*, Elsie Giorgi described anonymous threats from Watts doctors, one of whom threatened to burn the Watts center once construction finished.[76] The most vocal wing of the group, based in Watts, went beyond the initial demands and broke off into a formation called the Watts Medical, Dental and Pharmaceutical Society, and it excoriated the center for months. A local newspaper, the *Star Review*, published the group's statement, entitled "Why We Oppose the USC Health Center." "Most patients prefer going to their own private physicians or dentists," the group argued, before claiming that the center would be redundant anyway next to the new Watts hospital and existing county health centers. Furthermore, apart from medical care itself, the Watts endeavor would hardly "scratch the surface of the job problem in Watts" but would instead funnel residents into low-paid positions.[77] Worst, it was a symbolic and hypocritical affront from a university that "has cared neither about Watts nor the Black community in the past" but now wanted to "hoodwink Watts into thinking it cares more about the community than the $10 million and a training facility."[78] It represented, to the *Star Review*, racist invasion from a predominantly white institution: "What the proposed center and publicity about the many health shortcomings in Watts tends to create is an image which says to them, 'You black medical people have neither the talent nor the ability to do a damn thing for the health of the community.'" Now, it declared, "the ball is being thrown back to the community. It will have to ask 'what about the sacrifices made by individual physicians, dentists and pharmacists before the anti-poverty program money was available for health services in Watts'?"[79]

The opposition from the Watts physicians contained no small share of contradictions. At times, they appeared to oppose the center outright, while at other times they appeared willing to accept it if they were given full governance. Some of the oppositional stance seemed motivated largely by turf protection. Speaking in communitarian tones, the Watts doctors portrayed USC as a disruptive outside force that had manufactured a nonexistent problem with a solution for which there was no demand. It was a dubious depiction given the postriot data that Milton Roemer had amassed and the public support the Watts center had drawn even before it was built. But whatever the legitimacy of the Watts doctors' claims, they underscored the political contestation that existed around "community" as an anchoring concept for health services. The project now contained at least four clear potential lines of authority: OEO, USC, the CHC, and the Black Watts doctors. Each was claiming to act on behalf of the community's health interests.

Jim Bates, the Watts center's community organizer, was an acute observer of intraracial class dynamics, and he wrote sensitively and sympathetically about the dilemma faced by independent middle-class Black medical professionals amid liberal health policy reform. To him, the Black physicians in Watts were competing with white liberal reformers for the loyalty of the wider Black populace. He wrote at the time: "A man's imagination would have to be stretched to the outer limits to understand negotiations and debates between white professionals with guilt feelings and altruistic needs trying to gain understanding with freed Black professionals, who for the first time are trying to negotiate for their professional livelihood and for the Black masses whom they fear as much as the whites." "Two lost opposing group[s]," he continued, "are trying to reach a decision about an angry, hostile Black population that has just become visible to both." The "Black doctor in America has always been considered the pillar of leadership in the Black community," Bates observed, social status that the Watts initiative threatened to undercut.[80]

At the same time, Bates and others didn't hesitate to note the Watts physicians' hypocrisy. For all the talk of commitment to the area, a number of the physicians within the Drew Society, he noted, maintained practices outside of it altogether.[81] Bates wasn't the only one who picked up on self-serving tendencies. An anonymous pamphlet circulating in the neighborhood made similar observations, though in much more incendiary language. Written entirely in capitalized letters, the broadside was punctuated with the question, "Where Were You Doctor?":

Recently, I conducted a study. At random, I took 100 residents of our community of Watts. I asked each of them to give me the names of three doctors in the neighborhood. The results were shocking. Not to me but to you. Only three persons knew the names of two or more of the doctors and only nineteen knew the names of one doctor in the community. . . .

Lately, I've noticed more and more black doctors visitin in our neighborhood. All of you couldn't have practices in this neighborhood, else you would've been long fighting with each other over who has the right to cheat this or that brother. I know most of you are from fancy westside offices on Crenshaw Boulevard. You know the ones I'm talking about. The ones that whitey kept you out of until just recently. . . .

Where Were You, Doctor?[82]

Despite such skepticism, the Watts physicians threatened to create a serious crisis of governance. To avert it, USC administrators attempted negotiating with the Drew Medical Society but, unable to do so, brought in an outside arbiter, John Frankel, from OEO. Bates recalled the tense atmosphere under which talks occurred, writing that he witnessed "two opposing groups . . . [debated] on the behalf of the rights, privileges, and needs of the Watts community, still keeping in front of all their arguments, their financial interest and [thus] security in a subliminal sense. Out of all these negotiations, I scarcely can remember an argument being caused by any other premises than [vested interest] . . . to a point where they could no longer get together and discuss the project intelligently."[83] Deadlocked, the two parties turned to Congressman Augustus Hawkins, a supporter of the center who had remained in contact with OEO director Sargent Shriver throughout the planning process. Hawkins reaffirmed his support for the center and, Tranquada recalled, subtly signaled his contempt for the Drew Society's inflated claims of strong neighborhood connections by noting that he'd not gotten much sleep the previous night due to police sirens in the neighborhood.[84]

The negotiations resulted in a clear message: the Watts center would stay but would allow for some shared governance in the form of a professional advisory board, made up mostly of Drew Society physicians. The key difference, however, was that the board wouldn't have any final say and instead would issue recommendations to the Community Health Council, a radical challenge to how power flowed in the Watts medical landscape, such as it was. A major additional concession from USC was the hiring of a Drew Society physician: none other than Sol White, the longtime advocate for both a new hospital and Watts administrative boundaries. He would serve as co-medical director alongside Elsie Giorgi. Finally, USC agreed to add language to the OEO grant promising that the Watts project would "be specifically keyed to the supplementation of existing medical facilities and services" and, with few exceptions, would only accept medically indigent patients, easing the Watts physicians' fear of competition from the new center.

## Ribbon Cuttings and Rocky Beginnings

In October 1967, the Watts center opened with a staff of 230 and much fanfare, including an appearance from Sergeant Shriver, Congressman Hawkins, and Joseph English, head of OEO's health programs, a few years before he headed New York City's Health and Hospitals Corporation. They appeared with a giant pair of scissors for the ribbon cutting—Shriver peered through one of the huge finger holes—and the optimism offered an escape from behind-the-scenes governance battles that'd wracked the operation up to the final hour before opening.[85] They were equal parts interpersonal and political. Three months before, Elsie Giorgi had resigned after many office skirmishes over her role. Several staff had been on the receiving end of put-downs and insults. In a private memo, Tranquada spoke of "harangues" colored by "the theme that Elsie is right ('I told you so')." Besides calling members of the staff "stupid and ineffective," Giorgi had made homophobic remarks about them based on how "they talk[ed] and walk[ed]." Apart from demeanor issues, Giorgi chronically showed up late to important meetings and had failed to get a community outreach program running properly.[86]

Sol White's hiring as Giorgi's co-medical director in early 1967 had also created problems. Although Giorgi claimed to welcome him, when White came on board, she saw the tandem as undercutting her authority. The two got along poorly from the start, with Giorgi complaining about White's unilateral actions, writing at one point: "He repeatedly and is continuing to completely disregard the established table of organization and crosses divisional and departmental lines without going through channels."[87] In Giorgi's view, White was "very political in his approach" and "motivated towards self rather than the task," especially when it came to currying favor with the CHC, at one point leaking confidential information from the center's leadership.

This was no isolated interpersonal skirmish. Sol White had upset more people than just Giorgi. While still a candidate for the co-medical director position, White had promoted a contract with a local laboratory service, J & H, where he served as medical director, a conflict of interest he hadn't revealed to other Watts center staff. There was also the time White used center stationary to solicit funds from outside agencies for a training program of his creation. A final straw came during the center's first few days, when White had approved—without anyone else's knowledge—the presence of an outside ambulance company that received phone calls at the center. He was fired shortly afterward and hadn't even lasted a month.[88]

It would be easy to reduce the tumult to a war of egos. But there was more than that. A commitment to community health meant inevitable debate over what exactly that meant. Sol White, in particular, had long been invested in the area's health services, having proposed versions of the Watts hospital for years before the county moved on the matter. Giorgi had spent extensive time in Watts on related OEO programs. It wasn't entirely surprising, then, that they both would have trouble fitting into a structure where a perceived interloper like Tranquada was calling the principal shots, not them. Tranquada's association with USC only added to the potential for friction, especially with White.

National politics compounded the troubles. For the latter half of 1967, it was unclear whether OEO would survive a budget appropriations fight in a markedly new Congress, where Democrats showed up after the 1966 midterm elections retaining control but much less of it: forty-eight fewer seats in the House, three in the Senate, and much of the ability to pass Great Society and War on Poverty legislation now gone.[89] The uncertain fiscal context exacerbated psychological duress in Watts. Tranquada captured the mood in a report to the CHC. The budget impasse was "very nearly disastrous for the Center" and had "resulted in a three month period in which more than half of the time of the senior staff had to be devoted to problems related to budget."[90] The university advanced the Watts center temporary funds to stay alive as the situation dragged on. Shortly afterward, Tranquada decided to split his associate director position into two, perhaps because of all the demands, infighting, and stress that had accompanied the job in its first two years. He moved to a part-time position, while Clifton Dummett, a Black dentist in charge of the dental department, became full-time "associate project director–health center director." Although the addition of a Black administrator partly assuaged antagonism toward what some viewed as paternalistic white liberals, it also generated other suspicions. Dummett's issuing of directives from the dental department, which was spatially more removed from the rest of the facility, enforced the perception of a distant yes man, with staff morale declining.

Sensing problems, OEO initiated a "full scale site visit" in early 1968, which led to yet another radical shake-up in personnel. When OEO left, all parties involved with running the center agreed to convert the associate project director–health center director back to a single job and hire a new person to fill it. That sent Tranquada—the public (and white) face of USC at the center—back to campus. In his place was a Black pediatrician, Rodney Powell, who had just completed a stint as the assistant chief in the Bureau of Maternal and Child Health at the California State Department of Public Health. A native of Philadelphia, Powell had done his residency at UCLA and knew Los Angeles well. He'd also served as a Peace Corps physician in Ethiopia and Tanzania in the early years of the program, keeping him integrated within a network of people—up to Sargent Shriver himself—centrally involved in health initiatives of the War on Poverty era.[91]

Powell immediately struck a different chord than had his predecessors. When he accepted the job, the CHC had some real input, but true and final decision-making still rested with the actual recipient of OEO funds: USC. But Powell declared in the *Los Angeles Times* that if he had "to choose between allegiance to the community and allegiance to USC," he'd side unreservedly with the community.[92] Despite this professed position, the Watts center staff's initial reaction to Powell was lukewarm. Shortly before his formal assumption of duties, an ad hoc group of employees issued questions about the future of the center, particularly around USC's involvement. "What are the University's goals in this Center? What are the immediate and long-range plans?" read one. Another noted that "the University will derive millions of dollars in either direct or indirect benefits through the sponsorship of this program" before asking about "what . . . the University perceive[d] as its commitment to this Black community." One person captured both the recent past and the future that Powell was entering: "There has been some difference in philosophy between University and Center in regard to" community participation mandates. "How can the Center help the University to resolve this source of conflict?"[93]

Despite what he later called the "somewhat hostile milieu" greeting him, Powell worked with the CHC on a new division of labor to clarify power sharing. Powell proposed streamlining the structure of the Watts center and having the council operate as a board of directors. It'd set broad goals for the center and have the final say on major "program operations" but leave daily operations to others. He requested control of personnel, including the hiring of his deputy administrator, with the CHC approving only "key staff personnel" rather than micromanaging each hire. In Powell's view, as associate project director–health center director, he was in the best position to know the center's daily needs.[94]

The CHC agreed to Powell's suggestions, largely because of his efforts to reach out to it through multiple meetings: what he would later call "sustained, in-depth and even sensitivity-type sessions between the CHC and myself as well as, between the key program staff and the CHC."[95] His efforts contrasted sharply from the head butting that had marked the center experience back in the USC days. A key barometer of slow but increasing harmony came at the end of August, when the Los Angeles Police Department swarmed the summertime Watts Festival after a "minor civil disturbance." Powell recalled "the spectacle of heavily armed police, four and five to a car with shot guns and riot guns displayed in the car windows, patrolling the community in convoys of 4–5 cars," which left the entire area tense and worried about another possible uprising. The center had prepared for extended hours into the night, formulating an impromptu disaster plan in case events escalated. Although nothing ended up occurring, the events cultivated solidaristic feelings among those working at the center: "special knowledge," in Powell's words, "that a team had been born."[96]

Better relations boosted staff morale. After White's firing, the Watts physicians and their professional advisory board had gradually lost interest in the center, focusing instead on the new Watts hospital, yet to be built. With the decline in conflict came more time to focus on actual center programming. Long marred by the general inexperience of its members, the CHC instituted a formalized training program that built new members' skills in a variety of areas, including general parliamentary procedure, dealings with OEO, and budgetary management. Its members began receiving a stipend for attending trainings in administration. It was a gesture that addressed a largely unspoken assumption at not just the Watts center but OEO programs everywhere: that predominantly working-class members of community boards would want to conduct often grueling administrative oversight without compensation. This quality had roots, as historian Amy Offner has demonstrated, in OEO and the community boards' origins in Latin American self-help housing programs.[97] But the Watts project was now evolving into something beyond OEO architects' original designs. It had shaken off white patrons, and its council participants were now being paid to do their oversight work. Moreover, the oversight had real teeth to it.

Toward the end of 1968, Powell left Watts in good spirits, remarking that "the final benefit of this citizen control will be the acquisition of individual and community expertise, sophistication and strength in dealing with the legal, social, political, economic as well as health care issues that are the real determinants of individual and community destiny."[98] His experience demonstrated the importance of strong interpersonal skills when it came to managing conflict and realizing lay participation in War on Poverty health projects.

### The Watts Center in Context

Common critiques of neighborhood-level War on Poverty programs have honed in on their individualistic character, and as historian Alice O'Connor has documented, the pervasiveness of human capital cultivation as a chief goal across a number of programs. "Philosophically," in the words of one scholar, "the OEO addressed poverty as a problem of individual development and the social disorganization of poor communities rather than as a function of the distribution of existing jobs or employment segregation."[99] In some respects, the neighborhood health center experience in Watts fits into this tradition. Its founding advocates, after all, portrayed the facility as a job training opportunity and entry path to health careers. In the grand scheme, it amounted to little more than a single-site dent in Watts's unemployment problem. At the same time, unlike many War on Poverty experiments, the Watts center, like Gouverneur in New York, wasn't just a training site but an actual creator of substantial jobs itself. And beyond "the problem of jobs," it was part of a nationwide investment in permanent infrastructure, a political response to the crisis of medical maldistribution. Neighborhood health centers certainly didn't upend the occupational structure of Watts and Manhattan's Lower East Side, but they transcended the individual-level focus characteristic of many War on Poverty programs in other sectors.[100]

But the Watts center still bumped up against intrinsic limits. They were illuminated by Powell's 1969 presentation at a Harvard conference on "Medicine in the Ghetto." Powell meditated on his time in Watts and what he dubbed "the proper limits and proper realm of concern for medicine and other providers of health care." Facilities like his own, he suggested, "must attempt to deal not only in disease treatment and in traditional disease prevention but also must attempt to become relevant to the total needs of its community." With lay participation and local employment on health teams, the Watts center was a large step toward this vision. But there might be more: "In the deprived ghetto communities, a health care system must deal with 1. environment: housing, sanitation, food, clothing; 2. jobs: education, training, underemployment, unemployment; 3. vicious cyclical harassment ('law and order') resulting from the above; and 4. illnesses thus resulting from all the above that take their toll in the physical, social, and emotional well-being of the people."[101] He ended by calling for a "pluralistic approach" that'd link these elements.[102]

Powell based his remarks on regular exposure to problems in Watts. That same year, Powell traveled to Washington and testified at a congressional hearing on "Nutrition and Human Needs."[103] He reported seeing glaring physical manifestations of severe protein and vitamin deficiencies: "protruding abdomens," "angular lesions and cheilosis of the lips," "easily bleeding gums and atrophic, receding gingivae," and "children with wasted limbs and prominent shoulder blades indicating diets that are not only qualitatively inadequate but in terms of calories unable to satisfy daily energy needs."[104] Medical care was too late of an end point for tackling problems fundamentally rooted outside the clinic. Just a week before his appearance, Powell and a coworker had left the center for the day and "observed a child about 7 to 9 years rummaging in a wire mesh waste receptacle for food."[105]

The Watts center's shortcomings were fundamentally rooted less in the individualistic myopia of its architects than in the inherent limits of experimental programs in severely resource-deprived areas. Powell's remarks at the Harvard and Washington gatherings indicate that he and his attendees were well aware of these constraints and of how medical care could only do so much against a gamut of structural impediments to the realization of human health. Indeed, his own U.S. Agency for International Development background offers another window into such limits. Like international development programs, states and institutions that had neglected (at best) or actively participated (at worst) in the exploitation of entire regions and neighborhoods later sought to remedy the subsequent fallout.[106] But their efforts did not even begin to reorder the power relations that had created the deprivation in the first place.

## The Problem of Sustainability in an Age of Austerity

Powell was right to point to structures outside health facilities themselves. The county health system had been challenged by the foment in Watts, but it was now confronting something else altogether: the tectonics of the economy. If the story of Los Angeles in the immediate postwar years was one of contrast from a New York City public hospital system under pressure, by the mid-1960s, the situation had changed, and like its East Coast counterpart, Los Angeles was on its way to a similarly turbulent fiscal landscape: budgetary tightness, austerity, threats of cutbacks, ever scarcer resources.

An episode in May 1965 is illustrative. That month, residents at the County General Hospital, recently renamed Los Angeles County–USC Medical Center (LAC–USC), mounted a protest. The "heal-in" took an unusual form. The residents admitted extra patients with nonurgent conditions who normally would have been deferred for later treatment. Over the course of two weeks, they increased the daily patient census by as much as 500 patients, hoping to dramatize persistent pressures on LAC–USC's staff and their view that current compensation was incommensurate.[107] The residents' one-shot action was ultimately about more than wages. It was staged at an increasingly overburdened facility and was meant to highlight the larger sustainability challenges facing the county.

These pressures continued into the decade, fueled in part by the region's population growth, which had spiked from 1.5 million to 2.4 million from 1940 to 1960, an increase of 64 percent. The county's other major hospital, Harbor General, confronted challenges as well. The average waiting period there, according to Harbor's own assessments, was a little more than two hours. Fifty-nine percent of patients waited between one and three hours before someone saw them, and 21 percent waited even longer, at three or more hours.[108] The patient experience could be harrowing, like Bunnie Berry's time at Harbor General for a sore foot. She recalled arriving at 7:45 A.M. and staying until 4:30 P.M. before she saw a physician. While spending the day in the admitting room, Berry learned from other patients a method for discerning how many people preceded her and how much longer the seemingly interminable wait would be. At one point, she had realized she would miss the last bus, to which the waiting room clerk replied: "You're not paying for it what the hell do you expect." It wouldn't be the end of her ordeal. Repeat visits to the hospital by bus—and redirection to different hospital wings, from general surgery to orthopedics to the emergency room—occurred over the month for Berry.[109]

Other patients fared similarly. Joseph Spinazzola was taken by ambulance to Harbor and "pushed into a vacant room with only a sheet covering me and strapped on my back to a table or bed just big enough for me, for about three hours." "I kept calling for a nurse and no one would answer," he said. "I was very cold and I asked for a blanket which I never received." Three hours later, Spinazzola finally got X-rays before spending the rest of the night in a space next to the admitting room. By morning, Spinazzola wanted to be transferred to another hospital but couldn't find anyone willing to make a call for him and characterized one nurse's response to his request as "nasty." "I hope I shall never have the misfortune of being taken to the Harbor General Hospital again," he declared.[110] Another patient, Mary McShane, wrote of two visits to Harbor General and remembered receiving barbiturates after specifying that she was allergic to them. On another visit, McShane's foot swelled from a problematic intravenous fluid injection. When she woke up the next day and saw a "red streak of infection ... about two inches above the ankle," McShane told an attendant and waited two hours for a physician. When no one arrived, she found a doctor on her own, one who told her that she needed to elevate her foot while applying hot packs to it. After two more hours, McShane was fed up. She told the hospital staff that she wanted to leave and take care of the problem herself.[111]

County officials acknowledged the patient grief and overcrowding. "It is extremely difficult to maintain an orderly flow of admissions in County acute facilities," Alex Rogers, a county official, wrote in a statement to the board of supervisors. "Unlike their private hospital counterparts, receiving rooms at General and Harbor Hospitals have little control over the number of admissions to be processed in any given period of time."[112]

One contingent development—the passage of Medicaid in 1965—promised relief. Funded by a combination of state and federal appropriations, Medicaid held the prospect of an infusion of cash into the system that could then be used to hire additional personnel. In 1968, three years after the formation of the state Medicaid program—called Medi-Cal—the California Department of Health Care Services authorized a $10.5 million increase in county hospital spending, with $4.78 million marked for hiring 1,185 new employees at the county hospitals, especially LAC–USC, which received more than half of the positions, followed by Harbor General.[113] Furthermore, since Medicaid offered the uninsured a means of payment, it could theoretically thin some of the patient load if some enrollees decided to use private facilities or practitioners instead of county ones.[114]

The early years of Medi-Cal, however, proved to be anything but easy relief. As in New York, Medicaid's complex stream of funds created unexpected grief.

At its outset, the California program gave counties two options for attaining Medi-Cal reimbursement. Option one reimbursed counties for costs incurred by each of their Medi-Cal patients. Option two skipped a per diem approach and instead called for the county to pay its own contribution, helping match guaranteed state and federal appropriations. The county's contribution would be calculated from a constant "base": the total it spent on all hospital costs in 1964–65, with small adjustments for population increases.

In its first year of participation, Los Angeles County opted for option two, estimating that it'd provide an additional $8.6 million in revenue.[115] This was a bad choice, and it made county implementation of Medi-Cal anything but smooth. In May 1967, a county grand jury commissioned an audit and identified significant delays in getting the county its Medi-Cal money, blaming the difficulty of actually calculating the county's expected contribution. The audit expressed frustration over how long the state was taking to come up with the figure, with state and county eventually agreeing to small, stopgap "provisional settlements" for six months. Remarking on the situation, Caspar Weinberger, then serving as the chair of Governor Reagan's newly created Commission on California State Government Organization and Economy, quipped that the Medi-Cal reimbursement process "requires the services of several certified public accountants just to advise us how difficult it is to understand." Apart from noting administrative burdens, Weinberger warned of sharp increases in Medi-Cal costs to the county, citing a quintuple jump between the past fiscal year (approximately $7 million) and the next one ($35 million).[116] Medicaid budgetary flows, in short, were unpredictable, hardly optimal for an increasingly stretched county system.

Then there was the governor's hostility. In August 1967 Governor Reagan ordered a cut of $210 million in state funds, more than 25 percent, to bring Medi-Cal's budget under $600 million. Those working directly on the front lines accused Reagan—not without some justification—of pushing through cuts less out of true fiscal necessity than from an ideological desire to starve the program. One group of social work students from Sacramento State College noted that Reagan had failed to meet with the legislature to work out a budget compromise. The students emphasized the human side of the cuts: "Why should children who have trouble seeing the blackboard not get the glasses they need? Why should the elderly be forced to go without needed false teeth?"[117] The 1967 standoff was resolved only when the California Supreme Court declared Reagan's cuts illegal. After the court's ruling, Reagan briefly attempted to preserve the cuts in partial form by announcing that he would eliminate medical indigents from the Medi-Cal rolls. The move earned swift rebuke from the county, which had already allocated its budget for the next fiscal year and estimated that it would, at minimum, need to find an additional $8 million to offset lost revenue from such a reduction of rolls. One emergency possibility for filling the gap, a sudden property tax hike, would "approach the outrageous," in the words of county supervisor James Mize. Speaking as a whole, the county added that "it would be harsh treatment and totally unfair to the sick and injured medical indigents to transfer them summarily to county government which is not budgeted to assume their care."[118] Sensing a mounting political storm for his young administration, Reagan announced suddenly in January 1968 that the cuts would no longer be necessary.[119]

## Pressures on the Countywide System

For all its limitations, Medi-Cal still placed the county hospital system on more reliable fiscal ground. By the early 1970s, the county contribution to Medicaid—45 percent—became less unpredictable and more consistent.[120] In turn, Medi-Cal eased the overall patient burden. With some patients opting for noncounty facilities, the total daily census at LAC–USC dropped from 2,408 patients per day on average to 1,861 by 1970, a decline of 23 percent. New sources of funds enabled an expansion of the workforce. Staff physicians nearly doubled, from 212 to 384, while total residents and interns grew from 597 to 739. The total number of employees jumped from 6,700 to 8,221.[121]

But these bird's-eye metrics obscured day-to-day strains when one looked more closely. In December 1970, five internists held a press conference where they claimed that LAC–USC's conditions were unfit, even dangerous, for patients. They singled out emergency services in particular, stating that understaffing and associated delays had in some cases even resulted in death. "They die because it may take 10 hours for them to have emergency X-rays taken, or because there are not enough laboratory technicians, or because equipment is out of date, won't work or simply does not exist," said David Gans, one of the internists.[122] Thomas Brem, LAC–USC's director of internal medicine, spoke directly about the county's rising population and the ongoing challenges it presented, noting that the hospital received 36,000 patients per year, twice as many as Cook County Hospital in Chicago. Bed occupancy, he observed, sometimes hit 90 percent or above, and the figures for admissions to staff ratios were above those of typical institutions elsewhere in the country and state.

Like Harbor General, LAC–USC's admitting room was "terribly overcrowded" at all hours with poor triage and coordination. Inpatient services after admission were particularly compromised. Brem reported that the hospital was reducing lengths of stays, which posed risks to continuity of care. Summarizing Brem's remarks, county investigators wrote that "over a 4-day period, each ward has a nearly total turnover, a tremendous challenge to both the doctors

Table 3.2. Admissions-to-staff ratios at LAC–USC versus other major
California county hospitals, 1968–69

| Name | Total beds | Ratio: admissions to staff |
|---|---|---|
| LAC–USC | 2,992 | 12.6 |
| University Hospital of San Diego County | 398 | 6.4 |
| Sacramento Medical Center | 552 | 8.5 |
| Santa Clara Valley | 455 | 9.0 |
| Orange County Medical Center | 575 | 11.0 |
| San Francisco General Hospital | 918 | 11.6 |

*Source*: Los Angeles County Department of Hospitals, "Ratio of Admissions to
Staff: Urban Counties—County Teaching and University Hospitals, 1968–69,"
in Los Angeles County Committee on Emergency Medical Care, "Subcommittee
Report to the Board of Supervisors: Investigation of Charges Made by the Interns
and Residents Regarding the Quality of Patient Care at the Los Angeles County/
USC Medical Center," April 1971, 13–17, Box 3260 40.2 "County-USC Medical Center
10-6-70 to 5-28-74," Folder "#2 County-USC Medical Center-Outside Medical Relief
[unintelligible] 40.2 From: 10-6-70 To: 1-18-72," Hall of Records, Kenneth Hahn Hall
of Administration (Los Angeles County), Los Angeles.

and the nurses. Patients who are discharged early and who are still really ill, are
given outpatient appointments to continue their treatment, but it is an unfor-
tunate fact of life that over 50% do not return. Then when they get desperately
ill again, they return and may need treatment in an ICU [intensive care unit]."[123]
Resources were also often disproportionately distributed. For example, of the
600 beds in the medical department, only 6 were available for coronary care,
leading to rushed and compressed stays for those patients.

Similar problems existed in surgery, a department that otherwise boasted
many achievements, including a low 12 percent mortality rate for trauma and
emergency care. For other types of procedures, however, a small number of
operating rooms and a shortage of anesthesiologists and nurses made it unde-
pendable. The hospital had conducted no hernia operations for two months and
had "postponed dangerously," in the words of the investigators, "operations for
cancer advanced biliary cases." Room shortages led to disastrous scenarios. The
head of the department of surgery recalled being confronted on a recent Friday
evening late at night with "1 pediatric emergency, 2 stab wounds, 2 emergency
appendectomies, 2 orthopedic emergencies, and one neurological injury." For
adequate care, he stated, six operating rooms were necessary, not one. Even
some of the urgent procedures that Friday night had required twenty-four-hour
postponement.[124]

Understaffing was common. One pathologist estimated that laboratory
requests were six times the national average.[125] When coupled with the higher

Table 3.3. Interdepartmental variation in occupancy by median percentage, 1970.
(Departments/subdivisions with occupancy rates above 70 percent are in bold.)

| Department | Bed capacity | Occupancy median (%) |
| --- | --- | --- |
| Alcohol | 33 | **103** |
| Burns | 43 | 65 |
| Internal Medicine | 546 | **82** |
| General Surgery | 156 | **76** |
| Neuro Medicine | 67 | **80** |
| Neuro Surgery | 52 | **87** |
| Ophthalmology | 32 | 52 |
| Orthopedics | 201 | **76** |
| Otolaryngology | 32 | **75** |
| Renal | 23 | 63 |
| Thoracic Surgery | 24 (first half year) | 63 |
| | 15 (second half year) | **100** |
| Tumor | 32 | 58 |
| Urology | 58 | 64 |

Source: "Admissions (1970)," in Los Angeles County Committee on Emergency Medical Care, "Subcommittee Report to the Board of Supervisors: Investigation of Charges Made by the Interns and Residents Regarding the Quality of Patient Care at the Los Angeles County/USC Medical Center," April 1971, 13–17, Box 3260 40.2 "County-USC Medical Center 10-6-70 to 5-28-74," Folder "#2 County-USC Medical Center-Outside Medical Relief [unintelligible] 40.2 From: 10-6-70 To: 1-18-72," Hall of Records, Kenneth Hahn Hall of Administration (Los Angeles County), Los Angeles.

volume of patients, the consequences were serious. Hugh Edmonson, who directed the lab, explained that "many tests that the laboratory runs do not do anybody any good because after the test is done, the results do not get back on the chart in time for the doctor to see while the patient is still here." Shortages in clerks staffing the laboratories led to logistical errors. "Oftentimes the same test is done twice because the doctor does not know it has been done as the chart does not show it," investigators observed. With X-rays, the situation was similar. Requests for them had skyrocketed, even in a single year, from roughly 300 a day in 1969 to more than 700 a year later. But understaffing meant that they often did not reach a physician by the time he or she saw a patient.[126]

The roots of the hospital's sustainability problems in the 1970s were multi-pronged. Medi-Cal had recently suffered trimming from a reinvigorated Reagan, and though not as severe as the $210 million he had unsuccessfully attempted in 1967, the more recent round of cuts threw the county into panic. In 1971, LAC–USC's chief deputy director, Liston Witherill, estimated that the latest state rollbacks would increase the necessary expenditures for health services by a potentially unfeasible 30 percent.[127] As serious was a personnel freeze and 2 percent budget cut imposed by the county, a move prompted by a projected $59 million in county debt. Loopholes on business taxes and unexpectedly reduced vehicle taxes from low sales had contributed to the problem, as had the costs of an expanded law enforcement apparatus after the Watts riots.[128]

Care was compromised. By one estimate, even if the hospital were to fill all personnel vacancies—caused by hiring freezes and stagnant wages tied to the recent cuts—and increase the hospital budget by $8.3 million, it would "only restore the level of care which existed on July 1, 1970."[129] Worsening conditions forced the county to rethink the core assumptions of its entire health services program. A year earlier, a county health services planning committee had restructured the system entirely, consolidating fragmented agencies into a single "department of health services." In a report, it had also questioned the centrality of the hospital itself as a front-line point of access for care. The planning committee argued for more decentralization via the creation of satellite OEO-type health centers around a central hospital and an additional class of clinics devoted specifically to short outpatient visits. A new comprehensive plan for health services was a chance to see through an unrealized vision, and the county chose the eastern part of the Watts area as a site for another neighborhood health center in an OEO mold, hoping it might take some patient stress off LAC–USC and complement the imminent Watts hospital.[130] These facilities were small, intended to complement hospitals, not replace them. But while never criticizing hospitals outright, the focus on decentralized facilities implicitly questioned a hospital-centered path for the county. It made one wonder if a large county hospital and all its high fixed costs were the most effective means of delivering medical care.

The question was important, as the Watts hospital was about to finally open in a markedly different budgetary milieu than the one in which it had been planned. The early postwar period had been characterized by growth and liberal support of the health care sector, doubly enforced by Medicare and Medicaid in the mid-1960s. But a decade had made a critical difference. Governor Edmund Brown, a liberal Democrat, had been followed by Ronald Reagan, antagonistic to public medical care from its earliest days. County budget cuts, meanwhile, had affected LAC–USC considerably. It was a precarious environment for the new facility, called Martin Luther King, Jr. Hospital, to enter.

## The Tragedy of Martin Luther King, Jr. Hospital

In 1972, seven years after it was planned, the Martin Luther King, Jr. Hospital finally opened in Watts, after overcoming innumerable political hurdles. The 465-bed full-service hospital arrived amid enormous optimism. Elmer Anderson, its first medical director, characterized it as "the realization of a miracle."[131] Like the Watts center, the hospital was designed as a simultaneous solution to both the medical maldistribution problem and larger economic deprivation in the area. It would be part of a medical complex consisting of a new medical school, the Charles R. Drew Postgraduate School of Medicine, which would use the facility as a teaching hospital, and a paraprofessional training center. Its intertwined goals couldn't have been clearer: "to treat those diseases borne of poverty and economic depression by decreasing the level of under and unemployment."[132]

From planning to opening, however, the King project was deeply dependent on predominantly white institutions and locked into powerful establishment networks. In the earliest stages, county supervisor Kenneth Hahn had played a key role in raising funds from bond sales through back channels. Now, during its early years of operation, King continued relying on external support. Although the Watts center had decoupled from USC, not linking with an existing university was harder to do for a full-service hospital and upstart medical school. One priority was attracting personnel and faculty. Enter USC and UCLA. They had both provided crucial support for the Drew School of Medicine in the form of affiliations, parallel faculty appointments, and temporary office space for Drew faculty, and they would oversee recruitment of chairs for Drew departments.[133] These ties deepened when UCLA becoming the primary steward of multimillion-dollar annual allotments from the state ($2.8 million in 1975) that it dispersed to Drew.[134] But UCLA's middleman position, along with the general affiliation itself, meant something else, too: King and Drew were far from the autonomous "community hospital" envisioned in the early 1960s by figures like Sol White.

Governance questions aside, demands on King were large from the moment it opened its doors. An assessment of the facility two years after its opening found that a staggering 50 percent of its surgical cases were trauma cases. This high figure indicated a dearth of similarly equipped facilities in South Central Los Angeles for those incurring serious physical injuries. The hospital's hypertension clinic also saw an influx of patients. Noting the higher incidence of the condition among the Black population, Joseph Graves, the Watts health center's chief of internal medicine, speculated that this high rate was partly due to "environmental factors—such as diet, stress, culture, disease, economic and social security."[135] At King, those who staffed the clinic found that 65–70 percent of patients showed signs of hypertension.

King had also been sold, politically, as never exclusively about just *Watts*. Partisans such as Hahn and those won over to the cause had also seen it as a way to alleviate pressures on LAC–USC. Two years after King opened, county officials predicted a 39 percent decline in inpatient infrastructure at LAC–USC, from 1,636 beds to 999, and a 177 percent gain at King, from 228 to 408.[136] King was thus beginning its life beset by multiple demands. It received patients from the broader county *and* medically deprived Watts. But sanguine county officials thought that these pressures would be manageable. As in New York City, county officials foresaw an overall decline in inpatient hospitalization at public facilities. And they assumed (rather strikingly in retrospect) that some form of national health insurance would arrive imminently, providing patients with a ticket to private institutions. For Los Angeles County, this additional source of third-party payment from the federal government would allow some patients to go elsewhere for care, further relieving the load on county facilities.[137]

Officials were too optimistic. New structural constraints on the county were growing. King's long birth had come during a period of transition. The postwar health services construction boom had ground to a halt by the time building finished in 1972. And while Los Angeles continued to grow, that trend hardly trickled down into the world of social services spending. Following the 1971 budget reductions, the county fell into deficit, resulting in periodic service cuts. A half-decade later, these trends had worsened, leading Liston Witherill, the director of the county's department of health services, to write that "the fiscal situation is the gravest the department has experienced in recent history and the outlook for the future is similarly critical."[138] Among other contributions, Witherill pointed to the persistently high county contribution to Medi-Cal. The county had also become overreliant on appropriations of property tax revenue that were less than generous. And it now faced a world after the War on Poverty, where federal largesse for novel social services programming was plummeting and a new "austerity politics" had arisen, both in and outside of Los Angeles County. In the mid-1960s, many liberals continued to think that Medicare and Medicaid were stepping-stones to some form of national health insurance, and various flavors of it were proposed by everyone from Senator Ted Kennedy to President Richard Nixon in the early 1970s.[139] By 1976, though, it was clear that no form of it was coming, and worse, county officials noted that private physicians were rejecting Medi-Cal patients more frequently. Both developments resulted in continual pressure on the public system.

Utilization rates reflected the trends. King's capacity was 10.7 percent higher than budgeted for. In a single year, LAC–USC had experienced a 13 percent increase in new patients.[140] As Witherill put it, the "demands for increased services have come at a time when our resources have been seriously diminished." By that, Witherill meant a health services budget cut of $7 million, a loss of 450 positions, and another hiring freeze that had "brought staffing levels to a critical low point," even threatening the accreditation of some facilities. On the ground, "hospitals were forced to close intensive care units, consolidate wards," and "cope with extensive overcrowding," a daily grind for employees at all hospitals. Impromptu solutions were often devised to deal with the squeeze. Los Angeles County–USC obstetrics patients, for example, were transferred to King, yet another load on the already taxed new facility. Witherill issued a larger warning: "The public must realize that many of these conditions, translated into human terms, mean increased suffering for persons who cannot afford or in many cases obtain private care." Further, fiscal stringency within the sector could translate into political conflict. "As the gap between the expectation and the availability of health services widens, both the consumer and the health professional can be expected to step up their public actions," he remarked.[141]

It was a poignant statement, given that "public actions"—in the form of a riot—were what had given rise to King. Witherill's warning was prescient. A landscape of relentless scarcity exacerbated stresses at King. In May 1975, King residents commenced a one-week work stoppage to protest working conditions and quality of care in the facility itself. They called for an end to spending freezes, and they pointed to long wait times and delays in making appointments and receiving laboratory results, all attributable to an overtaxed staff. They further demanded increases in hiring: 50 percent for interns and residents, 25 percent for permanent physician staff, and 50 percent for nurses. Made in the name of "the community of patients and workers [who] want quality patient care at Martin Luther King Hospital," most of the demands were unfeasible, given the county's fiscal shape. But the work action attracted attention to the dire on-the-ground situation of county facilities. Soon, county officials acceded to the strikers' call for forming a task force. And the protesters moderated their stances, acknowledging that their "long term demands" were "complicated issues" requiring extended deliberation.[142] The task force ultimately agreed to minor tweaks in protocol rather than the sweeping expenditure increases the strikers had demanded. Two representative reforms, for example, reexamined how King distributed supplies and increased problem reporting procedures for the laboratory. But they didn't—and really they couldn't—tackle King's real problem in a punishing fiscal climate: too few staff and not enough funds.[143]

If the work stoppage and resulting task force didn't translate into many deep reforms, it certainly had unexpected political ramifications. Reaction to it revealed governance issues and several fault lines in the King Hospital's support base. The most vocal opposition to the action didn't come from county officials or King administrators, who'd responded in good faith to the strikers. Rather, it emanated from those who saw the negotiations as illegitimate, conducted by supposed advocates without long-standing roots in Watts. One critical voice was the Black Grassroots Caucus, started in 1972 by social service workers and welfare recipients in the area, and chaired by Callie Greene, a Watts community organizer. "Everyone is talking for and about the neighborhood people but not to them," Greene complained. Though Greene had always supported the King Hospital, she'd always done so cautiously. During early planning, she consistently questioned USC's and UCLA's involvement in shepherding the project.

She'd also put King's leaders through the ringer, subjecting them to scrutiny. At a 1970 conference, speaking on the new Drew School of Medicine, she praised its Black dean, Mitchell Spellman, whom she described as someone "who knows exactly what he is doing." Spellman, she added, had undergone "two years of DEbrainwashing, and he stood the test."[144]

As with the Watts center, Greene's comment on "DEbrainwashing" reflected intraracial fractures. Once again, tension existed between Black Watts constituents and Black medical professionals. Five years after her qualified praise of Spellman, Greene hit a far more critical note and repudiated the Drew School of Medicine, characterizing its conduct and the task force as an illegitimate action by those allied with Spellman and the school. To Greene, the task force not only pacified protest but allowed the Drew School to assert more aggressively its "control," in her words, of King's affairs. She counterposed the Drew School with an "entire Grassroots community" that would push to end "any and all contracts with the Charles R. Drew Postgraduate Medical School and to send all . . . chairmen along with Spellman on his Sabbatical Leave."[145] In Greene's eyes, the ideal setup was one disentangled from traditional academic medical institutions altogether, whether predominantly Black or white. Put another way, the optimal path was full independence. Yet given the fiscal realities of funding hospitals, it was a fundamentally symbolic wish. Still, the questions raised by Green persisted, especially as the Drew School and UCLA's relationship tightened. In 1978, UCLA and Drew signed an agreement expanding their agreement to create a joint program that placed forty-eight students at the King Hospital. It gave UCLA considerable power, requiring the medical school to consult with UCLA during its faculty searches.[146]

The deepening involvement of UCLA attracted further hostility because of a controversy from earlier in the decade. The university had caused an uproar when news broke that it was forming a center for the study of violence influenced by the work of Frank Ervin and Vernon Mark's *Violence and the Brain*. That book underplayed social contributors to violence and instead pushed biological explanations. As sociologist Alondra Nelson has characterized it, "Mark submitted his hypothesis that brain dysfunction caused urban violence," and he openly pondered whether the Los Angeles riots had been "carried out by unruly African Americans with diseased brains." Plans for the center dovetailed with national controversies around IQ and race, particularly those surrounding the work of Arthur Jensen, a psychologist proffering racist hereditarian explanations of intelligence gaps.[147] It all attracted enough enormous criticism—on and off campus—to kill the violence project but not without souring UCLA's reputation, especially among many Los Angeles Black activists.[148]

These prior developments fed later controversies over governance. In 1978, Drew appointed M. Alfred Haynes, a Black physician and professor, to the position of dean. Anticipating criticism, Drew School administrators conceded to a "community interview" of Haynes but, to many, didn't go far enough. Around the same time, the chairman of the school's psychiatry department, Frank Hayes, had fired John R. Seeley, an accomplished researcher, claiming school budgetary crunches. For one group of protestors, who identified themselves as a "coalition of organizations" invested in King, the action epitomized the school's lack of accountability to a wider Watts constituency. The coalition wrote that "we do not know Dr. Frank Hayes, for the community has never informally nor formally been introduced to him," before speculating that Seeley had been fired because of his criticisms of UCLA's violence project. The coalition took a clear stand on the future direction of the King Hospital and Drew School of Medicine and "protest[ed] the hiring of department chairmen and professors who have not met with and been interviewed by the interested community."[149] But how one adjudicated invocations and counterinvocations of community remained a question with an elusive answer. Compounding the issue was the changing racial composition of Watts itself, which had seen an influx of Mexican American migration, a trend noted by county officials as well as the 1976 strikers, who'd demanded Spanish-language interpretation for a changing patient census. By 1981, 53 percent of King's patients were "Spanish-surnamed," according to one county assessment, a stunning increase from its first years, when "less than 6%" of its patients would be classified as "Hispanic."[150] Who, indeed, was the community now?

In the end, however one worked through these dilemmas, did participatory governance matter? The battle over the UCLA and Drew School of Medicine appointment process took place in 1978, the same year that Proposition 13, a ballot initiative, passed with 65 percent of the vote. Proposition 13 capped property valuation at 1975 levels, limited rates to "1 percent of 'real cash value,'" and imposed stringent two-thirds majority requirements if the state legislature wished to raise property taxes in the future. For municipal budgets, the consequences of hundreds of millions in lost revenue were enormous. "Overnight," writes journalist Peter Schrag, "property tax revenues for local agencies declined by between $6 and $7 billion annually," about 27 percent of city revenues and 40 percent of county revenues, making these jurisdictions more beholden to the whims of state finances.[151] A few months before the election, Supervisor Edmund Edelman asserted that "within Los Angeles County government, the effects of Proposition 13 will be felt no greater than in the Department of Health Services."[152]

Edelman's predictions weren't hyperbole. Projected state allocations to the county became increasingly unreliable, and budgets often had to be scaled back. In the 1981–82 year, for example, an original budget of $906.7 million for health services was decreased by $65.2 million after a state budget review. That same budget resulted in 4,434 lost county positions, but 52.8 percent of them came from health services, even though the department accounted for only 19.4 percent of county funds. When disaggregated further, the health services budget looked even worse. Of five county health services districts that ran new decentralized ambulatory care centers, four suffered one-year budget cuts, with the two highest-poverty districts (28.4 percent and 23.1 percent) suffering declines of 11 percent.[153] And while health services spending did eventually increase again on a year-to-year basis, after precipitous initial decline following Proposition 13, it failed to outpace the upward trend in health care costs—propelled by a multitude of forces, from inflation to equipment pricing—with which municipal health systems were contending.[154]

But for those working in county health care, what historian Mike Davis later called the "Watts Riots of the Middle Classes" wasn't so much a sudden budgetary jolt as it was the culmination of a decade when fiscal tightness became the new normal. For the two Watts institutions, the consequences took on a tragic dimension as Proposition 13 took fiscal pressures to another level. Federal funds for many local social services had grown tenuous when OEO folded into the Department of Health, Education, and Welfare during the Nixon administration, with the last federal $5.4 million appropriation coming in month-to-month installments.[155] At the Watts center, which drew much of its financing from federal sources, administrators moved to convert the facility into a health management organization (HMO). It would be sustained by a contract with California and would primarily serve Medi-Cal patients, thus lessening its reliance on direct federal funds. Around that time, in 1973, the organization sat on $4.5 million in construction debt and reported trouble finding additional creditors to service miscellaneous operations.[156] Renamed the Watts Health Foundation, the Watts center's conversion into an HMO occurred in 1977 and prevented collapse. But it depended heavily on inconsistent and unpredictable Medi-Cal funding. In 1987, a 10 percent Medi-Cal cut forced the foundation to lay off 200 workers. As in New York, sustainability had trumped governance as a primary concern.[157]

Martin Luther King, Jr. Hospital's issues were even graver, including basic operations problems. One early example was lack of stable protocol for billing intake. A county assessment found that the hospital had failed to interview outpatients for Medi-Cal status or follow up on inpatient bills, especially accounts that were past due. The investigators estimated that unclaimed Medi-Cal reimbursements alone had resulted in $3 million lost.[158] Even more serious was quality of care. A passionate letter to county officials, written in 1977 by an anonymous employee, opened by stating that "patients call or refer to the hospital as 'Killer King,'" a moniker of dubious distinction that stuck with the institution throughout its existence. The writer then complained that "many times things come up each day that I think should be reported to make things work better. But, going to persons here at this institution is just a waste of time." He or she attached a list of thirty-four concrete complaints. Formal lists of personnel, the employee wrote, didn't reflect "the amount of actual bodies available." Inebriated workers or those using work time to watch television were rarely held accountable. Slow laboratory work and personnel shortages were common.[159]

Subsequent media scrutiny of King raised the question of why managerial laxity hadn't attracted attention sooner. One reason was simple: the charged origins of King and the political patronage surrounding it from the start. Criticism of the hospital could easily be interpreted as indifference to the chronic maldistribution that had given rise to the Watts riots or, more cynically, framed as an attack on what many thought of as a Black institution with huge political symbolism.

But in the end, focus on King's administration tended to treat the hospital as if it were an autonomous institution rather than one whose local fortune was dependent on multiple nonlocal forces.[160] This interpretive tendency was especially pronounced in the Los Angeles press, as the scholars Darnell Hunt and Ana-Christina Ramon have observed in their content analysis of *Los Angeles Times* coverage, which regularly framed King's mounting problems as a case study in institutional dysfunction and, at its worst, turned the hospital into a symbol for "black failure." Mismanagement was certainly real, but it needed to be analyzed in an era of immense fiscal strain, one where meetings on how to confront budgetary crisis occurred on the regular. In 1984, local members of the vaunted Southern Christian Leadership Conference, Martin Luther King's civil rights group, met in a King auditorium to discuss how Los Angeles County facilities would weather consequences of a $2 billion federal budget cut. Two years later, a veto by Republican governor George Deukmejian translated into a $29 million dearth of funds for county health care.[161] The consequences for day-to-day employees were taxing. As one employee of King-Drew put it to the *Los Angeles Sentinel*, one of the city's major Black newspapers: "There's just too much work at King-Drew, Harbor-UCLA and County-USC and too little pay for what you have to do. It affects the care you can give to patients and it affects what you think of yourself and the quality of your life."[162]

Yet it was King that bore the most racially tinged scorn and blame, with its head, William Delgardo, removed from his position by the county in 1989, ostensibly for "poor administration" and "major breakdowns" in patient care.[163] The move led to outcry from Watts activists. It prompted one *Sentinel* columnist to decry the myopia with which county authorities and the press assessed King's troubles. "There is little doubt," Larry Aubry wrote, "that what lies behind the statistics on the death rate, patient care and quality assurance, etc. is a policy of institutional neglect by the county."[164] Aubry was right to move blame beyond King itself. But he was also wrong to stop at the county. In fact, fiscal pressures at the state level, and contraction of funds from the federal government, contributed as much to King's plight and constrained its potential.

Martin Luther King, Jr. Hospital had the misfortune of opening in harsh circumstances that never quite let up, preventing it from achieving institutional stability, even as it absorbed other facilities' excess patient loads and did more with less. One alternative might have been construction of smaller satellite facilities similar to the original Watts center. Few asked whether building a hospital, with all its infrastructural liabilities, many of which could never be sufficiently met, was in retrospect a good idea. But in the wake of Watts, anything less wouldn't have possessed the symbolic power that a large county hospital generated.

When King did finally emerge, it faced fiscal circumstances far less hospitable than the one from which it was hatched, weathering fiscal tumult from the start. The toll it took on everyday operations and conditions was predictable, and it culminated tragically in 2007, when county authorities shut the hospital down after it failed federal inspections. It wouldn't reopen for nearly another decade. This was an outcome, if not foreordained, tragic and predictable enough.

Los Angeles air pollution control had been a success story, with conflict much more muted, if not exactly absent. The postriot health care experience, by contrast, thrust questions of power, control, and resources to center stage, much as in New York City, which entered the 1980s in similarly rocky budgetary territory. But racial reckoning was even more fundamental to the battles in Los Angeles. That was the case 2,000 miles away in Cleveland, too, where riots rocked a similarly resource-deprived and racially segregated neighborhood, setting off a parallel frenzied quest by the city's power brokers for explanations and solutions. The two regions bore many similarities: long histories of civil rights activism alongside brutal racism, two of the most high-profile riots in the 1960s, and soaring promises to do better in the aftermath. There were some differences, too. Cleveland was smaller and experiencing either population stagnation or outright loss, not growth—circumstances that helped it weather a recessionary world better than its coastal counterparts. And the nature of its medical exclusion was different. Instead of medical deserts, the East Side of Cleveland—its Watts—was surrounded by elite medical abundance that had attracted both national and world attention. It was elite medicine for some except those who lived immediately around it. In 1966, insularity would find itself on defense.

# 4

# Cleveland

### Health Innovation, Health Citadels, Health Ghettoes: Progress and Deprivation in Midwestern Medicine

If you drive or ride eastward today along Euclid Avenue, a thoroughfare in Cleveland, the landscape looks pretty much the same for dozens and dozens of blocks: a lot of mini office parks, a church now and then, the occasional upstart apartment building, and many empty lots of grass, some nicely landscaped, some not. It's not very dense, and little changes until you hit the high-eighty streets. Then suddenly, the multistory pavilions and glass structures come at you: the Cleveland Clinic, University Hospitals, Case Western Reserve, concentrated together as one of the most prestigious academic-medical constellations in the world. The buildings scream high tech and cutting edge, and they're flanked by banners, running for blocks, that let you know the various institutions are top ranked in the country for this or that specialty. It's hard not to feel awe, but it's hard also not to wonder who really gets to enjoy these resources and how much of it is really helping those who live around it amid residential segregation, high poverty, and overall extreme hardship. Drive just a couple blocks north or south of this area, and you'll see many abandoned dwellings, boarded-up buildings, the typical and depressing markers of disinvestment in a city riven with inequality. The tracks of history are all over this East Side medical mile and those pockets just outside it.

Like Watts, the area erupted in the 1960s, and in the aftermath, residents angrily pointed to powerful institutions' histories of negligence and exclusion. Executives certainly didn't expect to spend the rest of the 1960s wondering whether they'd be a target of rioters and if it might just be a good idea to pick up and go. Residents' rage was understandable. Cleveland hadn't undergone a medical expansion like Los Angeles. It had developed, however, a reputation as a site of innovation in both medical care delivery and medical technology itself—but it was for some, not all, especially Cleveland's low-income Black residents. The riots won major concessions from Cleveland politicos and its medical strong-holds. And thanks to seemingly mundane alterations in governance with roots in the 1950s, Cleveland's health care system wound up buffering it from the fiscal storms confronting larger counterpart cities elsewhere.

## The 1950s Restructuring of Cleveland Health Care

If the 1960s were eventful years for health care in Cleveland, the preceding decade was the opposite. While the New York City public hospital system was fraying, and the one in Los Angeles was booming, Cleveland, alas, was expe-riencing neither, and it treated its City Hospital with striking nonchalance. At least, that was the conclusion of Doris Reed and Thomas Reed, two consul-tants retained by the National Municipal League to examine City Hospital's state. In 1949, both expressed bewilderment at the informality of the operation, praising the quality of the facility while commenting that "strangely enough, it has reached its present proportions without a plan consistently adhered to for even its physical development and without any clear-cut determination of its functions and policies."[1]

The lack of structure worked for now, but the Reeds sounded alarms. Loose oversight of the hospital had led to a considerable amount of undercompensated and uncompensated care, which they estimated at 25 percent of the total cost of operation, caused "chiefly from the failure to realize all the income to which the hospital is entitled." The problem stemmed from the hospital's origins—like its counterparts nationwide—as a charity institution in the late nineteenth and early twentieth centuries. Now, it struggled to adapt to the mid-twentieth cen-tury, when its patient population transitioned, as writers Charles Rosenberg and David Rosner have shown, beyond just medical indigents but also those able to pay "whole or part" of the hospital's fees.[2] And yet, the hospital didn't seem to have a functioning billing system. "It is supposedly part of the hospital routine," the Reeds wrote, "that a bill be presented to the patient at a final interview with a member of the social service department before leaving the hospital. Many, however, get away without this attention."[3] Then there was the problem of reim-bursements for indigent patients. City Hospital hadn't devised a reliable means of receiving timely reimbursements from Cleveland's "relief fund." Many cases lagged for months. In one set of 275 inpatient cases for May 1947, for example, 40 were still pending an evaluation by October. Outpatients were no better. Only 19 percent of bills, after submission in May, had been cleared by November.[4] The result was regular debt each fiscal year.

The Reeds presented short- and long-term ideas for Cleveland that officials debated into the 1950s. Tighter billing and reimbursement procedures were obvious solutions. In the long run, though, the problems required something that stretched beyond both facility walls and city boundaries. For the Reeds, it was the transfer of City Hospital to Cuyahoga County's government. The most obvious appeal, as in Los Angeles County, was an enormous fiscal burden lifted off the city of Cleveland. In the Reeds' analysis, Cleveland residents had always been subject to a kind of double taxation when they subsidized hospitals in *both* the city and larger county boundaries. Why not, they asked, just redirect all tax dollars for hospitals to a single entity?[5]

But City Hospital's modus operandi meant anything but action. Into the 1950s, the Reeds' proposals languished, were visited periodically, then forgotten again. In part, that was because sustainability crises at City Hospital were never as severe as they were in places like New York City. Chronic yearly deficits didn't cripple day-to-day operations. One reason was that City Hospital never faced an overly burdensome patient load. In fact, the figures declined sharply over the decade from around 151,349 "patient days" in 1947 to 115,228 by 1955, and an overall occupancy rate of only 60 percent. The trends tracked that of the city, which would lose nearly 39,000 residents from 1950 to 1960, declining from 914,808 to 876,050.[6] To make up for debt, the city imposed minor hikes in daily rates charged to patients.[7] For a while, it worked. Debt may have been a nuisance, but it was hardly disastrous.

Personnel problems plaguing New York City didn't strike Cleveland, either. Like Los Angeles County General Hospital and USC, Western Reserve University and City Hospital had been affiliated since 1914. The relationship tightened during World War II. Western Reserve had become responsible for "nominations" of physician staff that the city had heretofore approved. Affiliation made City Hospital an attractive destination for prospective staff, preventing the exodus that New York City suffered at the same time.[8] The decline in patients spared city personnel, too, from the taxing workloads suffered by hospital labor in Los Angeles.

But in the mid-1950s, the tranquility ended and the loose management caught up with the city. Having failed to modernize its billing system, City Hospital's debt grew onerous by the mid-1950s, and it couldn't paper over it with tiny fee hikes. In 1955, the hospital had overspent by $194,000, resulting in increased appropriations to Cleveland's Department of Public Health and Welfare while "depriving some other departments of necessary income," warned a worried mayor Anthony Celebrezze.[9] The financial pickle ramped up pressure to act before the problem got worse. That action came in the form of a ballot measure for a hospital operating levy, but it failed. With no other options, the city implemented emergency salary cuts in November 1956. Physicians and city officials feared a staff exodus equal to that of New York City, noting that it had "happened at other teaching hospitals with subsequent decline in the caliber of medical care and teaching."[10] The situation grew still more urgent a year later, when the hospital characterized a nursing shortage as "critical."[11]

It was enough for a 1957 City Hospital committee to recommend transfer of City Hospital to Cuyahoga County, first proposed in 1949 by the Reeds in their report. City and county officials moved quickly this time, and they had pressure from civic elites. The Welfare Federation of Cleveland, which occasionally funded city health programs, devised a plan for executing the transfer, recommending that the county "purchase" City Hospital for one dollar while the city paid off its remaining debts as a condition of the exchange. The federation celebrated the shift to county governance in communitarian terms, arguing that it signaled a new city-county unity. The transfer foreshadowed "cooperation that the community can expect in the solution of the many problems which will face it as the community strives to develop more effective government for the Greater Cleveland metropolitan area."[12] In January 1958, Cleveland completed the transfer, averting a sustainability crisis at its flagship institution for public medical care.[13] County governance would have implications two decades later, when the city, like many counterparts on the East and West Coasts, confronted fiscal crisis.

## Organized Labor and Health Care Reform: The Community Health Foundation

But this was still the 1950s. Catastrophe averted, Cleveland developed a reputation for medical innovation over the next decade. City Hospital's troubles opened up space for advocates considering alternatives to both the classic public hospital model and the individual private, fee-for-service physician. In the mid-1950s, doctors connected with the Ohio American Federation of Labor and Congress of Industrial Organizations, and locals of the Retail Workers and Meat Cutters unions met regularly to discuss new ideas for provisioning health care in Cleveland. Unions were on an upswing in the city. In 1958, organized labor had defeated a right-to-work law in the state legislature, which would have allowed employees to work without joining a successfully recognized union. This was a critical win, given the proliferation of right-to-work laws elsewhere in the country, especially in the South.[14] A year later, even against fierce opposition from such physician lobbies as the Ohio State Medical Association, labor successfully mobilized legislative support for a bill authorizing experimental prepaid group practices, a reversal of a restrictive bill against them.[15] Energized, the advocates convinced the United States Public Health Service (USPHS) to study the benefits of a prepaid model, whereby a flat fee entitled subscribers to all of a facility's services. The USPHS concluded that group practice might be particularly appropriate for Cleveland. Health care in the city was getting expensive. During the 1950s, Cleveland's consumer price index for medical care costs had risen drastically, from 113.1 to 173.1, above national trends (156.2). And workers' insurance often wasn't very comprehensive, either. Only 50 percent of those surveyed were enrolled in plans that covered nonsurgical procedures, and there existed wide variation in copay rates and employer contributions to insurance costs.[16] By pooling all components of health care—doctors, equipment, physical plants, various specialized services—into a single institutional entity, prepaid group practice could not only bring down prices by reducing redundancy but also assure a fuller spectrum of services for patients.

In the early 1960s, the physicians constituted themselves formally as the Community Health Foundation (CHF) and brought on board three experienced health care consultants: Richard Weinerman, Glenn Wilson, and Avram Yedidia. Weinerman had worked as a consultant with the similarly minded Los Angeles Community Medical Foundation and health programs run by the United Auto Workers and United Mine Workers of America. Wilson had consulted for the United Steelworkers and United Mine Workers as well. Yedidia came from California, where he had played a key role in guiding the Kaiser Permanente Health Plan from its early days as a program for Kaiser shipyard workers.[17] All came out of the same orbit of health professionals, allied with strong labor unions, as Gouverneur's Howard J. Brown.

The trio's previous programs had come with obvious pros and some cons. The advantage of the union-connected initiatives was a ready-made membership based in union rolls. That meant sound fiscal footing, which in turn enabled full-time staffs and infrastructural investment. (The Los Angeles Community Medical Foundation, where Weinerman had also worked, lacked a sufficiently large membership base, contributing to its collapse.) But a union base was also a disadvantage, by definition excluding large numbers of the ununionized population from participation.

The Community Health Foundation was a chance to merge the best aspects of these models. Although organizers targeted a group of Cleveland unions from the outset, they reached out to other potential enrollees as well: a "wide cross-section of the community," in the organizers' words. Still, the unions remained a top target, and not just because of their high membership potential. In the late 1950s, some of them had developed a project, the Union Eye Care Center, built on prepaid group practice principles, which suggested a full-fledged medical practice along such lines could be successful in Cleveland. The eye center had become successful enough to expand to four locations within a half-decade.[18] By May 1962, seven Cleveland union locals, along with individual consumers and employers, had expressed interest in the CHF upstart. In addition to unions, foundation organizers reached out to Western Reserve

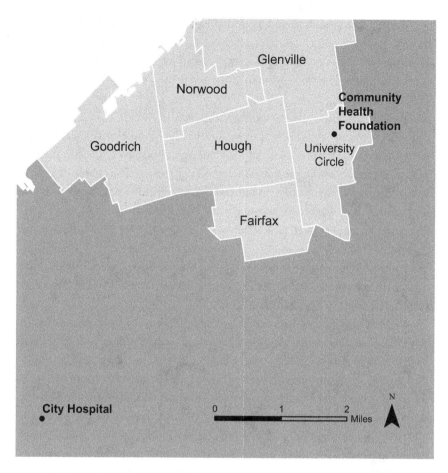

**City Hospital and Community Health Foundation sites.** This map shows the distance between City Hospital and East Cleveland (site of the first CHF Health Center), where a flurry of activity addressing medical maldistribution was about to take place.

*Source*: Author's cartography. In this and subsequent Cleveland maps, I geo-referenced Cuyahoga County "social planning areas" with 1970 U.S. Census tracts and achieved a 100 percent match of boundaries. The areas correspond to popular neighborhood names, except for Fairfax, which was formally named "Central East." The maps are commonplace in a number of official documents. See, for example, "Program for Consolidation: County Health Facilities," April 15, 1971, Dittrick Medical History Center, Case Western Reserve University, Cleveland, Ohio.

University. Like City Hospital, the foundation saw association with Western Reserve as a magnet for attracting staff and a means of resource sharing, particularly in-patient hospital referrals.[19] Rather than operate as an isolated neighborhood medical silo, the Cleveland facility's administration took steps to connect it to established institutions and ensure sustainability.

The first Community Health Foundation center opened on Cleveland's East Side; that site selection came after a foundation memo criticized myopic health planning that didn't consider a facility's accessibility and who might use it the most. The East Side was ideal. It had the largest density of union members in the city.[20] In the lead-up to the opening, the foundation had initiated a recruitment drive where staffers made personal appearances to discuss the program with potential members, especially at union locals. The foundation initially limited enrollment to the East Side and anticipated a membership of 13,000 in the first year of operation, with a projected increase to 22,500 within a couple of years.[21] More challenging than patient membership was recruiting physicians, many of whom had never worked as part of a medical staff under one roof and feared professional reprisal over association with group practice, still controversial within the mainstream medical profession, which perceived it as a transition away from fee-for-service medicine and toward "socialized medicine."[22] That apprehensiveness subsided when Eugene Vayda, a prominent Western Reserve physician, signed on as medical director.

Whatever political skittishness might have existed, the Community Health Foundation had no trouble attracting monetary support. In July 1964, it opened its first facility with $1.3 million borrowed from union locals and Cleveland business groups. The staff consisted of twenty physicians, plus public health nurses.[23] To cultivate stronger bonds between patients and administrators, organizers developed "health center committees" to represent enrolled patient groups at CHF board meetings.[24] The foundation's biggest innovation was at the level of patient experience, where it encouraged close connections between patients and practitioners, reinforced with principles of "health maintenance": that is, the notion that one's health was not a series of one-off treatments but a prolonged state of being to be monitored and upheld. Each enrollee was designated a "personal physician" who then directed the patient to specialty services within the facility as needed. The program's administrators saw the model as a response to fragmentation of care and poor planning that didn't gracefully match medical services to patient health needs. A few years after the opening, Glenn Wilson, CHF's executive director, wrote that the foundation was designed to reverse a typically "casual relationship to the physician." Too often, he observed, "when the patient decides that the illness is beyond the scope of the physician, the cure has not been immediate enough or completely by chance, the patient will go to another physician. Complex medical problems which the family doctor would likely have resolved if given an adequate opportunity are taken from his hands by the acts of the patient." That "increasing alienation between the patients and their family physician" might stem from increasing specialization. "On the one hand, he [the patient] wants all of the knowledge in the field of medicine made available to him—at the same time he is shunted—in his mind—from pillar to

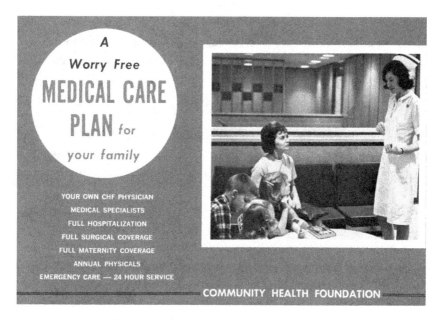

Community Health Foundation recruitment pamphlet, ca. late 1960s (from context).

*Source*: Box 40, Folder 257, Edwin Weinerman Papers, Sterling Memorial Library, Yale University, New Haven, Conn.

post, from specialists to specialists in a bewildering maze of referrals."[25] Moving everything into a common unit, and anchoring it with a personal physician monitoring a patients' movement through a system, prevented the "bewildering maze" that Wilson bemoaned.

Community Health Foundation membership grew, doubling to 25,000 by 1967. The foundation opened another facility on the West Side of Cleveland and signed agreements with four local hospitals for in-patient services. By 1970, administrators estimated, the CHF might hit anywhere between 70,000 to 100,000 members.[26] The program had grown prominent enough to attract plaudits in both the city and national press. Cleveland's *Plain Dealer* praised the foundation's approach, writing that its "object is to keep people in good health, not simply repair them." In addition to holding costs down, the foundation's centralized model allowed physicians to be "spared the cost of offices, private staffs and materials" and provided "the opportunity to stay abreast of progress in the profession. . . . The theory is that the doctor who is less rushed and is better informed is a more efficient physician."[27]

The foundation continued refining several innovations for "health maintenance." One program, targeted at chronic disease patients, was oriented around a "Basic Health Record" and periodic "Family Health Conferences." The record was no "usual diagnostic 'work-up' of the ill patient." Rather, the CHF empha-sized, it was "person- and health-oriented," not simply focused on disease itself. It contextualized a patient's "current health status" by breaking it into "physical," "emotional," and "functional" dimensions, and it linked personal health history with the patient's broader "social history," including birthplace and moves, level of schooling, work history, and housing status.[28] Each patient's health team gen-erated the record not just at an office meeting but at a "family home visit and evaluation," followed by "periodic medical control" and detailed conferences to plan regimens for "existing health problems and outline plans for improved management."[29]

The extended nature of these interactions and the group setting reflected the CHF's holism. One health conference for a diabetic and his wife and son, attended by a physician and two public health nurses, involved a detailed pre-sentation of the condition by the team, which noted that "both the patient and family were confused and fearful about prospects in Diabetes. . . . It was obvi-ous that neither patient nor family were yet ready to accept the full burden of knowledge of Diabetes." But "an optimistic attitude was accepted. Prognosis of patient is considered 'fair,' but presented to wife and patient in more favor-able terms." The team also discussed the patient and his family's "acceptance of medical regime" and whether a public health nurse should keep making home visits to monitor his progress. Another patient, who worked in the tailoring and dry-cleaning business but had been recently laid off, had learned the previous year of an ulcer that had probably existed for years. Despite this misfortune, he entered his conference with a copy of a popular health magazine and appeared "very alert and interested" and "actively participated." In a discussion of his "atti-tudes, understanding, problems, adherence to regimen," his health team noted his physiological condition before adding that he now "wonder[ed] if loss of job, which he had had for 15 years," might be linked to a stress-induced ulcer.[30] These three-way dialogues among health teams, patient, and family were striking. They anticipated by almost two decades subsequent movements, identified by histo-rian Nancy Tomes, that sought to empower patient agency in interactions with both practitioners and the medical system at large.[31]

Toward the end of the decade, the Community Health Foundation planned an expansion beyond the two Cleveland sites and into suburban Cuyahoga County. Its membership was becoming occupationally and geographically more varied. The foundation was now serving teachers, government employ-ees, workers in heavy industry (especially the automotive and steel sectors), plus retail workers and food processors, who'd been the first of the unionized workforce to support the program in its infancy. But the program's impressive strides masked limits. Foundation leaders, always careful of the potential polit-ical stigma that might surround prepaid group practice, never presented the

CHF as a challenge to the dominant system of employer-based benefits—what political scientist Marie Gottschalk has called "the private welfare state"—that was solidifying in the decades after World War II.[32] The CHF board of trustees included executives from the Kroger Company, the Greater Cleveland Growth Association, and the Cleveland Electric Illuminating Company.[33] Likewise, when it came to the city's fee-for-service landscape, the CHF ducked battles. Its leaders repeatedly emphasized that it was but one of many options available to Clevelanders. In 1965, its medical director wrote that "dual choice" was given to a patient each year so that "he can reselect his previous plan or choose another plan. This then is freedom of choice as to system of medical care."[34] The foundation was ultimately more vested in its service delivery innovations than in the political project of rethinking American health care.

The word "community" in Community Health Foundation highlighted another tension—namely, who truly constituted it. Located at East 117th Street, it was immediately adjacent to Glenville and Hough, two of the city's most economically depressed and racially segregated neighborhoods.[35] The foundation enrolled its members most frequently by employer groups, not unlike traditional employer-based insurance plans. And most of its subscribers were, in reality, those with access to stable unionized jobs or, if not unionized, working at employers who paid their dues. Consequently, few working people outside such circumstances encountered the CHF, even though it theoretically welcomed them. But, in practice the foundation did little to reach out to indigent patients such as those most reliant on City Hospital. It may have been an institution for working-class people but only of a certain kind.

The racial politics of Greater Cleveland marred attempts to incorporate Black Clevelanders in particular. The Community Health Foundation was already aware of the ire that prepaid group practice and union ties might draw. Racism directed at the project would have been even worse. It wasn't just speculation. In 1967, the foundation planned a small 128-bed hospital, mostly for inpatient needs, in Independence, a nearly all-white Cleveland suburb. The project required voter approval. "Unfortunately," the CHF wrote, during the campaign, "the hospital has become a race issue. Whatever the opposition's true objections to the hospital were, what probably started out as an auxiliary argument—the hospital would bring Negroes into the community—has crystallized as the key issue." The foundation reported that the hospital was confronting "racist-slanted objection" and that opponents were claiming it would result in a flood of "undesirables." It was an example of suburban racial gatekeeping, or racially reactionary "crab-grass roots politics," in the words of one scholar, and it threatened the CHF's expansion.[36] At the eleventh hour, the controversy became a moot point. Kaiser Permanente, a burgeoning health plan in California looking to expand its operations to Ohio, acquired the CHF and planned to build a $10 million facility in Parma, another neighboring suburb.[37] The showdown in Independence, though resolved, was suggestive of the backlash that CHF organizers feared they might incur if efforts to expand membership became too overt.

## "Ferment Is Seething": Cleveland versus the Clinic

Racism in Cleveland had already rocked the city before the events in Independence. A year after Watts in Los Angeles, in July 1966 the Hough neighborhood on the East Side exploded after a restauranteur had posted a sign containing racist antiblack epithets on his door. And just as in Watts, a justifiably angry crowd soon cascaded into a week of rioting that included not just robbery but arson and "firebombing" of mostly commercial establishments. The events resulted in the deaths of "four black civilians" while "injuries numbered in the hundreds," and the National Guard was called in by the city to quell the violence. It'd set off a decade of introspection, soul-searching, and solutions.[38]

As in Los Angeles, assessments of the event soon followed, but this time they took the form of *three* commissions, not just one. The first official analysis came from a Cuyahoga County grand jury, and it differed from other riot commissions convened throughout the decade. Rather than focus primarily on the sociological basis of the riot, the report instead suggested that the Hough uprising was the plot of Black nationalist and communist radicals.[39] "The outbreak of lawlessness and disorder," the grand jury wrote, "was both organized, precipitated, and exploited by a relatively small group of trained and disciplined professionals at this business."[40] Of the neighborhood's inhabitants, it wrote that "diminished incentives by repressed and neglected people" on welfare "enables the father to walk out of his 'marital arrangement' to escape his proper responsibilities." In turn, that led to "tragic deterioration of moral behavior, and the brittle, bitter, hypersensitivity which emerges therefrom."[41] The report's chief narrative of the riot, then, depicted a vulnerable and rudderless Black mass preyed on by a small band of instigators who incited them into action. Still, beneath all the conspiracist and racist moralism was an acknowledgment of material hardship: "inadequate and sub-standard housing," "charging of exorbitant rents by absentee landlords," "non-enforcement of the housing code," "sub-standard educational facilities as a consequence of long neglect," "excessive food prices," and "denial of equal economic opportunities." It was, in other words, what was becoming the standard list in riot commissions across the country.

Mayor Ralph Locher's "emergency committee" repudiated the grand jury's conspiratorial narrative. It drew a much more direct link between Hough's material conditions and riots. Run-down housing, the committee declared, "must have been a contributing, if not a causative, factor in the riots."[42] It also pointed to chronic unemployment in the area and called for expansion of federal employment programs along with housing rehabilitation and improved sanitation service.

The most unsparing and unadulterated of the Hough analyses, however, came from outside formal governmental channels. Cleveland was a rich hotbed of activism with roots in the Great Depression and organizations such as the Future Outlook League, which organized the unemployed and boycotted discriminatory establishments in the city. In the 1960s, Cleveland had a mix of highly active civil rights and neighborhood advocacy organizations, including the Congress of Racial Equality, the Urban League, the NAACP, and the Hough Area Council.[43] They came together to form an ad hoc Cleveland Citizens Committee on Hough Disturbances and held three days of public hearings to develop an alternative account of what'd happened. Like the mayor's report, the committee was focused on Hough's resource shortfalls and concluded that it was almost "inevitable" that "neglect and disregard . . . would finally burst forth in a destructive way."[44]

But the citizens committee went further. It didn't just talk about neglect and exploitation in a broad-brush way. It pointed its finger precisely at those it held responsible in the last instance: the federal government, city officials, and institutions around Hough. All had called for urban renewal— state-subsidized efforts whereby scores of neighborhoods were condemned by public authorities as "blighted," razed, and then replaced with housing and institutions typically catering to the affluent.[45] Daisy Craggett, a columnist for Cleveland's Black newspaper the *Call and Post*, was one of the first African American residents to move into Hough. She worked for the in-progress University-Euclid urban renewal program, named after one of two of Cleveland's thoroughfares, and saw its disruptive effects from within and firsthand. "It was quite evident from the moment this program was implemented that there was no real commitment to the people in Hough nor the Negro community," Craggett charged. "We have seen Urban Renewal actually come in and destroy what was once a good community along with the other problems that have encroached upon the people in our area." She didn't hold back: "We in Hough have come to the conclusion that the way this program is going, that this is just one more step in moving the Negro out; acquiring the land for some other purpose."[46]

Each of these committees offered different analyses of what spurred rioting, but all agreed that the everyday hardships of Hough played some role. But in contrast to the McCone Commission in Watts, none mentioned health care deprivation. That was because medical maldistribution took on a different form in Cleveland. In Watts, maldistribution was marked by facilities' *absence*. But in Hough, the problem wasn't *absence* but *access* to existing institutions. The area was home to a cluster of elite medical institutions in the adjacent University

Circle. All had varying levels of tension with those who lived around them. But of them, University Hospitals, Western Reserve's voluntary affiliate, was the least insulated from its neighbors, admitting a large percentage of indigent patients, many from Hough. In addition to a more open door at University Hospitals, Western Reserve had long overseen City Hospital's training program.[47] Western Reserve's motives, of course, weren't completely benign. The university was motivated by civic obligation but also clinical instructional needs—namely, a supply of diverse patients for training.[48] But one could not accuse it of walling itself off.

The foil was the Cleveland Clinic. Like the Community Health Foundation, it was also a font of medical innovation but of the high-priced, technologically intensive variety. Founded in the 1920s, in less than half a century, the clinic had expanded from modest roots in a four-story building on a single block to a citadel of medicine spanning from East 90th Street to East 93rd Street. It wasn't just any medical complex but the elite of the elite, famous for pioneering technology used in heart surgery, and it primarily catered to an affluent clientele.[49] By the clinic's own estimates, just slightly less than two-thirds of its patients came from outside not just Cleveland but greater Cuyahoga County.[50] As one advocacy group later put it, the Cleveland Clinic had "made no attempt to provide any type of services to the residents of that community." Beyond insularity, the pamphleteers pointed to the geographic politics of the clinic, writing that "the irony of a specialty hospital in the midst of a ghetto is extraordinary. The clinic with its extensive medical resources could, if it chose to do so, provide health care services to its surrounding community." It was part of a "hospital-based slum clearance" that had "reached city-wide proportions," part of "a coordinated effort to create a 'white corridor' of renewed areas through the east side ghettos." Medical institutions on the East Side, they wrote, were "repositories for large amounts of investment capital," "centers of real estate empires."[51]

Whatever one thought of the metaphor, the underlying factual claims weren't hot air. Glitzy medical complex and impoverished ghetto stood within walking distance of one another. Hough was the byproduct of multiple trends in the 1950s: an exodus of white residents from the city, an influx of Black residents, and entrenched housing discrimination that "trapped," by historian Mark Souther's rendition, most Black Clevelanders in just "several square miles of the East Side," not unlike Watts in Los Angeles. It all occurred atop larger economic turbulence, as cities with once-robust industrial cores saw them (and their jobs) dissipate in the 1950s when major firms shifted operations to tax-friendlier areas elsewhere.[52]

If much of Cleveland—Hough and otherwise—was looking at a troubling economic future, exacerbated by racism, the Cleveland Clinic wasn't. In the

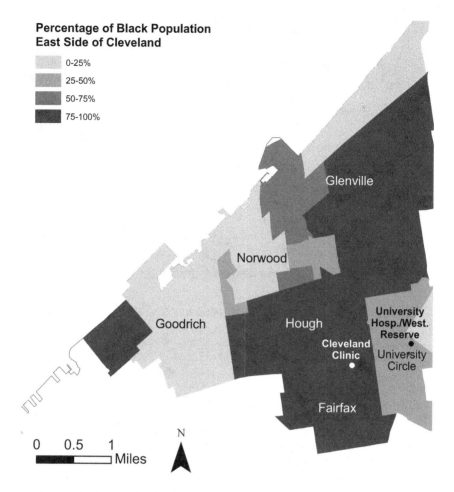

**Percentage of Black Population
East Side of Cleveland**

- 0-25%
- 25-50%
- 50-75%
- 75-100%

Glenville

Norwood

Goodrich

Hough

University
Hosp./West.
Reserve

Cleveland
Clinic

University
Circle

Fairfax

N

0    0.5    1
━━━━━━ Miles

**Segregation in East Cleveland and locations of Cleveland Clinic and Western
Reserve in University Circle/Hough area, 1970.**
*Source*: Author's cartography and calculations based on 1970 U.S. Census
data (National Historical Geographical Information Systems database, Minnesota
Population Center, University of Minnesota).

years immediately preceding the Hough riot, the Cleveland Clinic had become
a major player in the area's real estate transformation. It had actively lobbied and
conceived the University-Euclid urban renewal project that the Citizens Committee had attacked. Approved in 1961, University-Euclid's second phase would
enable the clinic to develop, with the aid of federal money, a "Health Sciences
Center." The clinic had developed elaborate plans to hold land plots for other
nonclinic entities, plus its own buildings. All of it would entail significant demolition. An earlier and smaller phase of the project had displaced 1,456 families,

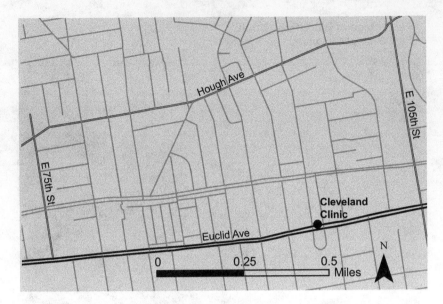

**University-Euclid Urban Renewal Project, Phase II.** The darkened streets are outlines of potential boundaries—extending as much as thirty blocks—for the proposed preriot University-Euclid Urban Renewal Project. Had it gone through, the
project might also have expanded a few blocks south of Euclid Avenue.

*Source:* Author's cartography based on Thomas Hatch to Richard DeChant,
memorandum on "Phase II of the University-Euclid Urban Renewal Program"
(binding), January 5, 1966, Box 3, Office Files, Clipping Files 1965–1966, Papers of
Thomas Hatch [semiprocessed], Cleveland Clinic Archives, Cleveland Clinic, Beachwood, Ohio; Thomas Hatch, daily journal entries, February 8, 10, 1965, Box 23,
Folder 3, Gottron Papers; Daniel R. Kerr, *Derelict Paradise: Homelessness and Urban
Development in Cleveland, Ohio* (Amherst: University of Massachusetts Press,
2011), 148–54.

70 percent of them "non-White" (and almost all Black).[53] The expanded phase
might displace many more, "1,600 structures containing 5,200 dwelling units"
and "21,000 people," by one estimate conducted at the time. Its boundaries
could stretch as far as East Seventy-Fifth Street westward and East 105th street
eastward, in addition to northward expansion by one or two blocks.[54]

Clinic administrators drew on familiar (and implicitly racial) imagery to
rationalize the project: an exodus of "professional and upper middle-class"
property owners, crumbling housing stock in their place, and rampant petty
crime. Just months before the riots, Thomas Hatch, its urban renewal coordina-
tor, declared that the clinic's expansion would "clear a blighted and deteriorating neighborhood" and "provide an improved environment where health care,
health education, and health and scientific research can be conducted effectively
for the benefit of the people whom we serve."[55] Hatch invoked a powerful trope

in twentieth-century urban planning whereby demolition was conceived as a health remedy—what historian Samuel Roberts has termed the "medicalization of blight"—via clearance of perceived health threats (often signified by "blight") and construction of medical facilities in their place.[56] It was, in short, to be medical Manifest Destiny.

The Cleveland Clinic was powerful politically, and few city officials dared challenge its plans. One exception was Leo Jackson, a Black Cleveland City Council member representing Glenville, which bordered Hough. In one meeting with clinic officials, Jackson stated that his constituents just wanted "decency and protection of present property," not urban renewal.[57] As the council's chairman, Jackson used control of parliamentary procedure to hold up approvals for the project, a standoff that continued into May 1965. It angered clinic administrators, who groused privately about council members who were otherwise sympathetic to its designs but "part of [Jackson's] Negro bloc" and therefore forced to oppose it.[58]

But then Hough happened, and it instantly put the clinic on the defensive. During the rioting, administrators communicated around the clock with city police officers and the National Guard, anticipating a possible attack on the "immediate vicinity" of clinic grounds. Two days later, a Cleveland Clinic employee expressed relief over momentary containment of the riot, stating that if not for the convergence of law enforcement in the area, "there would have been a real catastrophe" and "the Clinic itself would have unquestionably been involved."[59] Over the next year, clinic administrators delayed politicking over the University-Euclid project. The tone of many meetings was mixed, a fusion of administrators' frustration over stalled plans, befuddlement over what had taken them by surprise, obliviousness about neighbors' views toward the clinic and development, and resigned admission about the need to change course.

At the end of 1966, Hatch captured clinic officials' collective mood, writing of a "crisis situation in Hough—cannot overemphasize its gravity. Poor commentary on Cleveland community, which was once noted for good racial relations. These have deteriorated. Ferment is seething." He wondered whether the area was "on collision course with another Watts. All the ingredients are present—fuse is set—small incident, as in Watts, could set it off. Despair, cynicism, antagonism are abundantly present." But Hatch concluded that even the clinic's own self-interests meant that "massive efforts are needed" and that "timidity and half measures have not paid off." In the future, the clinic would have "to excite imagination of community" and "secure cooperation."[60]

Optimism didn't color subsequent clinic deliberations. Absolute fear did. Into 1967, leadership monitored rumors of future riots, speculating that "agents of unknown and subterranean leaders are at work, recruiting youths and young men and training them in guerrilla tactics, so that they will form effective striking forces." Its leaders questioned the reliability of intelligence from what it dubbed "responsible Negro leaders," who they suspected didn't know much about the designs of "militants." Fear was so pitched that the clinic crafted emergency plans in the event of another uprising. It would hire its own private "guard force" and an additional layer of "squad leaders" composed of "men with previous military service, especially combat experience," to complement any National Guard and police assistance. Clinic officials discussed creating strategic "withdrawal points" in case the facility became besieged, along with use of nonlethal weaponry: "fire hoses with 2.5 inch streams" that could thwart "the mob and drive it back," tear gas, and "riot guns, which are more likely to injure than to kill."

But in a worst case scenario, "ultimate weapons" would be needed, and they'd include "fire-arms, pistols, and rifles" aimed at anyone who entered a Cleveland Clinic building. One clinic official wondered whether it was all too over-the-top and really necessary, arguing that if the National Guard failed to contain rioters, then the game would pretty much be up anyway, and there would be little choice but "to turn the property over to the mob." "Armed resistance," by that point, could only "breed destructive retaliation that might involve loss of life and severe property damage." The official mused that, all told, an attack might not be so bad: "Suppose a mob stormed the place—what would it be likely to do once it got in? Probably try to find narcotics and food—but, it is hard for me to believe that even under the most imaginable circumstances, these people would harm patients or unresisting personnel. They would only hurt their own cause—and bring total, lasting retribution on their own [heads]."[61]

These remarks were a window into the split psyche of clinic leaders. They no doubt exhibited contempt and ignorance, reducing rioters to a drug-addled "mob." And many of their fears were a paranoid fever dream. Most rioters across the country were discerning with their targets, taking aim at egregious symbols of exploitation, particularly police departments and small-time shops that price gouged. They avoided many other structures, from schools to churches to corporate buildings.[62] But in characterizing rioters as people with a "cause," clinic officials admitted that substantive grievances did exist and were traceable to the clinic's own conduct. Its leaders were accepting what other analyses of Hough had as well. Behind the language of mobs and militants was an acknowledgment that their "attitude . . . is that conditions are intolerable, and they are anxious to precipitate changes in the social system which they feel holds them in bondage."[63]

## Clinic Concession: A New East Side Health Center

The riots had implanted perceptions of a grassroots threat that could rise at any moment. For the clinic, it meant realizing how much rage surrounded it and clipping its ambitions accordingly. Two of its partners in the expansion project, the Cleveland Health Museum and the Harshaw Chemical Company, expressed doubts about their commitment, with the latter pulling out altogether. Two years after the riots, the clinic pondered its loyalty to the city and outlined options: "gradually phasing out at this location and planning to relocate" or instead working to "improve the immediate neighborhood," and if so, "how far to go in 'relating' to surrounding areas."[64]

Beyond the clinic, the riots shook up city politics, too. They killed support for Mayor Ralph Locher, a member of the city's white ethnic Democratic machine. In his place emerged Carl Stokes, a Democratic Black state representative, who became the first Black mayor of a major American city, drawing national attention and the cover of *Time* magazine.[65] For the clinic, the victory was a well-timed blessing. During his campaign, Stokes had deftly positioned himself as an alternative to two political poles in Cleveland politics. He was neither a member of the white ethnic machine nor a Black politician in the mold of Leo Jackson, the clinic's primary opponent on the city council, who'd taken consistent—and very vocal—aim at the city's white leadership, urban renewal, and predations of the real estate industry. Stokes, by contrast, preached unity and was "somebody business knew they could work with." (His 1973 memoirs contained a chapter entitled "How to Get Elected by White People.")[66] By cooperating with Stokes, the clinic profited from the political symbolism inherent in supporting a ceiling-shattering Black mayor—especially in the aftermath of the riots—while never actually backing a political program that fundamentally challenged the basic thrust of the clinic's expansionist strategy. Stokes, in turn, could draw on clinic resources to advance his gentler version of urban renewal, which retained its fundamental assumptions but included some social welfare provisions that were previously absent. He called his program *Cleveland Now!*, and the clinic backed it enthusiastically. Three of its key planks reflected the postriot moment, pledging programs for job creation, youth, and health.[67] Yet radical structural reform it was not, and in fact, it allocated $61 million to existing urban renewal projects, even as Stokes sought to curb their worst abuses.[68]

Not long after *Cleveland Now!*'s launch, Stokes turned to medical maldistribution. In early 1968, he summoned clinic representatives to his office. Stokes discussed "great dissatisfaction among the poor people in the inner city over the quality and quantity of health care available to them," noting the burdensome West Side location of Metropolitan General Hospital (formerly City Hospital) and lack of public transportation to reach it. Pointing to tax credits that the clinic received, Stokes pressed the administrators to share their institution's resources with the city. The political stakes increased again in July 1968 when a shootout in Glenville, an East Side neighborhood about a mile north of Hough, resulted in another uprising and the calling of the National Guard.[69]

The Cleveland Clinic responded to Stokes's request immediately, offering to oversee an East Side health center for outpatient services. The plan called for the city to finance building and land costs and to handle inpatient hospital care at Metropolitan General. The clinic, meanwhile, would handle staffing by recruiting physicians in the area and providing clinic employee status, and it'd share its personnel. The plan was a win-win for Stokes and the clinic. Stokes could respond to public clamor for proactive political response to the conditions that had precipitated the 1966 events. The clinic could shed its reputation as a private and isolated medical fortress unconcerned with the health and welfare of its neighbors, protecting itself from possible future hostility, which it still considered a very real possibility. Clinic officials displayed keen political savvy throughout the process, with one commenting that the plan would allow the institution "to provide moral support for his [Stokes's] efforts and by so doing to benefit from the good public relations which might ensue. We think that the Mayor could profit by the support . . . whereas the Clinic can benefit by jumping on the bandwagon rather than being dragged in by the heels." He continued: "The public relations aspects could conceivably even take on national dimensions due to the Mayor's prominence and popularity on the national political scene."[70]

The clinic had other motives, too. Ohio was about to launch its Medicaid program, and the clinic had been worrying over, in its words, "a great influx of local Medicaid patients in our existing Clinic structure."[71] The new facility offered a way of rechanneling that "influx." The clinic's discussions of the facility's precise location reflected careful calculation, self-interest, and more than a little racial dog-whistling. Although the events of 1966 had taken place in Hough, on whose southern boundary the clinic was located, facility planners proposed instead to build in Fairfax, a neighborhood to the immediate south. Fairfax's racial demographics were not hugely different from those of Hough's. But subtle contrasts existed, and the clinic had carefully studied them. The clinic's internal assessment of the Fairfax area characterized it as a "stable community" with a high prevalence of home ownership. It noted that a city ordinance banning multiple-family occupancy into single-family buildings had enabled Fairfax to avoid "the fate of Hough and other sections where excessive over-crowding took place." It was one of many observations laden with value judgments. Fairfax, the report continued, had largely avoided midcentury Black migration because it "was already filled with a 'higher class' of resident" and, at least in the clinic's view, was a bright spot that possessed many "values" amid "the deteriorated appearance of the east-west through streets."[72] The neighborhood was what urban historian Todd Michney has elsewhere called a "surrogate suburb": a Black middle-class enclave, within a central city, that self-imposed strict "respectability" norms, comprising everything from stringent property upkeep to purposive displays of manners and "moral" behavior.[73]

For the Cleveland Clinic, the Fairfax site selection served multiple ends. Though the clinic could no longer wall itself off from the rest of Cleveland, via strategic location, it could still screen and filter who was most likely to come through the doors of its new extension. Then there were its future plans. The clinic's evaluation of Fairfax noted larger economic restructuring in Cleveland, principally the decline of the steel industry, and speculated that the city was transforming into a "center for education, medicine, culture and the several arts." It continued: "Qualifying for a place in these fields is the price the Fairfax resident must pay if he intends to find a place for himself in the Cleveland community." Hosting the clinic's satellite center was a way for Fairfax to remain part of the process.[74] The clinic, in turn, established a beachhead for later expansion. It could fulfill "a feeling of moral obligation" while aiding what it dubbed the "protection of our interests in the local community."[75]

## "Yet They Share No Responsibility": The Limits of Postriot Concession

All the planning for the East Side center bumped up against a problem familiar to those in Watts: delays, delays, and still more delays. The city kept pushing off allocation of the land and construction of the building, its end of the bargain. Although Stokes was reelected in 1969, his second administration became politically besieged by critics and an obstructionist city council, and, exhausted, he chose not to run again in 1971. These political developments had distracted from mayoral obligations, including the stability of the city's health department.[76]

The clinic, however, never dropped the project entirely, despite the city's fumbles. It might have were it not for a fortuitous event. In 1971, Cuyahoga County officials pushed for a major overhaul of the county system, part of a long-standing attempt to coordinate city and county operations. One component of the plan called for the construction of "primary care health centers" to relieve severe outpatient pressure on county facilities, especially Metropolitan General Hospital. Health centers were a way to decentralize some outpatient functions, and the East Side center could help fulfill that role.[77]

The clinic saw an opportunity, a chance to hand the chief reins of the East Side center to someone else. It negotiated a new role with Cuyahoga County and did so in a much less volatile climate than had existed just five years earlier in the heated aftermath of the riots. Whereas the clinic had been the chief catalyst in moving along the previous version of the project, by 1973, government and clinic had reversed roles. This time, Cuyahoga County, not the clinic, drew up the bulk of formal plans before asking for the clinic's commitment, which came mainly in the form of personnel, lending its imprimatur, and contributing

$100,000 annually for the first two years and assuming 50 percent of annual deficits (but capping the obligation at $200,000), a relatively modest financial obligation.[78] Although the Cleveland Clinic remained aware of the public relations benefits attached to involvement with the center, that benefit was less important now that more time had elapsed since the riot, and the clinic even wondered whether to make its role public.[79]

Other players joined in the East Side center's development, too, as the Cleveland Clinic receded from a central to a complementary role. Besides Cuyahoga County itself, another player drumming up support for the East Side center was the Fairfax Foundation, a philanthropic organization composed of Cleveland businesspeople, religious leaders, and civic boosters. In the hands of this consortium, the charged symbolism of the original project—a check and reversal to the Cleveland Clinic's decades of neglect, even exploitation of those around it—fused with something much more politically palatable: the rhetoric of economic development and uplift, with a health facility as a key spark. Health was part and parcel of a larger program that addressed, in the words of one Fairfax Foundation representative, "improved housing . . . a need for jobs, improved educational and recreational facilities, new shopping facilities, improved transportation, and access to ambulatory health care." "The whole community needs and deserves rejuvenation," the official concluded.[80]

In 1976, the Kenneth Clement Center, named after a prominent Black Cleveland physician, finally opened in this new political climate. The liberal *Cleveland Press* edition that published a day before the ribbon-cutting asked—and then answered—a question: "Who pays for care of poor? Not the Clinic." The headline captured the long-standing perception of Clevelanders toward the institution. At the same time, the accompanying story granted that the clinic had made strides in accruing a "record of community service," however modest, and named the Clement Center as an example, followed by praise from Cleveland civic figures who noted the shift in the clinic's orientation. Still, some East Side residents, including the Reverend Charles Rawlings, expressed skepticism. "Every time they broke ground they kept promising they were going to offer some kind of primary health care for the neighborhood—and they reneged," Rawlings remarked. "They illustrate how health care in this country derives from the power of the dollar."[81]

At the same time the Clement Center opened, the clinic rebooted expansion of its main campus in the late 1970s. It wisely did so, however, in the opposite direction, eastward toward East 105th Street, home to a flamboyant Black entrepreneur, Winston Willis, who presided over a neighborhood empire of eateries, retail outlets, bars, and adult theaters, all while antagonizing the clinic with obscene billboards that derided it as a racist institution. Unfazed, the clinic lobbied for the area to be condemned, invoking eminent domain successfully in the late 1970s and early 1980s.[82] It was less concerned with the collective political reaction that it might have met a mere decade before, when it'd feared Molotov cocktails being thrown into its windows and exploding in its halls.

A turning point was the city's 1978 fiscal crisis, which further reopened the frontiers of expansion. Like New York City, Cleveland found itself hamstrung by years of bond-financed borrowing and the inability to pay it back when it came time. Much of the debt ($88 million) had been racked up by Ralph Perk, the Republican successor to Carl Stokes, who'd used specially allocated bond money to cover general operating expenses and had overseen generous tax abatements for commercial developers. When Perk lost his seat for office in a three-way primary, he'd actually dodged a bullet. Instead, the tattered fiscal house he'd built—and the task of fixing it—was left in the hands of a brash thirty-one-year-old populist Democrat named Dennis Kucinich. After the so-called boy mayor failed to attain a federal bailout or approval of a tax increase to cover the debts, banks stepped in with an offer: if Kucinich sold Cleveland's public electric utility, they'd roll over the debt and provide more favorable loan conditions. When Kucinich refused, it led first to a $15 million default, then to a narrowly failed attempt at recalling him from office (supported heavily by the city's banking interests), and finally, to his ouster in the next mayoral election.[83]

As with New York City, Cleveland's fiscal crisis ushered in emergency restructuring of multiple municipal functions, all undertaken to refinance debt repayment. Private revival efforts surged, too. That same year, the Greater Cleveland Growth Association, Cleveland's version of the chamber of commerce, proposed expansion of University Circle on the East Side, with medical facilities as its center of gravity. "Today, medical research here continues to provide opportunities for local industrial and commercial growth, yet these too may be lost unless mechanisms are identified and established to attract or nurture production and distribution ventures," the association wrote, before advocating a three-year plan whose basic outlines the city followed to the end of the century.[84] Mayor Kucinich's successor, George Voinovich, a mainstay in the white ethnic Democratic machine, proposed that the clinic play an integral part in a development effort in East Cleveland between East Fifty-Fifth and East Seventy-First Streets. Calling the clinic "the single most important institution within this economic vitalization target area," the city announced "blight studies" and suggested additional roles for the clinic that included attracting private medical firms backed by venture capital. The clinic took part with aplomb. In 1982, it advocated for its own and other institutions' expansion projects along Euclid Street, including an "Institute on Man and Science" reminiscent of the "Health Sciences Center" it had plotted in the mid-1950s.[85]

But the clinic's rediscovery of expansion came with well-chosen benign alterations. In addition to the Kenneth Clement Center, it pushed for clinic employment of "targeted populations" and "planning an on-going strategy to inform and involve, as appropriate," what it called "the Minority Business Community." These gestures were a testament to the Hough riots and their residual impact. When it came to medical maldistribution, the Clement Center wasn't inconsequential, either. A little more than a majority, 54 percent, of its new patients in 1984 were medically indigent. And against the clinic's initial desires, it actually drew patients from all over Cuyahoga County, with 62 percent of county census tracts sending at least one new patient there that year.[86]

The Clement Center implemented several innovative practices, too, many of them borrowed from—or similar to—neighborhood-level medical care experiments elsewhere in the city and country, including the use of health teams; focus on health maintenance; training of staff to take into consideration patients' sociological contexts; and more generally, softening the hierarchical and impersonal nature of medical care delivery. One year, for example, the center listed as annual goals a new "emphasis . . . on patient respect, satisfaction, and responsiveness," which entailed administrator meetings with all staff "to identify the current interpersonal tone and to elicit ways that we can improve it for both the patients and employees." An infant mortality program, prompted by the problem's high prevalence in Cleveland, screened pregnant women for delivery risks and turned the center into a major source for "high risk" obstetrics care. It became especially important for obstetrics patients who often missed appointments at Metropolitan General Hospital due to its West Side location.[87] A hypertension program, similarly created because of high prevalence in Cleveland, tracked and followed patients with elevated blood pressure during regular screenings and expanded throughout the decade. And an initiative on geriatric health enrolled about 40 percent of the age sixty-plus population in Fairfax, offering moderately priced home care to an increasingly aging East Cleveland population. Much of the care wasn't even explicitly medical but a way for patients to experience "social and/or psychological" support and less isolation.[88]

In the grander scheme, the Cleveland Clinic's efforts were a minor remedy. It hadn't even been the ultimate driving force in the Kenneth Clement Center, as Cuyahoga County officials had eventually performed most of the work to bring it to fruition. The center came to rely heavily on federal, state, and local government funds, which dwarfed the clinic's drop in the bucket in the low six-digit range. With fear of neighborhood reprisals declining, pressure from below for the clinic to take on a monetarily deeper commitment, and of wider scale, had dwindled. The clinic responded accordingly and was scorned—this time not by protestors on the streets but by suits in the beltway. More than a decade after Hough, Henry Manning, president of the Cuyahoga County Hospital System, appeared before a 1980 federal congressional committee on "financially distressed hospitals," which hosted medical care administrators from around the country. Senator Howard Metzenbaum, a liberal Ohio Democrat, accused the clinic of "stand[ing] out like a sore thumb in Cleveland for not accepting a share of responsibility." After Manning quickly mentioned the Clement Center, Metzenbaum continued to chastise the clinic for not making more efforts to serve more medically indigent or low-income patients, arguing that there had not been enough "peer pressure" by other medical providers in the area. The overall concern over the problem of maldistribution had flagged, observed Metzenbaum. The clinic was "right square in the heart of the area where it should be, they are extremely well-off financially, and I have been told by the former director, they are unquestionably one of the most profitmaking operations of any hospital in the country. Yet they share no responsibility."[89]

Senator Metzenbaum's observation about the gulf between the Cleveland Clinic and its surroundings resembled the observations clinic officials had privately made among themselves immediately after the Hough riot, when they acknowledged, at least at that historical moment, that they could no longer remain a glitzy medical "sore thumb" amid rampant poverty, hardship, racial exclusion, and displacement in which they'd been complicit. The Clement Center and other outreach efforts were certainly bridges connecting the clinic to some of the broader neighborhood, shedding the reputation of the fortress. But an island was still an island.

## Oh, Medical Governance Battle, Where Art Thou?

The reform impulse in Cleveland medicine differed in one glaring respect from similar experiments in health services provision elsewhere: a decidedly smaller emphasis on participatory governance. Cleveland was a hotbed of labor, left, and civil rights activism in the twentieth century, so the absence was surprising, and it may have stemmed from timing. By the time the Kenneth Clement Center actually got off the ground in 1976, the demand for community control was hardly at the same level that it had been in the 1960s. Moreover, the Cleveland Clinic didn't have to answer to any legal requirements, like the "maximum feasible participation" clause, since the Office of Economic Opportunity (OEO) hadn't funded it. Although it created a "community advisory council," it was much smaller and less powerful than those at neighborhood health centers outside Cleveland, such as Gouverneur or the Watts center, and it mostly relegated members to advisory roles and a single board seat. A few months after the center opened, the council complained of poor communication with the clinic's board of governors and questioned the center's hiring practices, pointing specifically to the dearth of Black physicians on the staff.[90] There is little evidence, however, that these disagreements (or others) led to protracted struggles over governance.

Clashes over governance were mostly absent, too, at another facility, the Hough-Norwood Family Health Care Center, which unlike the Cleveland Clinic project, was planned with OEO dollars. Created by the city's own health department, Hough-Norwood began operation in 1967 out of an existing health center on the western edges of Hough at East Fifty-Fifth Street in an existing and dated city health center, with plans for later movement in the early 1970s to a permanently constructed home.[91] Though its medical services were similar to the Clement Center's, Hough-Norwood, like the Watts center, displayed a stronger orientation toward job training and career development for people who lived around it.[92] Much of the training was on-site, as paraprofessionals supported three-person health teams, composed of a pediatrician, an internist, and a dentist assigned to each patient.[93] These trainees participated in programs overseen by a "Neighborhood Health Committee," Hough-Norwood's community council, which besides serving as a channel between neighborhood and organization, supervised a team of community health workers. Hough-Norwood administrators took far greater pains than did the Clement Center to devise a way of creating a body composed "of genuine present and potential consumers of the Center," though it tended to pick, in its own words, "the most frequently named and most acceptable community organizations and leaders" rather than use the more elaborate community representation mechanism devised in Watts.

Such a skew toward the "most acceptable" people might've produced some initial concern, even conflict, in other locales. But in Cleveland, it didn't. Hough-Norwood organizers expressed surprise over how wider neighborhood interest in governance tended to spike, then decline just as rapidly, expressing concern over an "understandable but alarming fall-off of interest in the community."[94] Housing in temporary quarters in its early years may have given those potentially interested in larger governance roles a sense that there was less at stake. Then there was location. Hough-Norwood sat at the borderlands between heavily Black Hough and two neighborhoods to the west, Norwood and Goodrich, which consisted of white European ethnics and recent Appalachian migrants. This demographic fracturing impeded cultivation of more obvious communitarian sentiment that could then channel its collective energy into administrative affairs. Last, Hough-Norwood wasn't affiliated with an academic medical powerhouse that received federal funds, eliminating the possibility of fierce head butting between elite administrators and lay representatives.[95] Its leadership instead rested in its own board of trustees overseeing a nonprofit corporation.

Ultimately, however, the lower priority given to governance by the Neighborhood Health Committee may have been due to the different programmatic

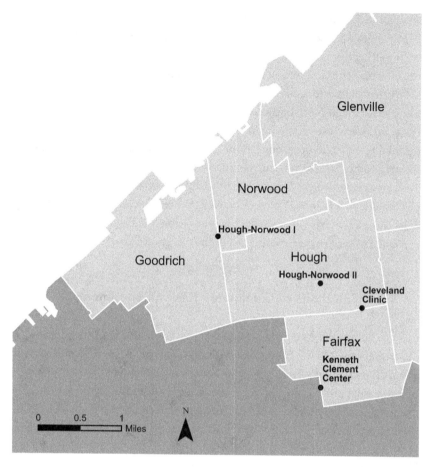

**Two Hough-Norwood facilities and the Kenneth Clement Center, 1976.**
*Source*: Author's cartography.

focus set for it from the start. Its members spent their energy primarily on neighborhood outreach, moving door to door around Hough-Norwood to spread word of its functions. Anna Bell Boiner and her team eased new patients into the center by preregistering them while describing Hough-Norwood's services further. Some of the residents were initially recalcitrant. Boiner detailed the demeanor required in such interactions: "We don't rush them. This way it won't make them think we came for just one thing. When we ask them a question, they give the answer, and if they want to talk about it, we listen to them. When you listen to them, you learn more information than what you came for."[96] The work required considerable interpersonal skill, as Boiner elaborated: "When we go into a person's home we tell them our names, and what our job is because some of the people resent us for asking how much is their family income. We tell them it's for research purposes. Some of the people think we're welfare, or we're getting this information for the welfare. We don't forget to tell them that the information is just for the Health Center's record."[97]

By many indicators, the efforts of employed organizers such as Boiner were a success. Hough-Norwood's new building, which was located thirty blocks eastward, was close to the heart of Hough. When it moved, administrators decided to maintain operations at the old facility as well and, in 1978, planned for yet another facility in Glenville, site of a shootout and riot a decade earlier. The three centers formed the kernel of what became an extensive regional prepaid health plan targeted at low-income patients that continued to draw most of its core patient base—around 75 percent—from the East Side area, even as it expanded to serve larger numbers from the county at large.[98]

## The Limits of Community Health Experiments

In 1963, before the riots, Mary Wheeler of Cleveland's sanitary engineering department took to the pages of the *American Journal of Public Health* to write about Hough. She discussed an exploitative housing market that the new wave of Black migrants to Hough faced, along with the health hazards they confronted on an everyday basis. "Overcrowding is a definite problem," she began. "One short block of apartment buildings is reported to house 1,000 youngsters! One apartment building with 12 four-room units has 84 children. Communicable diseases, especially tuberculosis and the venereal diseases, have a high incidence. Rats feast on overspilling garbage cans and raise their families in refuse piles and broken-down garages."[99] Unfortunately, these conditions fueled the solution that the city pursued into the early 1960s: building condemnation and clearance in the name of urban renewal.

In the same year, the Urban League of Cleveland released a report situating the city's health problems against larger social forces. But its take on where to go next differed from Wheeler's essay in one key respect. As it noted Black inmigration and overcrowding, along with its associated health effects, the report questioned the city's approach, writing that "inevitable urban renewal programs bring about a shift in the population from one gray area to another, creating large pockets of economically, socially and educationally deprived groups. These areas become breeding places of apathy, physical and mental illness, and hopelessness." These images contained no small measure of moralism anchored around images of concentrated disease and despair, an enduring mark of the Urban League's middle-class roots.[100] But at its core, the report contained a social critique pinpointing what ailed Cleveland's most vulnerable. After providing a battery of statistics on Black-white health differentials, the report declared that the problems that it documented were rooted in "poor living conditions and a lack of adequate food," plus "failure to use present public health facilities and services, inadequate as they may be." "The ghettoized segments," the writers concluded, must receive "the best services," overseen by those who understood "the relation between low socio-economic status and social problems."[101]

If health was inextricably social, as these two reports argued, the Community Health Foundation, Clement Center, and Hough-Norwood were attempts at providing "the best services" called for by the Urban League. But what did successful localist forms of delivery mean when evaluated from a wider perspective? This was a question anyone involved in the trenches of health services reform had to ask. In the mid-1960s, the Welfare Federation of Cleveland, one of the city's largest philanthropic organizations, launched an ambitious multiyear project to come up with health goals for the city. But the project soon struggled to settle on what "health" even meant, and the definition grew ever more elastic, including "enough of the right food," "liv[ing] in a clean and safe house in an attractive and safe environment," "good education," a life "free from prejudice and bigotry," and engagement in "productive employment and creative pursuits."[102] Publications explored these multiple areas in depth. An analysis of nutrition, for example, pointed to its economic bases, noting that 38–58 percent of Hough children were below the lowest quartile in typical height and weight development. Another section connected infectious disease's prevalence to "the quality of housing" and argued for new housing regulations that'd mandate proper waste disposal and protection from various animal vectors for disease.[103] It was a catalog of local risks—but it also indicted underlying systems that produced them.

The Hough-Norwood Center was familiar with the challenges of providing medical care against this backdrop. A few years after its operation, center staff observed that "an inseparable part of providing comprehensive health services" was to learn about the settings from which patients came. "We have found," they continued, "that our patients must face a discouragingly high level of hazards to health, including appalling poverty, bad housing, high crime rates, frequent fires, and excessive injury and death from accidents."[104] Those who worked in Cleveland's medical care experiments reported much success, but they discovered parallel competing demands in the lives of many of their patients, which sometimes interfered with their use of services, such as the follow-up appointments monitored by health teams. Innovative medical care at the local level, in short, existed in a matrix of health-influencing processes beyond it. It couldn't always transcend them.

## Weathering Fiscal Crisis: Restructuring
## in an Age of Scarcity

Like its coastal counterparts, Cleveland faced fiscal turbulence in the 1970s. Unlike New York City and Los Angeles, its health care facilities weathered the turbulence far more effectively.

It didn't seem that it'd be that way in 1978, when the city found itself on the precipice of default, just as New York City had in 1975. But even before Cleveland's crisis moment, there were signs of instability throughout the decade. The transfer of City Hospital to county control in 1958 had solved the facility's sustainability problems only temporarily. Continuing fiscal pressures took a toll, and they sounded familiar to those from other parts of the country. One 1962 report on both major county hospitals, Metropolitan General (located in Cleveland) and Highland View Hospital (located in suburban Warrensville Township) declared them "deteriorated and substandard." "Service areas were far too small," and "these and other conditions hampered the attempts of dedicated staffs to provide decent patient care, and to conduct vital teaching and research programs."[105]

County oversight of public hospitals was supposed to assure sounder budgetary foundations, and Metro General's problems would have been much worse had it remained in city hands. But county governance was no miracle, either. By the early 1960s, the city of Cleveland confronted population flight and a depleting tax base, and between 1960 and 1970, it would lose more than 100,000 residents, declining in population from 876,050 to 750,903. Although population growth in Cuyahoga County remained steady overall, the rate of growth seemed to be slowing as well. Between 1950 and 1960, the county's population had grown from nearly 1.4 million to 1.64 million, but from 1960 to 1970, it grew only from 1.64 million to 1.72 million.[106] County authorities stated the implications plainly, writing that "the financial needs of the hospital have been increasing at a much faster rate than the increase in taxable revenue." Another contributor to the problem, besides a shrinking tax base, was a general uptick in medical care costs themselves during the decade, not just in Cleveland but in New York, Los Angeles, and elsewhere around the country, propelled by a mix of factors hotly debated by health economists and observers who had yet to settle on any singular consensus explanation.

As in New York City and Los Angeles, Cuyahoga County improvised its response to an emerging sustainability crisis. In 1963, the county had implemented a temporary one-year salary freeze alongside the floating of a successful hospital bond levy, with a second one passing a few years later, raising $32.5 million in money for upgrading facilities.[107] Officials realized, though, that systemic solutions would be necessary alongside stopgap bandaging. In 1970, an ad hoc planning task force for the county system debated consolidating suburban Highland View and city Metropolitan General. Both offered the same types of services, though Highland View specialized in chronic care. Merging the two facilities, the task force's members argued, wouldn't just address sustainability. Apart from financial costs, it would make for a smarter operation and would allow better coordination of services, bringing Highland View's hallmark chronic care program into a single facility with the county's other institution.[108]

But the task force's proposal raised a thorny issue. It suggested a graceful transfer of disparate operations into a single plant, implying that one facility would be marked for either an overhaul of its functions or outright closure. The accompanying data made clear which one: suburban Highland View. Using data on patient admissions, lengths of stay, and occupancy rates, the report calculated projected bed needs for each facility, and Highland's remained constant or trended downward while Metropolitan General's increased. Highland View reported a projected bed surplus of sixty, versus Metropolitan General's shortage of twenty.[109]

The rationalizing impulse running through the proposal bore a resemblance to the logic that fueled affiliation policy in New York City. But when news of Highland View's future was announced, political reaction in Cleveland couldn't have been more muted by comparison. One reason was its location in the affluent Cleveland suburban belt. The typical resident there was far less likely to use the facility than was the case in Cleveland for Metro General, the only public hospital serving indigent patients in a city with entrenched poverty. Cleveland suburbanites, in short, had much less of a stake in Highland View.

However the public viewed it, the consolidation would cost money to carry out, and in 1971, the county floated yet another bond levy for it. Campaign materials stated explicitly that the funds would be used "to consolidate the county's health facilities into a unified system." It didn't mark Highland View for closure but instead planned for it to become an exclusively "long-term restorative care center."[110] The levy's supporters privately discussed barriers to passage. Overall, there was little knowledge among the "general public" about the county system, which was alarming in the face of "powerful real estate interests which have succeeded in part in raising war chests to defeat issues costing tax dollars." Hospitals got lost in the shuffle of other needs, some more immediately pressing for people in day-to-day life, such as schools.[111]

The most incendiary of the roadblocks recalled the fury that had greeted the Community Medical Foundation's proposal for a small hospital in suburban Independence. The bond levy's supporters discussed racialized stigmatization that had become associated with welfare provision. Public hospitals weren't an exception and were "tied up with 'welfare,'" and "underneath was the racial issue."[112] The concerns were overblown. Any racial animus conjured by the levy failed to defeat the measure, which passed with 53.1 percent of the vote, following a campaign that hit on communitarian themes. "Every one of these men, women and children—including YOU—at one time or other may require the services of the County Hospital system," read one ad.[113]

Consolidation may not have encountered public opposition, but there was internal debate within Highland View itself. Some feared that "staff amalgamation" would "result in a shifting of staff from one institution to the other and the inevitable dominance of one over the other." Many worried about finding their "proper place" in a new consolidated unit. Some speculated about the "disappearance of the Highland View program" in chronic disease and the loss of institutional identity. Many personnel at Highland View griped that they had long felt like an orphaned institution, ignored by Cleveland's academic medical complex, which focused its training programs on Metropolitan General. Austin Chinn, a consultant hired by the county to assess the consolidation proposal and interview staffs at both hospitals, wrote that at Highland View, "for whatever reason, communication has been almost non-existing and the staff . . . has grown increasingly defensive. It has struggled virtually alone to maintain a vital place in the community." For Chinn, consolidation as a cost-saving move was a sound idea only if Highland View's existing programs were preserved in the process and resulted in a "clear geographic and program identity of the chronic disease section of the hospital" that'd ensure Highland View's signature initiative wouldn't disappear.[114]

County officials went forward anyway, taking impressive steps to ensure as seamless a transition as possible. Metro General's use rate, they noticed, hovered around 75 percent, low enough to suggest redundant infrastructure. There were now more inpatient beds than needed, a decline officials attributed to the fall in infectious disease hospitalizations. Before the big transition, the county reduced inpatient beds from 1,444 to 1,087, converting the difference to equivalent outpatient capacity.[115] In 1978, the consolidation was complete. Highland View's old facility was closed permanently in 1978 and its patients were transferred to a new building in Cleveland, part of a rechristened "Metro General/Highland View" complex.[116] Crucially, the entire staff and its chronic disease program were preserved, thus avoiding the pains that often came with consolidations and closures elsewhere.

Consolidation brought Cleveland back full circle to developments of the early midcentury period, when City Hospital had transferred to county control in 1958. That looked, in hindsight, like an ever wiser move. In stabler county hands, Metro General was immune from the city's 1978 default and fiscal tightening imposed on Cleveland to fund payments to debt-holding banks.[117] Moreover, strong county oversight ensured, as in Los Angeles, that the city's problems were also the county's and that a mostly white and affluent suburban belt wasn't completely walled off from an urban core.

County governance became a layer of protection as Metropolitan General/ Highland View entered the 1980s, where rough fiscal waters awaited. "Federal retrenchment will be the hallmark of national policy," one county study on future concerns correctly foresaw, projecting more stringent reimbursements for Medicare and Medicaid and possible cuts for Medicaid in particular.[118] Medicaid cuts would be particularly devastating, given continuing spikes in health care costs. The Federation for Community Planning, a Greater Cleveland philanthropic organization, found that between 1980 and 1982, Medicaid expenses in Cuyahoga County had almost doubled from $114.5 million to $214 million, even as the number of recipients mostly held steady, increasing by only 1 percent.[119] This meant that funding cuts were likely. A parallel problem was an aversion to Medicaid by fee-for-service physicians, which threatened to swell the region's hospital facilities. That threat was made even worse by the growing numbers of uninsured, particularly following a spike in unemployment throughout the northeast Ohio area. By one federation estimate, 6.5–15 percent of Cuyahoga County residents fell into this category, simultaneously ineligible for Ohio Medicaid cutoffs and unable to obtain private insurance, thus requiring $73.8 million in county subsidies for public care by 1983.[120] Where would Cleveland's most marginal residents go, and how well would—and could—they be covered for the expenses they incurred?

And yet, the picture wasn't all gloom and doom. A set of idiosyncratic and local developments had unfolded over the past few decades, leading to a countywide medical care infrastructure that had evolved in response to a host of previous crises and wound up mitigating many of the worst feared effects. When the increase in outpatient demand came, for instance, enough county infrastructure existed to absorb it because of bed conversions during the consolidation plan, to say nothing of the Clement Center and Hough-Norwood, both mentioned by the federation as models for decentralized medical care networks. Other proposed solutions for cost containment, including regional prepaid group practices, were enacted and had their roots in prior local reform efforts as well—namely, the Community Health Foundation, since folded into Kaiser Permanente. On top of it all was limited county population growth, and actual decline in Cleveland proper, which curtailed the possibility of catastrophic patient overflows. A confluence of local transformations—a move to county governance, new facilities in the 1960s, a smartly executed consolidation, and population trends—thus shielded Cleveland and Cuyahoga County's health care infrastructure from a potentially turbulent future. Prior crises of sustainability and maldistribution had the effect of cushioning fallout from future ones that followed.[121]

It compared well to the other two metropolitan health systems we've seen. In the 1970s, New York City had too many facilities and too few resources to sustain them. The budgetary ax—spending freezes, service cuts, even closures—and the consolidation of affiliation followed. In Los Angeles, the story was similar, but with more pathos. Facilities birthed to reverse decades of racist neglect ended up hamstrung by new pressures placed on them and a new crisis of sustainability. Cleveland was hardly free from bumps—the city defaulted, after all—but local uniqueness buffered health care in the region from the worst ravages of the economic turmoil around it.

These three metros, for different reasons, had entered the national spotlight during the 1960s and 1970s. So did a place that, in other times, was much more insulated from the modal American's mind. But whatever surface differences existed from its urban counterparts, Central Appalachia, too, was home to local battles around environmental health and medical care, political contests whose trajectories were shaped by federal developments and initiatives below them.

# 5

# Central Appalachia

### Powering America on Other People's Bodies: Strip Mining, Environmental Health, and Human Suffering

The world of Wallins Creek in Harlan County, Kentucky, was changing rapidly in 1967, and people were panicking. Heavy machinery had taken up a regular presence: a phalanx of cranes, auger drills, tractors, and bulldozers were removing forest, vegetation, and the Earth's surface to uncover coal seams beneath. Blasting and shaking were now part of the sensory landscape. Immense ecological disruption had resulted, too, and many so-called strip mine operations spanned hundreds of acres. Panic was the right reaction for another reason. Of all the coal reserves in the United States, the most common—nearly 45 percent—was high-grade bituminous coal, whose volatility was second only to anthracite coal that was available in ever dwindling supply, accounting for less than 5 percent of total deposits by that point. And the mother lode of the bituminous variant was in Central Appalachia, in two states, West Virginia and Kentucky, which together in 1960 had more of it than any other region in the United States.[1]

The 400 residents of Wallins Creek didn't sit still, though. In 1967, they got together and signed a petition that eventually made its way to the U.S. Department of the Interior. The document spoke of "the dangerous condition brought about by unbridled strip mining . . . which has destroyed timber and has created a serious flooding problem by filling the beds of the stream with rock, dirt and other debree [*sic*]." "It is our wish," the petitioners continued, that authorities step in "to prohibit the further strip-mining or augering of coal" where they lived.[2] Not too long before and not too far away, Alice Slone, the director of a small school in Hazard, shared similar sentiments with President Lyndon Johnson. "We can never hope for security and prosperity with such hopeless destruction to our homes and property," she wrote. "More paupers are being made from stripminers than can ever be reclaimed through government funds."[3]

People all over Central Appalachia, like the people of Los Angeles County a decade earlier, quickly realized that the transformation around them might harm their health. They petitioned against, wrote about, and protested over hydrologic defilement by acid and minerals; mudslides and floods that required them to flee; improper disposal of refuse and waste; and general threats to their property and well-being. It wasn't for naught. But scientific recognition of their suffering came much more slowly because they lacked a coalition of politically powerful advocates like those who'd advanced the antismog cause in Los Angeles. By the early 1980s, the nation's energy infrastructure became even more entrenched in and bound up with the strip mining of coal. It reflected a collective choice to electrify the nation at the expense of Appalachian health and welfare.

## The Rise of Strip Mining

The people of Wallins Creek, and people like Alice Slone, wrote in the mid-1960s. They were trying to comprehend the emergence of a new energy infrastructure in the United States that'd leave an even larger imprint in the two decades to come. Removal of coal had long occurred through traditional deep underground methods, whereby miners extracted and transported coal from below the Earth's surface. Deep mining was the stuff of inedible imagery: hard hats, shafts, dusty faces, dangerous and dark conditions.

But by the 1960s, deep mining became less and less dominant, as surface—or strip—mining of coal escalated rapidly. A decade later, most coal came from the Central Appalachian region, consisting of eastern Kentucky, southern West Virginia, and a little bit of eastern Tennessee, and home to persistent double-digit poverty rates in the postwar period.[4] Nationally, after accounting for a little more than one-third of coal extracted in 1960, strip mining overtook underground mining by 1975 as the most frequent mode of extraction.

At the local level, the changes were striking. That same year, twenty-seven of thirty-two counties in eastern Kentucky reported that a majority of their total annual haul was strip-mined, up from only seven in 1955. Within some individual counties, the rise of strip mining was enormous. In Bell County, strip mining accounted for 72.7 percent of all coal mined in 1975, compared to 19.6 percent just two decades earlier. In Clay County, the trend was similar: an increase from 13 percent to 59.8 percent. In Jackson County, strip mining replaced underground extraction almost entirely, jumping from 7.9 percent to 99.6 percent usage within the same 1955–75 period. Even in counties where underground mining was most commonplace, usage of strip mining increased significantly. Letcher County, for example, had no strip mining presence in 1955, but mine

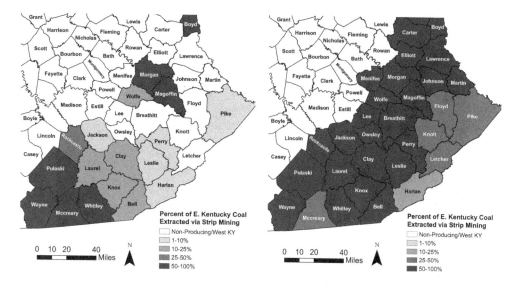

**Historical geography of eastern Kentucky strip mining, 1955–75.**
*Source*: Author's cartography based on James C. Currens and Gilbert E. Smith, "Coal Production in Kentucky, 1790–1975," *Kentucky Geological Survey Information Circular*, 10th ser., 23 (1977).

operators there attributed 29.9 percent of extracted coal to strip mining by 1975. Floyd County saw a similar trend, from no strip mining to 44.4 percent.[5]

Yet strip mining's predominance was as much a social as a technological outcome. Beginning in the 1960s, coal extraction would transform into a top-heavy business, dominated by a few dozen subsidiary firms that had acquired hundreds of independent local operators. Between 1965 and 1970, the percentage of total land leased for coal mining by "independent corporations" dropped from 55 percent to 44 percent, the first such decline in the postwar period, while that of "subsidiary corporations" rose from 30 percent to 37 percent. Appalachian pamphleteering of the period regularly deployed such phrases as the "forty thieves" to inveigh against not only concentration but absentee ownership and headquartering in regions outside Central Appalachia, casting such outsider firms as economically parasitic.[6] Consolidation had other consequences. It provided much more capital for investment in expensive, high-capacity methods of extraction. Throughout the decade, technical articles in such trade publications as *Coal Age* and *Mining Congress Journal* touted the virtues of novel techniques, boasting of "larger and more efficient mechanical equipment including drills, haulage or transportation equipment, and excavating machinery, as well as improvements in explosives." These "new machines, tools, and techniques," one author for a trade journal wrote, "make it possible to rip successfully many materials that previously defied tractor-ripper combinations." An ad boasted

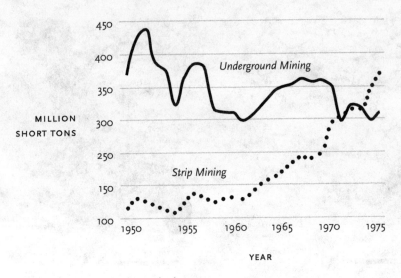

MILLION
SHORT TONS

*Underground Mining*

*Strip Mining*

YEAR

**National coal extraction by method, 1955–75.**
 *Source*: Author's calculations from U.S. Energy Information Administration,
*Annual Energy Review*.

not only of horsepower but of durability, writing of a dragline that worked for twenty-one hours per workday. These trade journals provided operators, too, with highly specific technical notes on terrain differences across localities and estimates of cost. In their pages, one could see strip mining's maturation.[7]

Technological transformations, in turn, influenced the social relations of extraction. During the Great Depression, the United Mine Workers of America (UMWA) had become one of the most politically influential unions in the United States, with a militant approach to bargaining that it wasn't afraid to wield. Union president John L. Lewis played a founding role in the Congress of Industrial Organizations (CIO), enjoyed the ear of Franklin Roosevelt, and conceived of organizing tactics replicated by other emerging unions. But by the end of World War II, organized labor's new power fell under rapid threat. The Taft-Hartley Act of 1947 imposed a gamut of restrictions on unions that made organizing campaigns and legal recognition much more difficult, to say nothing of a renewed hostility to good-faith bargaining from employers themselves.[8] Less than a couple of decades after the New Deal, labor was on the defense. It no longer had an ally in the White House. It faced new legal constraints. And it did so in a changed political era that historian Landon Storrs has called "the Second Red Scare," where fighting for protections in the workplace, expanded social services, and civil rights could soon have you appearing before a board probing for disloyalty and sympathy for the Soviet Union.[9]

Coal operators were no exception to the counterreaction faced by mid-century labor. Firms began to search for ways to undercut the United Mine

Workers' militancy. They found a solution by literally replacing union members with technology in the 1960s. Naturally, threat of automation alarmed the UMWA, which publicly discussed the issue and evaluated the threat strip mining posed to underground mining and to the workers who did it. But the union's resistance to strip mining was tempered by speculation that strip mining might produce new types of jobs for equipment operators. And from a strict *occupational health* standpoint, when compared to deep underground mining, surface mining could even be preferable. In 1962, the *United Mine Workers Journal* wrote that "increased mechanization, one of the most important changes affecting accident frequency, reduced both the number of hazards and the amount of human exposure to them."[10] Gone might be the days of roofs collapsing, freak injuries, permanent disfigurement, and respiratory disease. These considerations underpinned the UMWA's vacillation between occasional (if cautious) support of strip mining and opposition to it.[11] That ambiguity, along with internal organizational tumult in the 1970s over corruption in the union, prevented the United Mine Workers from serving as a reliable barrier to strip mining's fast adoption.[12] By the 1970s, strip mining was entrenched.

A final development came from land use law and coal companies' revival of the so-called broad form deed. Signed by residents' ancestors in the late nineteenth and early twentieth centuries, these deeds drew a legal distinction between coal itself and the surface around it. It granted the right of coal seams—closer to the Earth's surface—not to landowners but to prospectors. Put another way, if you were a property owner, everything within the perimeter was yours except for the coal you might be sitting on. Given the prevalence of underground mining—and the different locations of those sites—these deeds weren't a point of controversy for most of the century.[13] But now, with the advent of strip mining, they allowed coal companies to prospect widely and lay legal claim to previously untapped land. Massive ecological change soon followed.

## Everyday Experience and the Making of an Environmental Health Threat

As strip mining accelerated, laypersons struggled to make sense of their changing environment.[14] During the initial onset of strip mining, from the early to mid-1960s, they focused on incursion into private space, threats to self-sufficiency and autonomy, landscape desecration, aesthetics, and violation of multigenerational ties to land. Consider the following episode. In 1961, a local television program interviewed residents of Beefhyde Hollow, located in southeastern Kentucky in Letcher County, site of a strip mine under construction. An eighty-year-old man named Elijah Wright remarked: "It just ruined the whole thing, the whole thing. Just look all about. You couldn't get back up in the fields, you couldn't tend to nothing." A teenager named Buster Stewart discussed the relocation that the mine had caused: "Well, all the people has moved out of here. Since they started stripping, they all moved out. They had to all move out. They had to go." Buster ended by relating to the interviewer some more direct and personal property damage to his home. "They shot one rock through the house," he said. "A rock went through your house?" asked the reporter for clarification. "Yes sir," Buster confirmed.[15] One G. W. Burke, who ran Beefhyde Hollow's general store, described the waste the strip-mining operation was leaving: "Well, they put the rock and dirt down over the hill, you know, and threw the timber and big stones off to the bottom . . . and took down the timber . . . then it slips down all the time and just practically runs it all over the land. You can't get above the stripping on account of the height [created by the refuse]."[16]

The aesthetic damage wrought by strip mining wasn't the only issue. So was property destruction. Two years later, in 1963, in Whitesburg, Kentucky, the *Mountain Eagle* chronicled the travails of the Jones family, who lived on a mountain below a U.S. Steel strip mine. In the past three months, they'd experienced three mudslides. The third one, Mrs. Jones said, "sounded just like a jet airplane." The family decided to move after noticing "a section of debris from the strip mine covering more than two acres that threatens to burst loose any moment." "Fred and I have worked hard all our lives, and we've put everything we had into this place," Mrs. Jones said. "I don't know what we're going to do." A neighbor remarked that the Jones family was "just the first to go." "One by one," he continued, "we'll all have to move out."[17] The sense of a deep violation of place in the utterances of the Jones family—and those of Elijah Wright, Buster Stewart, and G. W. Burke—stemmed from what historian Chad Montrie has identified in the region as a deeply ingrained "concern for small-scale, private poverty and insistence on its importance as a foundation for independence and self-reliance."[18]

The mid- to late 1960s saw this continued focus on affronts to property and the sanctity and beauty of the landscape. But as with environmentalism in the twentieth century more broadly, residents' worldview expanded beyond this fundamentally conservationist impulse. Now, as strip mining encroached on their worlds, residents thought more along the lines of their counterparts in Los Angeles during the worst years of smog. More and more, they interpreted topographic change as a threat not just to aesthetics but to bodily welfare and to health.

Take Madge and Paul Ashley, two residents of Knott County, Kentucky, who wrote to the First Lady, Lady Bird Johnson: "As I'm writing you this a bulldozer and shovel are in the process of stripping the hill close to our home. As a lover

*Bertha Field*

# The MOUNTAIN EAGLE

IT SCREAMS!  Whitesburg, Kentucky, Thursday, March 1, 1962  Vol. 54, No. 42  10 cents

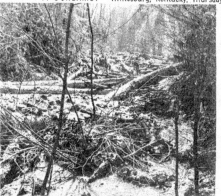

This river of mud, carrying huge trees and boulders, pushed down the side of Black Mountain at Blair, forcing the Fred Jones family and their son to leave their homes, which were in its path. The mud came from an extensive strip mining operation higher up the mountain. (Eagle photo)

## South-East seeks new UMW pact

A spokesman for South-East Coal Co. said today the firm hopes to negotiate a new contract with its employees which would retain present hourly wage scales but contain changes to permit the firm to operate profitably.

It is not true, the spokesman said, that the company wants to break away from the United Mine Workers of America union.

The company, he said, would like a new contract with the union—"one everybody can live with."

South-East, the spokesman said, is willing to continue paying its employees their present wage rate but can no longer afford to pay the 40-cents-a-ton royalty on coal used to finance the UMWA welfare program.

The spokesman said he did not know whether the UMWA would be willing to negotiate this type of contract with South-East. He said he recognized South-East is asking the UMWA to break its national pattern of contracts.

South-East is in a difficult coal marketing situation. It finds itself about the only remaining union mining operation in the Kentucky River valley. The company must sell its coal on the open market in competition with coal produced by non-union operations which do not pay the 40 cents royalty and in many instances pay wages equaling half or less than half the wage level maintained by South-East.

"Our non-union competitors are able to mine and sell coal for a price that in many instances is $1.00 a ton or more lower than our cost of production. During the past few years we have lost numerous contracts which would have kept our mines running a full five-day schedule because of this price differential.

"Our problem is simple but nonetheless serious. We must be able to cut our price on coal if we are going to meet competition and stay in business.

"Our company has made every possible effort in recent years to economize and maintain the lowest possible per ton cost on production. I might say that we have done well in this respect, but despite every economy we can achieve, we continue in a very difficult competitive situation when it comes to selling coal.

[...] for a new contract containing more realistic provision.

"We took this step with the greatest reluctance. We are not non-union in outlook, but to the contrary we feel that we have benefitted about as much as our men from the UMWA contract. We have known what to expect from the men, and the men have known what to expect from us.

"We feel that if we can negotiate a new contract containing the necessary changes, we will be able to market our coal and operate our mines on a full five-day week schedule, assuring full pay envelopes for our workers and a reasonable, although not large, profit for ourselves."

South-East wrote each man on its payroll January 15, telling each that circumstances had compelled the firm to notify the UMWA that it was terminating its labor contract 60 days after January 4.

(Continued on Page 8)

## Family flees strip mine slide

By TOM GISH

Mr. and Mrs. Fred B. Jones and their son, Haskell, were forced Friday to move out of their homes at Blair in the Cumberland River valley by a giant slide of trees, rock and mud from a U. S. Steel Co. strip mine high on Black Mountain.

"Fred and I have worked hard all our lives, and we've put everything we had into this place," Mrs. Jones said. "I don't know what we're going to do."

Furniture from the two Joneses' homes was loaded into trucks, with destination uncertain. Mrs. Jones said a coal company official had told her the firm would find a place for them to store their belongings in Lynch and said the firm would try to find a house for them.

Hundreds of tons of mud and giant trees up to two feet thick roared down on the Jones residence during an avalanche that started at noon Thursday and continued several hours.

"It sounded just like a jet airplane," Mrs. Jones said.

Mrs. Jones said this is the third and worst in a series of slides from the strip mine that has threatened her home since Dec. 22. Bad as it has been, the Joneses fear the slides so far are nothing but a warning of things to come.

The Joneses and their neighbors agreed there is a section of debris from the strip mine covering more than two acres that threatens to burst loose at any moment and come roaring down upon their homes.

Residents of the area said that if the threatened big slide comes enough trees, dirt and stones will roar down the mountain to cover the Joneses' home, cover U. S. Highway 119, and dam up the Cumberland River.

"We're going to have a dam across the river whether we want one or not," one observer said.

Residents also fear that if the threatened big slide does occur, it might have enough force to open up sections of the underground mines which honeycomb

Black Mountain, loosening millions of gallons of water which has accumulated in the mountain.

The homes of the Jones family are located at the mouth of Wolfpen Creek at Blair, near Cumberland and just across the Harlan County line from Letcher County. The usually wide Cumberland River valley narrows considerably here, so that the valley contains room for the Joneses' home, the river and the highway — and not much else.

The creek extends about one and one half miles from the rear of the Joneses' place up to Black Mountain, which towers in the background.

The swiftly descending creek is clogged with small, dam-like accumulations of logs and mud, each some 15 to 20 feet wide and from five to 25 feet in height and each holding back temporarily another slide. Looming several hundred feet above it all is the gigantic accumulation of overburden from the strip mine which threatens to break loose.

Mrs. Jones said she had not had a good night's sleep since the first slide in December. She never knew when she went to bed, she said, whether she and her home would be swept away during the night.

She said a representative from U. S. Steel had been inspecting her property and the threatening slide twice daily since December. Each morning he would tell her whether it was safe for her to remain at home during the day, and each evening he would tell her whether she could spend the night at home.

Friends and neighbors by the dozen stopped by the Jones home during the day to inspect the damage. There was general agreement that similar slides threaten at numerous points along the river.

"Fred and his wife are just the first to go. One by one we'll all have to move out," said one neighbor.

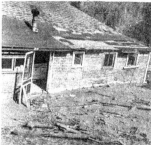

Mud oozes into the back door of the Fred Jones residence at Blair. Workers moving the family's belongings had to wade in ankle-deep mire which surrounds the house. (Eagle photo)

## Estill Blair heads seal sale

Estill Blair of Whitesburg, will serve as chairman of the 1962 Easter Seal appeal for crippled children in Letcher County.

Contributions received during the annual campaign, which opens on March 22 and continues through April 22, will be used for care and treatment given physically handicapped children by the Kentucky Society for Crippled Children.

## DEATH DELAYS PAPER

Publication of this week's Mountain Eagle was delayed because of the death in Lexington of E. A. Burnett, father of Mrs. Thomas E. Gish.

Mr. Burnett, 68, died Monday night at Good Samaritan Hospital in Lexington. He had been ill since October and critically ill for the past two weeks. Funeral services and burial were at Lexington.

## Jasper Pigman dies

Funeral services were conducted Tuesday at Thornton Regular Baptist Church for Jasper Pigman, 71, of Whitesburg. The Rev. Ray Collins, the Rev. Robert S. Owens Jr. and the Rev. Charles Carter officiated. Burial was in Thornton Cemetery.

Mr. Pigman died at his home, 8:20 p.m. Feb. 24. He had been ill for a long time. He was born at Pine Top in Knott County and was a son of Hiram and Sallie Franklin Pigman. He was a retired coal miner. He was a member of the Regular Baptist Church. Survivors are his wife, Mrs. Myrtle Martin Pigman; six sons, Delmas, Audra and Paul Pigman, all of Whitesburg; Ray Pigman, Melton, and Walker and Bill Pigman, both of Neon; four daughters, Mrs. Newton Comert, California; Mrs. Bethel Frazier,

Whitesburg; and Mrs. Emma Jean Kenny and Mrs. Arbadella Franklin, both of Cincinnati and a sister, Mrs. Sinda Swisher, Whitesburg.

Craft Funeral Home handled funeral arrangements.

## Library supporters will meet Monday

Persons interested in the growth of the Letcher County Public Library will meet at 7:30 p.m. Monday at the library to discuss ways of improving the book collection and library service.

Mrs. Harry M. Caudill, chairman of the library board, said Whitesburg residents especially are invited to attend.

The meeting is open to the public.

---

Local coverage of strip mine mudslides.
*Source: Mountain Eagle* (Whitesburg, Ky.), March 1, 1962.

of beauty I appeal to you to help us to keep the scenic beauty of our mountains intact."[19] This seemed similar enough to testimonials from the early 1960s that focused on disruption to land ties and landscape. But the second half of the Ashleys' letter took a thematic turn, moving away from the exclusive landscape emphasis. They wrote that "after the mountains are stripped[,] the streams and wells polluted, the garden plots covered with slides, even homes destroyed with slides and water, we will have to leave to find new homes."[20] Forced relocation became not just a violation of a tie to land; it was, rather, situated within ecological transformations manifesting themselves in multiple ways, including pollution and mudslides. A month later, Paul Ashley wrote another letter, this time to the president himself, that took on a similar cast. It opened by noting that Ashley had fought in World War II and that coal companies' impinging on his and his neighbors' property "denied the very rights for which we so bitterly fought." But he then turned to water pollution, writing: "They have turned sulfuric acid water into our streams killing all the fish, but they stated in the newspaper they didn't have to pay for any damages done unless they wanted to."[21]

Overt references to *physical* harm became more common. Ida Vass, a resident of Fayette County, West Virginia, wrote to her senator, Robert Byrd, "for help to curtail the destruction of our mountains and trees by strip mining in this area." She continued: "My house has been damaged, my garden destroyed and bridges washed out not to mention fear for *my safety* every time it rains. It isn't heavy rains either. The trees have been cut and graders cut away the mountains so much that very little downfall causes the creekbed to overflow because they're filled immediately with loose dirt, rocks and coal."[22] Urgency pervaded many of these communications. Albert Lopeg's widow, a former resident of Red Jacket, West Virginia, felt shaken by the memory of a "giant boulder that crashed through . . . and landed close to a window," where a neighbor was sleeping. She wrote two letters to President Johnson about the matter within the span of two weeks and added that "we had no floods before the strip mines got under way."[23] William Harold Headen of Goody, Kentucky, enclosed "pictures of the burning mine refuse piles which are affecting the lives and property of the citizens of the Goody, Kentucky, and Williamson, West Virginia Area." He continued: "Seven houses are in immediate danger with approximately 30 additional houses close by which are also subjected to fumes from the same fires. The entire community is constantly bothered by the harmful fumes from these refuse dumps."[24] The health threat wasn't subtle: "We have had one family of four persons hospitalized after being overcome by these fumes. We have had three boys hospitalized as a result of burns suffered while trying to push over a burning [barrage] that had ignited by fire from this burning dump. Our insurance policies are being cancelled because of the danger involved, and this is a constant menace to every person who inhales these fumes."[25] Headen's account ended with a plea to the president: "Our people realize you are burdened with the tension of International Problems, however, we realize you are presently making a fight to stamp out this type of pollution. We feel our community problem with our pollution is a good example of what you are attempting to erase. Therefore, we are coming directly to you for help."[26] It was a cry to focus away from global geopolitics and to the local nightmares Headen's family was living through. That it occurred in the area that President Johnson had toured shortly before launching the War on Poverty made it all the more poignant.

Pollution became even more frequent a topic toward the late 1960s, especially when linked to hydrology. The words of Kenneth Galyen of Muhlenberg County, Kentucky, to his senator, John Sherman Cooper, sounded much like writers from earlier in the decade, but the frequency of letters like his increased: "The pollution to our rivers, streams, and land is unbelievable. Erosion of stripped property continues to fill our rivers and streams while flooding and drainage covers fertile soil with the acid contents from the stripped areas."[27] Paul Staton, from Rumsey, Kentucky, urged Cooper to visit the area and "take a close look at all the copper and acid water, which there is *no escape* for." "It is practically pure acid and copper [as] water," he concluded.[28] Roy Fields's wife implored: "Why don't you do something to stop this disaster to our land? We talk about pollution, what is Strip Mining but pollution. It ruins the streams, it destroys the timber. The land can never be replaced, we need the land, and the land needs us to care for it."[29]

Health metaphors entered many descriptions, too. As had many others, Gerna Campbell and his wife used the life-death cycle to characterize the state of nearby rivers and streams, in this case the Cumberland, Kentucky, and Big Sandy Rivers: "They are already *sick* and smell like cesspools with aquatic life virtually gone. Silt is building up their bottoms which will cause flooding. We observed the Cumberland River this morning not only *swollen* from recent rains, but thick with silt and coal dust. If acid content were measured, we feel confident that the water wouldn't meet any established standards."[30]

The experiences of Mr. and Mrs. Harvey Kincaid are worth examining at length, for they were seeped with all the themes, images, and motifs discussed previously, with health—both metaphorical and actual—occupying a prominent place. They wrote while watching the arrival of "the strippers [who] came four years ago with their big machinery and T.N.T."[31] Daily life was marked by displacement and fear of a terrifying and changed world enveloping them. They began by describing the sheer force of the strip-mining process: "If their engineers make a mistake in locating the coal they just keep cutting away until they locate the seam of coal. When the rains come and there isn't anything to stop the drainage, the mountains slide and the highwalls fall down to the next highwall and so on until the whole mountain slides. There is a small creek in the hollow and when the spring rains come, its banks won't hold the water.[32] They described the immediate consequences:

> So where does it go—into people's yards, into their wells, under and into their houses. You have rocks, coal and a little bit of everything in your yards. When the strippers came they started behind our house in the fall sometime before November. There was a hollow behind our house and we asked them not to bank the highwall the way they did because we knew what would happen when the spring rains came. . . . But the rains came in the spring and the highwall broke and the water and debris came onto our property everytime it rained—into our well house, under the house everytime it rained.[33]

After short-term impact came residual health effects: "Then the damage comes to your house because of so much dampness. The doors won't close, the foundation sinks and cracks the walls in the house, your tile comes up off your floors, your walls mold, even your clothes in the closets. Then your children stay sick with bronchial trouble, then our daughter takes pneumonia (X-rays are taken, primary T.B. shows up on the X-ray). This is in July of two years about for a year this child laid sick at home."[34] Their living quarters grew uninhabitable: "So what do we have to do? Doctor's orders, move out for child's sake and health. We sell for a little of nothing—not for cash, but for rent payments." They wrote about moving somewhere else only to find that strip mining was hard to escape: "The same strip company comes up the road and puts a blast off and damages the new house—$1,400 worth. When they put one blast off that will crack the walls in your house, the foundation cracked the carport floor straight across in two places, pull a cement stoop away from the house and pull the grout of the ceramic tile in the bathroom."[35]

People like the Kincaids started mixing firsthand experience while pondering larger economic context, all as they thought about the plight of those who lacked the resources to move as easily. The Kincaids' sorrows mixed desolation and resignation: "To think of the poor people who have worked hard all their lives and can't start over like we did. They have to stay in these hollows and be scared to death everytime it rains. I know by experience the many nights I have stayed up and listened to the water pouring off the mountains and the rocks tumbling off the hills."[36]

A native of Floyd County, Kentucky, named Floyd Davis echoed these sentiments in a rhetorically scorching letter that spoke of "the themes of ecology, conservation, and pollution," before turning to underlying politics: "Greater than either the economic shock or the destruction of the land is the effect strip-mining has upon Eastern Kentucky's people. We must sit helplessly by while we see out-of-state companies destroy in a few days or weeks what it took our

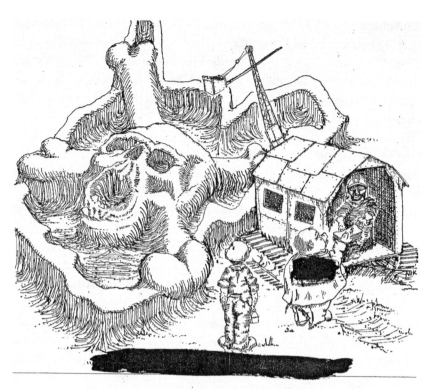

## Can strip mining be legally abolished?

Image from "Citizens to Abolish Strip Mining," pamphlet, February 1971.
*Source*: Box 22, Folder 1, Caudill Papers, Papers of Harry Caudill, Special Collections Division, Margaret I. King Library, University of Kentucky.

fathers and grandfathers generations to build." He concluded: "Eastern Kentucky's wealth has flowed into railroad cars, and has been hauled away, leaving us with only the slate piles, sludge dumps, and half forgotten dreams of a once beautiful land and a long ago proud people." Davis's words captured—without using the terminology explicitly—a growing political critique in impoverished sections of urban and rural America that made direct analogies between their residents' plight and those of colonial subjects.[37] The Appalachian variant borrowed from civil rights insurgents and characterized the region's relationship to the larger United States as economically predatory and "internal colonialism."[38] Like the health activists in New York City who dubbed private medical centers' exploitation of public hospitals a local form of "empire," those uprooted by coal mining believed that plunder didn't just end outside the borders of the fifty states.[39]

This outrage soon boiled into collective mobilizations that joined scattered individual pleas and cries. Health risk was a core concern of these incipient formations.[40] An ad hoc group of residents from Knotts County, Kentucky, drafted a petition to their representative, Democrat Carl D. Perkins (of "Perkins Loan" fame), in the late 1960s. They asked for help in stopping "damage being done to our homes, land, timber" and "in polluting our streams."[41] The Harlan County Emergency and Rescue Squad wrote a founding resolution centered on health hazards. It spoke of "irreparable damage," "surface miners . . . pushing literally millions of tons of loose soil over the edges of strip and auger mine benches causing the soil to wash down the steep slopes during periods of heavy rainfall," and "silt and sulfuric acid from surface mining practices" that "have been washed into the natural streams to cause the streams to be so polluted that aquatic life cannot be supported because of the destruction of the natural cover and the acid content of the water is too high."[42] The Pond Creek Citizens' petition declared that "the burning gob pile and slush ponds" created by a nearby strip mine were "a threat to our health, safety, and property."[43] And a larger group, Save Our Kentucky, issued a petition that referenced large swaths of the state's having "been laid to waste by mammoth earth moving machines" alongside condemnation of "the damage caused to Kentucky's streams by acid mine drainage, sedimentation and siltation," which resulted in "mud slides and floods."[44] Direct actions, influenced by broader political tactics occurring in the country at large, became more commonplace, as in Floyd County, where in 1972, members of the Eastern Kentucky Welfare Rights Organization delayed the opening of a strip mine operation by periodically walking past armed guards and onto the site.[45]

These were laypersons' cries for help, expressed in individual and collective forms. They explicitly framed strip mining as an environmental health concern; in this, Appalachians displayed a prescience far greater than that of scientists and elected officials.

### Science as Cuetaker

Scientific investigation in the region would eventually parallel the trajectory of lay response. But it occurred at a slower pace—more of a dribble—compared to Los Angeles, when a wide swath of agencies, municipal governments, businesses, professional associations, and even industry rallied around cracking the scientific puzzle of smog. In the first studies of strip mining, published in the mid- to late 1960s, health ramifications weren't even explicitly mentioned, though the material conditions they documented came with obvious health risks in retrospect. One such study, conducted in eastern Kentucky from the late 1950s into the mid-1960s, documented the reverberative effects of striking land alterations. Researchers with the Department of the Interior studied how spoil banks—accumulated waste from strip mining—eroded excessively and their byproducts worked their way into the Cane Branch Basin and its tributaries, altering their ability to facilitate runoff during heavy storms. That caused rapid "downcutting," which deepened the floor beneath streams by more than twenty feet. It all led to a thousandfold increase in sedimentation within a three-year period, and it resulted in changes in the "mean concentrations of chemical constituents" from acid drainage traceable to mines, especially sulfuric acids. "Strip mining of coal," the report concluded, "has significantly increased the acidity and mineralization of surface and ground water and increased the sediment content of streams in the mined area. These effects, in turn, have reduced or eliminated aquatic life in the streams."[46]

A 1968 U.S. Fish and Wildlife Service report found much the same. It drew together state-by-state assessments of mine acid drainage into streams. For both West Virginia and Kentucky, it estimated 25 percent—or 287 miles and 145 miles, respectively, in each state—of stream affected by acid could be attributed to new strip mining, listing a number of fauna and species severely endangered by the process. The study assessed, using value-neutral language, the status of revegetation efforts to date, concluding that almost all efforts as currently practiced had been "piecemeal." More generally, it pointed out that "few Appalachian States have geological formations which alleviate the deleterious effects of surface mining" and that future reclamation would require more technically "intensive treatment." The study's authors cautioned against "the loss that will occur by exploitation of one resource without regard for others."[47]

Other analyses discussed human health effects more directly—but hardly highlighted them. A 1967 U.S. Bureau of Mines report, which synthesized a number of smaller studies, exemplifies this. It contained a section on "environmental effects" that discussed acid drainage and water pollution at greater length. "Acid drainage is but one of several adverse chemical effects caused by surface mining," its authors wrote. "Even in minute concentrations, salts of metals such as zinc, lead, arsenic, copper, and aluminum are toxic to fish, wildlife, plants, and aquatic insects." It found that in streams receiving runoff from strip mines, 31 percent exhibited "noticeable quantities" of these precipitates. Its authors used the word "pollution" numerous times, which the earlier studies had not, in one instance stating that "water discoloration was recorded at 37 percent of the streams adjacent to the sites observed, suggesting chemical or physical pollution." The report discussed flood risks, too, possibly linked to "erosion and sedimentation problems." And in one of the few appearances of the actual word "health," it discussed the hazards posed by improperly disposed waste from strip mines, which many of the residents in the region had complained about during the decade.[48]

These were only three studies, and in each one, health was not a central topic of concern. But by the 1970s, the human health toll became a central part of scientific studies on surface mining. One catalyst? An escalating numbers of floods in the previous decade. Several government agencies initiated inquiries into topographic alteration by strip mining and its potential association with flood risk. Among the earliest was a March 1963 flood in Harlan County, which from 1955 to 1965 recorded an astounding 625 percent rise in strip mining, one of the largest increases in Appalachia.[49] The *Louisville Courier-Journal* characterized the flood itself simply as the "worst . . . in history." More than 25,000 people were displaced, and the *Harlan Daily Enterprise* estimated that the flooding affected half of all homes, placing residents at risk for typhoid in addition to forcing their involuntary relocation.[50] Recalling the scene from a helicopter, Sy Ramsey, a reporter for the *Associated Press*, wrote: "Muddy, swift water covered everything we could see as the copter circled the town of 42,000 looking for a dry spot on which to land and swinging away from deadly power lines." He described the "sight of two weeping women looking at flooded houses on lower ground. The husband of one held a small child and smiled at us in embarrassment."[51] The situation in nearby Pike County was similar. There, according to one account from the *Mountain Eagle*, "some houses were almost buried under mud."[52] The floods didn't stop. In December 1972, severe mudslides occurred during three weeks of heavy winter rain in Cumberland, Kentucky. Socrates Collins, a man forced to evacuate to temporary housing, remarked: "I don't have no place after that."[53] A catastrophic April 1977 flood resulted in $100 million in damage and raised, front and center, the question of whether the flooding was somehow attributable to sedimentation, erosion, and landscape alteration from strip mining.[54]

The most thorough work on the flood question came from the U.S. Forest Service's Berea, Kentucky, research station. Studies written between 1971 and 1977 did not identify a simple one-to-one association between floods and strip mining. In one, for example, investigator Willie Curtis examined streamflow data in Breathitt County, Kentucky, on April 1977, around the time of the flood, and noticed that *unmined* areas actually yielded greater streamflow.[55] In two other locations, however, Curtis discovered the opposite result, plus greater sulfate and magnesium composition in water. In another study, he wrote that "the flood potential after surface mining in Appalachia becomes more and more important with the increase in percent of land disturbed." This was because mining altered water trajectories and the ability of existing watersheds (near larger rivers, lakes, or streams) to absorb them. "If a number of small drainages in a watershed are mined," he cautioned, "flood potential in the watershed may be increased greatly."[56] Curtis noted that these problems were particularly pronounced on steep surfaces. "We must find ways to manage surface mining not only to reduce on-site damages but also to minimize harmful effects on the water sources," he concluded.[57] But Curtis was a circumspect scientist. Interviewed by the *Louisville Courier-Journal* about the studies, Curtis eschewed easy

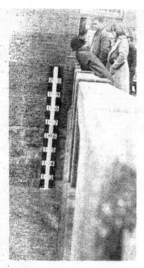

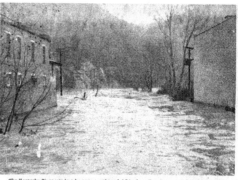

The Kentucky River was in a hurry to get through Whitesburg Tuesday morning, and the swift current churned the water almost into whitecaps. This view is looking toward Solomon Road from the bridge on Main Street. The line of utility poles at left marks the road, which was under several feet of water most of the day. All roads into Whitesburg were blocked for a time Tuesday morning. Water stood three feet deep across Kentucky 15 at the west end of Whitesburg. A woman who had fallen had to be carried down the railroad track to be transferred from one ambulance to another in order to get to the hospital from here.

The water had already started to recede when this picture of the Whitesburg river gauge in the North Fork of the Kentucky River was made about 9 a. m. Tuesday. The river crested at 13 and a half feet about 5:15 a. m. and began to fall about an hour later. The gauge shows it at 12 feet here.

## FLOODWATERS--AND WHAT THEY DO
### (Eagle photos)

Many bottomlands--priceless treasures in Letcher County-- were badly damaged by floodwaters this week, County Agent Jim Kendrick reported. Those which were covered with silt may be reclaimed, he said, but reclamation will be hard and slow for fields in which the water deposited sand. The field at right is at the mouth of Dry Fork. Many home gardens also were ruined.

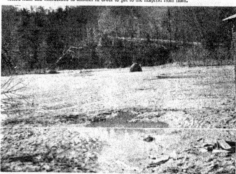

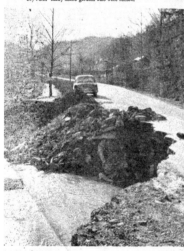

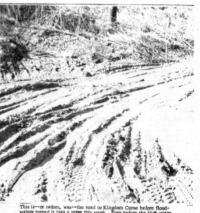

This is--or rather, was--the road to Kingdom Come before floodwaters turned it into a mire this week. Even before the high water residents often had to use jeeps to get in and out, and officials say it will be weeks before the road can be made usable again. At left, swirling waters of Rockhouse Creek undercut the highway to a depth of about six feet. Similar undercutting of paved roads was reported throughout Eastern Kentucky; many roads are expected to give way. (Eagle photos).

**Pictures of local flooding.**
*Source: Mountain Eagle* (Whitesburg, Ky.), March 14, 1963.

associations between strip mining and floods, at least in straightforwardly positive or negative directions. While one of his studies had shown *less* overflow in a strip-mined area, he cautioned that this was simply one site: "I would hate to say that this same thing happened all over the areas where we got the storm. I've done some other research (in stripped areas) that gave higher peaks (of water flow) than unmined ones did."[58] Still, in the same *Courier-Journal* piece, another researcher from the U.S. Geological Survey, Russell Flint, said that "he thought runoff would generally be greater in heavily strip mined areas," notwithstanding local variations here and there.[59]

Whatever additional nuances to the flood question remained—and there were many—by the late 1970s and early 1980s, potential human health risk from strip mining was no longer in the shadows. In 1979, the Presidential Committee on Health and Environmental Effects of Increased Coal Utilization published a series of reports over two years examining the health effects of increased coal use. Although the reports focused most heavily on emissions from coal plants during combustion, their authors also gave some attention to the extraction phase, especially the hydrologic consequences that people such as Willie Curtis and the U.S. Forest Service researchers had studied.[60] Soon afterward, in 1981, the National Research Council commissioned a similar multivolume study of strip mining, focusing on waste disposal. Its authors wrote that "hazards to human safety and health and degradation of the environment were slow in being recognized as warranting governmental attention."[61] They specifically named the high-profile Buffalo Creek mining disaster in West Virginia as a turning point. There, a Pittston Coal Company dam had burst in 1972, flooding a number of Logan County hamlets with waste, killing more than 100 residents, and leaving others isolated in temporary housing for months.[62] Though the incident occurred at an underground mine, it had catalyzed national attention to coal and its discontents more generally. The National Research Council report noted that smaller-scale accidents related to coal waste were commonplace, including piles of refuse regularly left burning. And it reviewed evidence of hydrological damage, mudslides, and surface runoff, including of minerals—"sulfate, calcium, magnesium, aluminum, manganese, iron, and zinc"—that cumulatively led to "adverse water quality conditions" that were "expected to continue." "Water quality," it elaborated in a section on serious threats to fish and wildlife, "can be severely degraded if toxic or acid-producing spoils are improperly placed in fill material." Although broadly sympathetic to continued strip mining, the report simultaneously was confirming—and at the most elite and the highest of scientific levels—things that Appalachian residents had been experiencing, writing about, and protesting against in the preceding decade. The National Research Council's imprimatur was significant, bolstering the legitimacy of questions about the environmental health effects of strip mining.

But what accounts for the drift into more scientific recognition of coal mining's health effects? The typical internal dynamics of scientific discovery—the phenomenon exists, it gets defined as problem, interest grows around it, scientific inquiry begins and eventually coalesces—were only part of the story. The other was the lay suffering and its expression via simple correspondence, newspaper articles, petitioning, and more escalated activism. The Forest Service flood studies, along with major funding increases for the Berea, Kentucky, forest station, had been ordered by Kentucky senator John Sherman Cooper after he heard from frightened constituents.[63] A July 1977 congressional subcommittee investigating "Strip Mining and the Flooding in Appalachia" followed the station's studies. Presiding over a hearing, Democrat Leo Ryan (who tragically would be assassinated the following year), stated: "There is a substantial element in this country that believes there is direct connection between strip mining and the destruction caused by floods, especially in Appalachia." Its members devoted significant floor time for an activist from the Appalachian Alliance to speak and show a film the alliance had produced on land alteration. The representative, a mining engineer as it were, proclaimed: "Current techniques utilized by the coal industry in the removal of coal by strip mining do not adequately protect the welfare of people and communities in Appalachia. Damage to homes and property by flooding, landslides, sedimentation, and blasting have become commonplace.... The people of Appalachia who live along the creek banks and up the hollows, on the ridge tops and in the small towns, are being continually subjected to severe and even life-threatening disasters caused by strip mining."[64]

Outside of rarefied scientific bodies and beltway hearings, there existed more cooperation between health scientists and laypersons. After the April 1977 flood—and two others in October and November of that year—a group of scientists formed Appalachia: Science in the Public Interest (ASPI). It was modeled after Science for the People, a nationwide network of scientists that sought to translate academic findings to a broader public and highlight critically the social downsides of uncritical technological innovation, often while working in concert with activists.[65] The scientists conducted a review of existing literature on the strip mine–flood issue (in addition to their own analysis of National Weather Service data). In two areas within Harlan County—Clover Fork and Cranks Creek—runoff had been particularly heavy, and they focused their attention there. They'd been spurred by interactions with residents in the region. The eventual flood report, the authors noted, was compiled only after "much time ... spent in the country, walking through the hills, creeks, and hollers, and talking with the people to gain from their experience and knowledge" and to identify affected areas.[66]

Though first and foremost written for local residents, the report displayed analytical complexity. It took to heart much of what Forest Service scientist

Willie Curtis had said about the importance of understanding specific local topographic characteristics and variations in assessing the strip mining–flood association. In fact, some of the report cautioned against too simplistic a causal account. To take one example, in a careful review of Harlan County topography, ASPI's report delved into the precise state of local vegetation and climate during three 1977 heavy rainfalls. It noted that a drier September month preceding October had allowed for more water containment than might have otherwise existed, thereby preventing a more severe flood. The report concluded that "rainfall runoff factors and watershed characteristics . . . have served to both increase and decrease the flood levels of 1977 to some degree," though more precise conclusions would depend on future research. Nevertheless, there existed enough evidence for some association between "land disturbance" and elevated flood levels under certain conditions. In light of ASPI's findings, the report called for better emergency response and more studies to clarify what those certain conditions were. Most bold was the report's call for a preemptive approach, even before all the evidence was fully in: "immediate cessation" of all strip mining within the county, not just because of potential flood risk but because ravished topography made it inhospitable to revegetation.[67]

Apart from research on floods, ASPI conducted a number of studies on related topics and hosted local workshops to disseminate its results. One workshop centered on "Surface Mine Blasting and Public Policy" and educated residents on reducing "off-site vibration" caused by extraction. The overt conceptualization of strip mining as a human health issue, not just an extreme irritant, was evident in the organization's call for "a continuing dialogue and the development of a public coal policy which ensures the integrity of the human and natural environment."[68] Other ASPI publications, such as a *Citizens' Blasting Handbook*, reflected input of residents themselves and were designed to communicate scientific knowledge and possible recourse in an understandable fashion.[69] Such lay-scientific collaborations around environmental health issues presaged "community-based participatory research" and "popular epidemiology" before those terms—and practices—were embraced in formal public health practice two decades later.[70]

## Slow Violence and the Rise of the Coal Consensus

These dual lay and scientific concerns over strip mining and population-level health risks generated some policy maker response, including the funding of the Berea research station and congressional hearings. And momentum emerged, at least in some quarters, for more concerted scientific inquiry and precautionary policy. In this sense, there were similarities to the 1950s smog experience in

Los Angeles, also home to impassioned residents clamoring for recognition by scientists and politicians.

But the similarities ended there. Coal policy proceeded in a markedly different direction. By the early 1980s a "coal consensus" formed in American energy policy—that is, the largely uncontested acceptance of coal, now heavily strip-mined, as a predominant and central (not simply additional) energy source for powering up and lighting the United States.

The coal consensus was shared by policy makers at all levels of government, the energy industry, and the general public (excluding much of the Central Appalachian population). It was the American piece of what political scientist Timothy Mitchell has dubbed "carbon democracy," whereby "political possibilities were opened up or narrowed down by different ways of organising the flow and concentration of energy, and these possibilities were enhanced or limited by arrangements of people, finance, expertise and violence that were assembled in relationship to the distribution and control of energy."[71] The coal consensus transcended party lines and ideology. By the late 1970s, Democratic representative Carl Perkins voted against and publicly criticized the first federal regulations eventually passed to introduce more rigorous constraints—at least on paper—on strip mining.[72] Democrat Robert Byrd, an otherwise stalwart defender of environmentalist causes in the U.S. Senate, persistently adopted coal-friendly legislative positions. This policy consensus, in turn, led to reliance on coal—particularly strip-minded coal—as a key American energy source, a development that embedded strip mining structurally into the U.S. economy's very operation. Reflecting on it, one feels a sense of inevitability. How else, indeed, was one to power the nation into the late twentieth century?

But how did such seemingly intractable development occur in the first place? One intuitive analysis interprets the coal consensus as fueled primarily by powerful and aggressive coal interests—the sociopathy of King Coal—running roughshod and exploitatively over those with few political and economic resources. There is much to substantiate such an analysis, as the human accounts here demonstrate. The coal industry mobilized extraordinarily in the court of public opinion to constrict terms of debate in its favor, often in disingenuous ways. And it adopted strip-mining technology in part to undercut labor and fatten its profit margins. Yet energy firms' venality was only one propeller. It dovetailed with several other trends and outright unexpected events. Their confluence made the coal consensus.

Nonetheless, it is true that the coal industry defended its economic interests vigorously, beginning with the aggressive consolidation and technological adoption analyzed earlier. It followed with a public relations front, responding to incipient concerns over strip mining by laypersons and subsequent collective action that had led to prominent discussions in regional and national

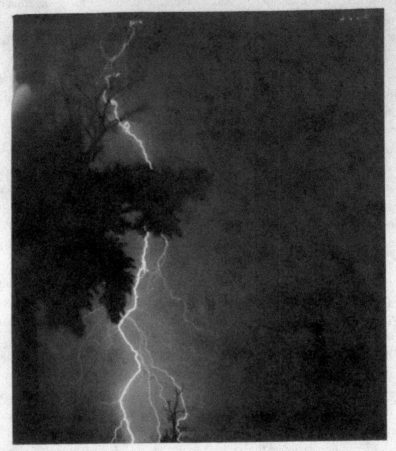

**Our hottest client**

Generating electricity is big business for the coal industry. About half of all coal mined in this country is sold to electric utilities. Conversely, more than half of our electricity is generated from coal. In addition, millions of tons of coal go into making steel, cement, chemicals, paper, food products—you name it. Your youngsters may think of coal as a merry old soul in a nursery rhyme, but don't you make that mistake. The future of our economy is bright but the basis of that future is black. Black as coal.

For further information, write 1130 17th St., N.W., Washington, D. C. 20036.

**Coal for a Better America**

"This advertisement sponsored by National Coal Association is one of a series appearing in *TIME* Magazine, *WALL STREET JOURNAL*, and *FIELD* and *STREAM*."

**"Our Hottest Client" (reprint), National Coal Association, ca. 1967.**
*Source*: RG 70, Records of the United States Bureau of Mines, Division of Environment, National Surface Mine Study Policy Committee, General Surface Mining Study Files, 1963–1967, Box 24, Folder "Appalachia-Correspondence-1967," National Archives, College Park, Md.

media. Most notably, a critical 1964 article by the *Louisville-Courier Journal* had launched a series on strip mining that culminated in a 1967 Pulitzer Prize for public interest reporting.[73] In response to the new spotlight, the National Coal Association, one of two industry trade groups, ran ads in popular periodicals ranging from the *Wall Street Journal* to *Time*. The ads downplayed strip mining's effects, suggesting instead that revegetation and reclamation of disturbed land were easy and routine processes. One ad featured a color photograph of a couple paddling in a riverboat, obscured by plentiful trees and vegetation. Beneath it were the words "Eyesore" in large print, followed by a paragraph that read: "This was a strip coal mine. Reclaimed by a coal company. It's the finest recreation spot for miles around. Note the phrase 'reclaimed by a coal company.' Some people believe that all worked-out strip mines are eyesores. But then some people don't know the coal industry has an active program to beautify mined land and restore it to beneficial use. It has, you know. After all, it's our country, too." Another, entitled "'Clean Air' Is a Relative Term," claimed that the industry was "putting time, effort and millions of dollars against the problem of air pollution."[74]

But a second message came with even greater ideological ramifications. It emphasized the growing centrality of coal to American daily life. "Our Hottest Client" reminded readers that "generating electricity is big business for the coal industry. About half of all coal mined in this country is sold to electric utilities." It continued: "Your youngsters may think of coal as a merry old soul in a nursery rhyme, but don't you make that mistake. The future of our economy is bright but the basis of that future is black. Black as coal."[75]

This theme surfaced, too, in a splashy multipage advertisement that appeared a few years earlier in the *New York Times*. Formatted to resemble a legitimate newspaper, "The Invisible Power of Coal" featured a run of short lookalike articles that responded to ecological concerns by ensuring readers that the coal industry was proactively attending to them—and successfully so. The most gripping section of the spread, "Coal Is All around Us," introduced the most frequent public message the industry would later push on coal. It identified automobiles, household products, and manufacturing plants as necessities powered by coal energy central to a booming postwar nation. Images of domesticity and family life adorned the advertisement's cover.[76]

Outside the world of public opinion, a behind-the-scenes examination of the Bureau of Mines's ongoing study of strip mining in the mid-1960s demonstrates how its authors framed policy options in terms of economic growth potential (or lack of it). In doing so, they accepted much of the coal industry's terms of debate. In an exchange with Appalachian Regional Commission cochairman John I. Sweeney, the bureau's Henry Caulfield explained that the study wouldn't push for complete reclamation of mined sites, despite its virtues, in part because "the potential for economic growth must be considered one of the most

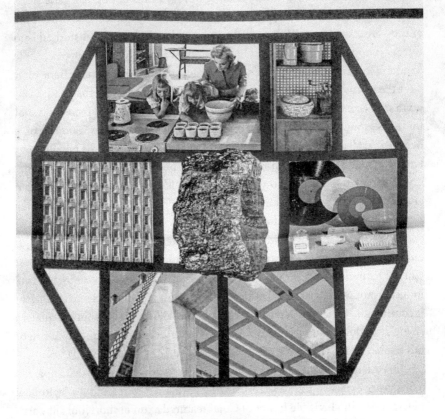

**"The Invisible Power of Coal" (advertisement).**
*Source: New York Times,* June 14, 1964, sec. 12. From The New York Times.
© 1964 The New York Times Company. All rights reserved. Used under license.

important criteria for evaluating individual project proposals."[77] At other times, there existed a reluctance to question the coal industry head-on. Responding to a resident's complaint, Walter Hibbard, the Bureau of Mines' director, wrote back: "We are aware that mining frequently results in environmental damage but we recognize also that alleviation and prevention of such damage must be achieved without serious disruption of the national economy."[78]

The Bureau of Mines released its eventual report in two parts: an interim study in 1966 and a final version, one year later.[79] Both contained exhaustive tabulations of total acres spoiled by strip mining. The final report summarized findings on landscape damage. Most notable was its stance toward reclamation. The bureau acknowledged several impediments. It suggested that existing means for reclamation, along with explicit standards about what it ought to entail, required significant improvement. It spotlighted the high cost for a comprehensive rehabilitation, $1.2 billion, and noted that the sources for funds, whether from operators themselves or the government, were hardly clear. According to its final report, only 34 percent of disturbed land had been reclaimed as of 1965—a contrast to the industry's public claims in advertisements and elsewhere. The quality of existing reclamation was another matter, too.[80]

But despite the uneven efficacy of landscape reclamation efforts, policy-wise, strip mining was going to stay. Even though research on its negative impacts was accumulating, however slowly, the report didn't suggest more regulation that might slow strip mining's adoption. A section of the final report, in fact, focused on the relationship between large-scale strip mining and the "economic potential of a nation." It stated that the United States was "blessed with a wealth of natural resources, needing only to import a small portion of its total mineral requirements," and, like the industry's own pronouncements, pointed to coal and other raw materials' increasingly integral role in both the energy supply and everyday consumer life.[81] Two years later, in 1970, Earl T. Hayes, a deputy director at the bureau, sympathized with a constituent's letter describing the "undesirable effects" of strip mining in Lovely, Kentucky. He added, however, that there was an unavoidable tradeoff with the "economy as a whole" and that "the recovery of our mineral resources is absolutely essential to the maintenance of our economy, and to our national security. Surface mining is one of the most efficient and economic ways to get these essential raw materials."[82]

And yet there were forks in the road ahead, and alternative possibilities were floated. Outside and inside government, discussions on taming strip mining— including an outright ban—took place. Nationally, public outrage followed the 1972 Buffalo Creek coal waste disaster. And in addition to on-the-ground grassroots activism, debates occurred in formal political arenas. In 1971, West Virginia congressman Ken Hechler introduced a bill to ban strip mining altogether, attracting almost ninety cosponsors. A year later, presidential candidate George McGovern campaigned on a strip mine ban.[83] Up through the early 1970s, then, there was still no fully solidified coal consensus. But activism around strip mining also lacked a critical element present in cases like Los Angeles: absent were enough influential elements, including factions of the nonindustrial business class and the Los Angeles County Medical Association, willing to join a broader coalition. In Los Angeles, the economic growth imperative had accommodated environmental regulation. In Central Appalachia, the former superseded the latter. The Appalachian experience missed two elements identified by the sociologist Connie Nathanson as critical for "active state intervention in public health": "the presence of politically savvy public health entrepreneurs" and "the strong support of highly placed political allies."[84] There were no Central Appalachian

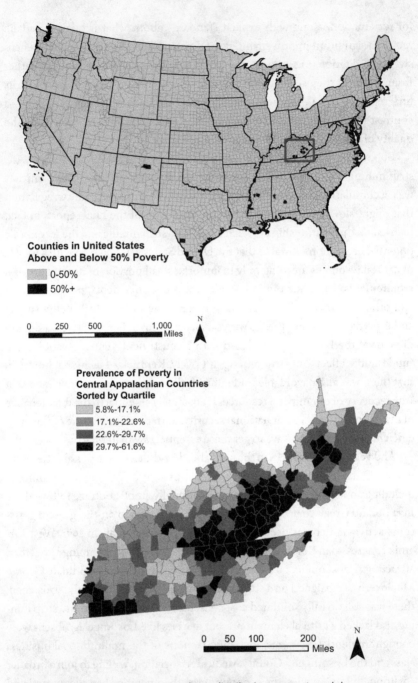

**Counties in United States
Above and Below 50% Poverty**

0-50%

50%+

0    250    500    1,000
                        Miles

N

**Prevalence of Poverty in
Central Appalachian Countries
Sorted by Quartile**

5.8%-17.1%

17.1%-22.6%

22.6%-29.7%

29.7%-61.6%

0    50    100    200
                      Miles

N

**Regional and national poverty prevalence distributions, 1970.** I used the 1970
Census because it was the first to incorporate a poverty rate measure. I relied on
the Social Explorer database's "Poverty Status for Families" variable, recalculated
from the original manuscript census.

*Source*: Author's cartography based on 1970 U.S. Census (Social Explorer
database and National Historical Geographical Information Systems database,
Minnesota Population Center, University of Minnesota).

analogs to either Los Angeles's aggressive air pollution control agency or the wide, if uneasy, consensus it had managed to build behind its program.

Timing was also everything. Into the 1960s, an overall postwar public policy shift, at regional and federal levels, coalesced around stimulating robust and steady economic growth. Places with little of it were no exception, and Appalachian policy makers' desire to jolt the economy was further catalyzed when the region received national attention after the publication of two high-profile books: Harry Caudill's *Night Comes to the Cumberlands: A Biography of a Depressed Area* and Michael Harrington's *The Other America: Poverty in the United States.*[85] The Appalachian economic deprivation that these authors chronicled took the particular form of not only persistent double-digit poverty rates but also chronic unemployment, limited diversity of economic sectors, out-migration, and low tax bases, among other indicators, and resulted in a multipronged search for some spark that might reverse these trends.[86] The area's economic plight was endemic and extreme, both when examined within its own borders and relative to the nation at large. The overwhelming majority of counties in the region reported double-digit poverty prevalence in 1970. And the region was home to thirteen of only forty-four counties in the *entire United States* with that much poverty.

Faced with this material reality, regional policy makers embraced what historian Robert Collins has identified as the era's hegemonic "growth liberalism"— that is, a commitment to constant acceleration of economic growth. For Central Appalachia, coal was more than a miracle economic fix; it'd keep the region in tandem with the rest of the nation's goals.[87] This embrace, in turn, explains why so many debates around coal and its potentially deleterious effects—health or otherwise—persistently circled back to whether potential policies did or did not impede "economic growth."

One should thus not view the coal consensus as simply the product of pandering politicians and coal executives' base self-interest alone. Coal policy's evolution fit neatly with prevailing policy parameters of the time. Moreover, if one measures real-world consequence, Central Appalachia did experience some tangible, if very short-lived, coal-related gains, with some "new jobs, in-migration, and small-business growth."[88] These short-term indicators resulted, too, in occasional support for strip mining from the UMWA.[89]

But was this enough to entrench the coal consensus? Another crucial development, and one more contingent, arose from the two oil shocks of the early and late 1970s. The sudden spikes in energy prices and shortages—captured best by now iconic photographs of automobile lines waiting for gasoline—sparked national conversation about decreasing dependence on foreign energy sources, including through synthetic fuel production from coal. In the early 1970s, this initially led to some discussion on comprehensive energy legislation and the need to invest in alternative energy sources.[90] But serious pursuit of them was quickly marginalized by a policy push for the most abundant—and readily available—domestic energy sources, including coal. The rhetoric of energy independence then opened up a political opportunity for the coal industry and its partisans to exploit. Kentucky representative Perkins said as much in a letter to two constituents, writing in 1974: "I must tell you in all candor that the job of passing effective strip mine legislation is going to be more difficult now that the energy crisis is upon us."[91] By the end of the decade, as Perkins had become an even stronger public proponent of strip-mined coal, he defended his position by declaring that "we need to eliminate our dependency on foreign oil. We will never be able to solve this crisis if we continue to strangle the industry which is capable of producing the energy for our domestic needs."[92]

Coal operators and their allies proceeded along these lines, too. In 1974, Hilton Davis, of the U.S. Chamber of Commerce, wrote to Perkins pushing for lighter regulation that would prevent "curtailed coal production that would make [the] nation more dependent on foreign energy sources."[93] And at the state level, the Kentucky Power Company's Waldo La Fon wrote similarly to Perkins, claiming, "The nation would be more dependent on foreign oil" with increased regulation or curtailment of strip mining and coal, which he characterized as a "vital domestic energy resource [that was] needed more than ever."[94] That same year, in a letter to Representative Morris Udall protesting stricter regulations, the National Coal Association's Carl E. Bagge referenced a speech given by President Gerald Ford on energy independence and declared that "energy is now a central issue of our world posture and the strength of our economy: what affects coal affects our foreign policy and, in the long run, world stability."[95] Following vigorous lobbying and publicity stunts from the coal industry—in one memorable set piece, a caravan of "six to seven hundred" coal trucks entered Washington, D.C., after traveling through Appalachia—President Ford promptly vetoed two regulatory bills, foreshadowing a shift in federal policy.[96] Such actions were in sync with the times. In the 1970s, coal and electricity became ever more symbiotic, with coal rising as the dominant source for powering the United States and electricity becoming its primary end use. The tight connection between coal and everyday American life that the industry had been promoting was becoming an infrastructural reality, as researchers Gregory Elmes and Trevor Harris have shown in their study of widening coal interstate trade routes following the industry's mass penetration into electricity markets, with electric utilities almost doubling as an end use between 1965 and 1975.[97]

The policy climate became even clearer after President Jimmy Carter's Commission on Coal issued its findings at the end of his term. Chaired by liberal West Virginia governor John D. Rockefeller IV, the commission explored "the acceptable replacement of imported oil with coal," and it made repeated reference to the oil crisis, concluding:

Even under the best of circumstances, it will take many years to overcome the constant threat that is posed to national security and to economic stability by continued reliance on foreign oil. It is, therefore, imperative that the Nation continue to pursue aggressively those courses of action designed to reduce dependence on imported oil.

It is the view of the Commission that coal can make a significant contribution toward this objective.[98]

As in the Bureau of Mines study published more than a decade before, economic imperatives assumed center stage. The commission did discuss "environmental and health consequences" but limited the bulk of its analysis to combustion, the phase of energy production *after* extraction, noting that "emissions from coal . . . contain nitrogen oxides, sulfur oxides, and particulates that have been linked to respiratory disease and to the increased acidity of rainfall and of lakes." And anticipating climate change, it continued: "There is concern among scientists that increasing atmospheric concentrations of carbon dioxide—resulting, in part, from the burning of fossil fuels—could result in warming of the Earth's atmosphere toward the middle of the next century."[99] When it did touch on extraction, the commission's report noted that a newly passed Surface Mining Control and Reclamation Act (1977)— much weaker than two federal bills President Ford had vetoed—remained "in the process of being implemented" and that "disturbance to ground and surface waters must be kept to a minimum." Yet despite these concerns, the commission's overall thrust was overwhelmingly optimistic; coal was less problem than solution, especially in the wake of the 1970s energy crises. The commission's stance differed little from everyone else's in mainstream American politics.

Consequently, the twin goals of economic growth and energy independence— both via coal—became firmly rooted in the late 1970s and early 1980s Appalachian policy making. One 1978 economic development report for Kentucky stated that a "specific development objective" was to orient all other social infrastructure spending around "coal-producing activities."[100] Another mentioned that "Kentucky's response to the national energy issue is constructed around a proposed improvement in the level and technology of coal production."[101] The Appalachian Regional Commission characterized Kentucky as "looking to an active coal industry to serve as the catalyst for broader expansion and diversification of the Region's economic base."[102] The state's 1982 five-year development plan declared that "for the short-term the coal industry must be supported since it is the dominant economic factor of the region and its major employer," even though coal-related employment had begun declining drastically by the end of the 1970s due to industry automation. Coal did increasingly little for the actual people of Appalachia. The same development plan that touted it, for instance, showed a double-digit drop of 10.3 percent in coal industry employment between

1978 and 1979 alone, a sharp fall that would continue into the twenty-first century.[103]

By the early 1980s, the coal industry's politicking solidified the coal consensus still further. Nowhere was this more evident than in Kentucky, when a Coal Policy Council formed by Governor John Young was chaired by none other than William B. Sturgill. Sturgill had appeared in the same 1961 news program that opened this chapter, in which Beefhyde Hollow residents Elijah Wright, Buster Stewart, and G. W. Burke had vividly described the destructiveness of the strip mine around their homes. In the two decades since the program aired, Sturgill had become one of the most successful coal operators in Kentucky, ascending to executive positions at a number of firms. His presence on the Coal Policy Council and later appointment as the state's secretary of energy extended his power from the industrial realm into the political. So, too, did the presence of other coal industry executives on the council, who occupied seventeen of its thirty-five seats.[104] At a press conference announcing his council, Governor Young declared: "Coal, without question, is going to be the No. 1 thrust of this administration."[105]

The Coal Policy Council passed multiple resolutions criticizing federal regulations on emissions and Clean Air Act amendments, claiming "inhibit[ion] of industrial activity" and criticizing the "shift [in] regulatory decision-making from States to the National Government."[106] And with respect to strip mining specifically, the council opposed attempts to increase the federal authority of the newly created Office of Surface Mining (OSM) in the permit and regulatory process.[107] In reality, OSM's powers were hampered structurally by delegation of many powers to state-level regulators. Under the law that created it, the office would intervene only if it found a state plan inadequate. The ability to assess inadequacy, however, only was as good as the good faith of political appointees overseeing OSM, to say nothing of adequate budgetary resources.[108]

Fortunately for the Kentucky Coal Policy Council, it had an ally in President Ronald Reagan. In his first term, the number of OSM inspectors dropped from "a high of 211" in 1980 to 97 just two years later. Violations predictably trended in the same direction, declining by 57 percent between 1979 and 1981.[109] It reflected Reagan's overall hostility to environmental regulation, as exemplified by attempts at rolling back—either in the form of regulations themselves or in the execution of them—the activities of the Department of Interior, most famously in the Environmental Protection Agency.[110] As strip mining's expansion continued apace, increasingly lax regulation at both the federal and state levels meant that the coal policy debate was effectively over.

When it came to Kentucky, it'd be tempting to characterize Sturgill (and figures like him in the other Central Appalachian states) as the primary driving force behind the coal consensus and politicians like Governor Young, who appointed him to the Coal Policy Commission, as mere pushovers and pawns in the process. But in truth, coal hegemony was a historical outgrowth of larger, long-term developments that transcended political actors alone. These developments included the search for regional catalysts that could end economic stagnation, a national commitment to economic growth, and the political lure of "energy independence" during the 1970s, all propelled by a national consumer economy dependent on coal energy. Taking this into consideration, it becomes harder to pass moral judgments on convenient coal industry villains alone.[111] Larger societal dynamics operating in tandem—perhaps clearer in hindsight than at the time—were as responsible for coal's eventual entrenchment.

The postwar expansion of a coal-powered energy infrastructure was a form of what environmental writer Rob Nixon has called "slow violence," whereby exploitation occurs not in the form of an immediate and acute episode but as a phenomenon that unravels over a protracted time, barely noticeable initially, but then becoming chronic, systematized, and entrenched right under society's nose.[112] By the early twenty-first century, Appalachia had ceased being the chief supplier of coal for the United States—states such as Wyoming now had that honor—and many celebrated as the United States began weaning itself off coal altogether. But the damage from slow violence had already been done. Because for much of the postwar period, Central Appalachia had provided most of the country with its coal—and relatively cheaply. And the local people of Central Appalachia paid for it—and with their bodies. National growth rested on local pain.

The divergence with the Los Angeles environmental health experience was stark, and it could be explained by how wide a swath of people were affected by the threat and how much powerful people did or didn't care. In Los Angeles, no part of the basin—urban core, suburban belt, rich, poor, everywhere in between—was untouched by the problem, contributing to a universal language of community that knit otherwise disparate denizens together around a common community health cause. In Appalachia, only those living in a belt of counties felt that stake. Their homes were in areas that were the poorest, the most remote, the least able to alter fundamentally coal politics, from the local to the national level, despite the occasional concession. It was thus no surprise that the analogs to Los Angeles's antipollution stakeholders were absent, along with the political capital and sway they brought with them. It explained not just overall political unresponsiveness but the slower pace of scientific inquiry. The full force of universities from the get-go—USC, UCLA, Caltech—was absent in the Cumberlands.

These local contrasts mapped onto respective national images of the two regions. In many ways, 1950s Los Angeles was the Cold War reboot of frontier ideology and its westward dream, right down to the racism, and it occupied a central place in midcentury American aspiration. Appalachia was the foil—its resources to be plundered, its people (at best) to be pitied, but ultimately out of sight and so very much out of mind.

# 6

# Central Appalachia

### Pork-Barrel Medicine and Poverty:
### Devolution and the Problem of Elite Capture

Since its inception, *Science* has published peer-reviewed research of wide interest across specialties and reports on major trends and frontiers in scientific research. It is not a publication that has typically concerned itself, then or now, with local political battles, least of all those in remote Kentucky counties with a total population of 41,000. Yet in 1972, *Science* dispatched a reporter to Floyd County to learn why a federal Office of Economic Opportunity (OEO) health project had failed so spectacularly, complete with accusations of funds misallocated and promised services never rendered.[1]

The Eastern Kentucky Welfare Rights Organization (EKWRO) had long beaten *Science* to the story. A year before the reporter's arrival, it'd plastered a striking poster all over the county that asked: "WHAT HAS HAPPENED TO $$$$$$ MILLIONS $$$$$$ HERE IN FLOYD COUNTY"? It answered: "The local doctors, pharmacists and politicians have taken control of the Comprehensive Health Program and have kept THE POOR PEOPLE FROM SETTING UP CLINICS AND HIRING THEIR OWN DOCTORS. So far they have managed to keep all the money for themselves!!!!"[2] The Floyd County activists were onto what development economists would later call "elite capture," the process by which federal programs shot money to decentralized areas—ostensible communities—where the entire governing apparatus, from courts to schools, was controlled by a coterie that quickly gobbled up incoming resources.

It was doubly tragic, not just because of resource allocation but because conditions in the region had catalyzed much of the War on Poverty in the first place. Hard-hitting books and reports had brought Appalachians' plight to national attention, and President Johnson himself had toured Martin County, Kentucky, posing for an iconic photo of himself gazing with purpose while squatting on a resident's porch. But the Floyd County experience demonstrated that local power could provide a formidable check to the ambitions of a federal program targeted at undeserved areas. When a half-victory finally followed a bitter crisis of governance, the welfare rights activists who'd wrestled control from a corrupt small-town political machine faced a different problem: how much that triumph mattered against a landscape replete with health threats that ranged from endemic water-borne diseases eradicated elsewhere to ecological devastation caused by a national energy transition reliant on the area's natural resources.

## Medical Care and the Coalfields

On the surface, Central Appalachia was a world away from the large cities that came to be associated with the War on Poverty in the public imagination. But the region was riven with medical maldistribution, and it'd long been of interest to reformers. In the mid-1950s, major studies presented readers with exhaustive charts and maps detailing low medical practitioner-to-population ratios and the relative undersupply of medical care facilities in the majority of counties. One reported that of the 257 counties studied, only 3 percent contained a "specialized multiple service health care center," the most comprehensive of five health center types. A full 47 percent contained no health care center, period.[3] Three years later, another social survey of the region, led by the eminent rural sociologist Rupert Vance, reached similar conclusions. "There is evidence of serious overcrowding in over 50 per cent of the general hospitals of the region," the report concluded, along with general calls for increases in per capita medical care spending, new facilities expansion, and personnel.[4] The message, boiled to its essence, was simple: there was scant medical care for those who needed it, and when it did exist, it was hard to access. A decade later, another analysis mentioned the persistence of "traditional barriers," including "geographic isolation" and "manpower shortages."[5] The most striking sections of these reports used cartography as visual rhetoric, showcasing contrasting shades and orbs of different sizes to convey the uneven distribution of physicians and hospital beds. They reflected an entry of medical care into the region that'd always been imbalanced, with a spate of construction occurring in the Progressive Era, followed by a stunting of infrastructural growth in the decades that followed. The consistent takeaway: too few facilities that were located too far away. Watts and Central Appalachia may have been different in dozens of ways, but not when it came to medical deserts.

Yet by the 1960s, the medical care imperative was back, much of it stemming from larger national concerns over maldistribution. Reports and surveys on shortages actually translated into policy, and from Washington, OEO funded a number of neighborhood health centers for the region. The Appalachian

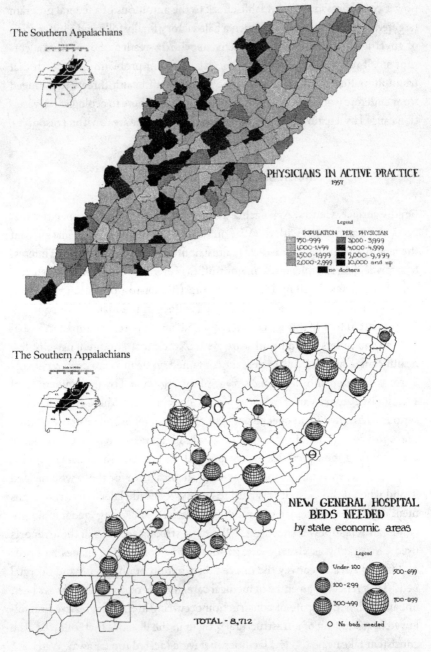

The Southern Appalachians

PHYSICIANS IN ACTIVE PRACTICE
1957

Legend
POPULATION PER PHYSICIAN
750-999       3,000 - 3,999
1,000-1,499   4,000-4,999
1,500-1,999   5,000-9,999
2,000-2,999   10,000 and up
no doctors

The Southern Appalachians

NEW GENERAL HOSPITAL
BEDS NEEDED
by state economic areas

Legend
Under 100      500 - 699
100 - 299
300 - 499      700 - 899

TOTAL - 8,712          O  No beds needed

**Conveying maldistribution, 1957.** These maps conveyed—with striking cartography—the gravity of an Appalachian physician and hospital shortage. In the first map, the darkest shading represented severe physician maldistribution in certain Appalachian regions, especially eastern Kentucky. The second map did the same using orbs of different sizes, with larger ones representing increased need.

*Source*: C. Horace Hamilton, *Health and Health Services in the Southern Appalachians: A Source Book* (Raleigh: North Carolina Agricultural Experiment Station, 1959), Berea College Special Collections and Archives, Hutchins Library, Berea, Ky.

Regional Commission, a new multistate developmental agency, bankrolled the Southeastern Kentucky Regional Health Demonstration Project, targeting eleven counties in the "hard-core problem area" of eastern Kentucky. It'd fund dozens of medical care projects into the mid-1970s, including construction and training programs.[6] Planners presented the initiative as a cure for the region's "fragmented, uncoordinated" medical care resources and a model for "demonstrating development through" careful regional planning.[7] State officials became part of the medical infrastructural push, too, and drew on the same kind of rhetoric. In 1967, the stated goals of the Kentucky Development Plan were "to help incapable persons become capable," "to help unproductive persons become productive," and "to help nonviable areas develop viable economies," listing health as one of four developmental priorities.[8] Medicine and development were intertwined.

Policy makers weren't the only ones seized by the allure of medical care. So were ordinary people. The Hazard and Perry County chapter of the Jaycees youth group "recognize[d] the immediate need for improved and expanded medical care facilities," pushing specifically for twenty-four-hour, full-time physician staffing at a nearby hospital.[9] From Louisa, Kentucky, Patricia Lee wrote of the need "to accommodate patients from a seven-county drawing area," claiming that two small propriety hospitals in the area were overburdened and ill-equipped for the task.[10] When pilot projects began to get rolling, a resident from Menifee County in Kentucky grew impatient. She wrote to her U.S. House representative, Democrat Carl Perkins, complaining about the slow pace of moving from blueprints to projects. "We are a poor area, but we know that our sick people can't wait on another survey or a State Advisory Council next year or five years later.... All levels of government are stymied with 'expert' planners who can talk a good game, but in the meantime, the medical situation worsens each and every day," C. M. Brand remarked.[11] Her comments came amid a larger multicounty effort to rehabilitate a small facility, Jane Cook Hospital, where "crowded conditions" had created "urgency" resulting from "illness" and "unusually severe winter weather."[12]

One problem was the instability of the most established health care network in the area: the ten Miners Memorial Hospitals of the United Mine Workers of America (UMWA). Located as they were in larger towns, the UMWA hospitals were already inaccessible enough to much of the Appalachian population. But when the UMWA's firebrand president, John Lewis, retired, the union became embroiled in a series of corruption scandals, financial woes, and internal infighting brought on by Lewis's successor, Tony Boyle. At one point, the union's travails led it to consider partial closure of the hospitals. Eventually, in 1963, they were sold and transferred to the Appalachian Regional Hospitals (ARH), an ad hoc nonprofit funded by the Presbyterian Board of National Missions.[13] But whether the ARH would find secure financial footing wasn't clear.

In some places, the problem wasn't lack of medical infrastructure. In the Red Bird Valley of Clay County, Kentucky, workers with the Appalachian Volunteers, a War on Poverty project, noted that the area contained plenty of medical facilities, particularly in maternal and child health services, at least compared to other Appalachian areas they had visited.[14] But residents' interactions with medical institutions were irregular and mistrust of them was common. "The fact also remains that in any area no matter how large or how good the health services the people will not use them unless there is a will or desire for these services," one report read. "There is in the project area a religious feeling that what will be, will be and that if it is God's will it will happen. If not, it will not.... This in itself is one factor that contributes to the health situation in the project area."[15] Engaging local worldviews required the work of knowledgeable laypersons as much as medical professionals.[16]

Unfortunately, outsiders' observations about lay Appalachian health beliefs could be class inflected and often hinged on a stark dualism between backwardness and modernity. Leaders in the Appalachian Volunteers, for example, told participants that they were working somewhere with privies, dirty water, and "lower health standards than those of the middle class in our country," and which "serves as a breeding place for flies."[17] Kenneth Osgood, a medical student from the University of Cincinnati, spent time with "Granny" midwives in Clay County, Kentucky, and wrote of them dismissively, noting that some hadn't undergone formal training. Of two such midwives, for instance, he observed that "both related strong religious guidance. For example, one of these 'Granny' midwives told this interviewer that the first time she was called to a delivery, the mother-to-be cried, 'I'm going to die.' The midwife said, 'No you're not: God don't say so.' She then related that not knowing what to do she yelled out to God and under his leadership she rotated her hands on the woman's abdomen and the baby 'was born.'" Osgood's condescension wasn't veiled. After one midwife told him she wore gloves, he added, "that these gloves are in no way sterile. No further evidence was related indicating any other attempts at practicing aseptic technique."[18]

But medical care attained enough of a toehold by the end of the 1950s, and reformers aimed ultimately for some syncretism between formal medical care and lay practices. Osgood himself noted as much. Midwives such as those he'd observed were "leaders of their respective hollow communities" in the Cumberland Plateau "to whom many people go for advice on medical and social problems." "It seems apparent to this observer that channeling a constructive medical or social program through these women would greatly enhance its chances of success."[19] His analysis exemplified the revived confidence in bringing medical care to Central Appalachia during the 1960s, even with all of the epistemic tensions—sometimes acknowledged, sometimes not—that it entailed.

# The Localist Imperative

Addressing medical maldistribution came with a simultaneous commitment to expanding governance.[20] The Southeastern Kentucky health project hoped to "demonstrate an approach to development of the health service system in which responsibility for planning and implementation is effectively exercised at the local level," and three health planning councils would be "structured to assure . . . broad representation, involvement, and leadership." They'd include "leaders from professional groups—particularly physicians, dentists, nurses, and hospital administrators—and representatives of the general public, with the latter," perhaps most critically, to comprise "the majority of the members."[21]

Many facilities embraced this new push for local participatory governance. In the late 1960s, the 9,000-person town of Evarts, Kentucky, housed only one medical practice, overseen by a single physician who had recently resigned. The Clover Fork Clinic, designed to replace it, mandated from its founding in 1969 the active involvement in the planning process those who would use it in the future. Further, its chief physician was required to live among and interact with those residing in Evarts, and like its New York and Los Angeles counterparts, the clinic hired as much of its nonphysician staff from the surrounding area as possible. In addition to providing medical services, Clover Fork also provided basic social services, including counseling and assistance with day-to-day tasks.[22] Early on, its board members reminded themselves that it was "easy to assume that we know the problems of this area and that our methods are best suited to meet these problems. However, we need to constantly be open to the community's own self-understanding." It discussed "extended" nurses and a "pastor-counselor" to serve as conduits for "criticism and positive comment from the community" back to administrators.[23] "We cannot really function without this community regulation," the Clover Fork board noted proudly.

No other project tested these principles more than a high-profile facility set up principally with OEO funds in southeastern Kentucky. It was called the Floyd County Comprehensive Health Program in 1967, and its struggles raised questions about the prospects for new medical care projects in the region. There were the obvious challenges: low financial resources, spatial distance from clientele, and infrastructural deficiencies. But in Floyd County, an additional barrier was political, not physical. Conflicts over governance in New York City and Los Angeles had resulted from the flow of medical care funds into academic medical centers, which then administered the programs, with varying degrees of recognition for lay input. In Appalachia, the big difference was that dollars flowed not to single academic institutions but to county governments, long dominated by political machines made up of tightly connected judges, local politicos, superintendents, small-time proprietors, and landowners, with some occupying more than one role. Political machines, of course, were hardly exclusive to Appalachia. But in large metropolitan cities, their power was centered in neighborhoods, and their influence was further diluted by competing blocs. The power of Appalachian political machines, by contrast, wasn't diffuse but concentrated. It was lopsided rule by local power elite that had a chokehold on county governance structures that were small and bureaucratically simple, allowing for wholesale dominance over entire programs with little in the way of checks and balances.[24]

The unique qualities of Appalachian local politics shaped the Floyd County health program from the start. Unlike the analogous projects in New York City, Los Angeles, and Cleveland, OEO funds *didn't* go toward construction of new medical care facilities. Instead, the funds just subsidized a transportation network that shuffled patients to small private hospitals and about two dozen fee-for-service physicians, some of whom had received positions with the county health department. Lack of new facilities meant lack of fresh personnel that would've staffed them. It preserved the county's tightly guarded medical circles, and critics of the program later charged that its initial structure was conceived precisely to avoid disrupting the status quo in any way.[25]

What new construction there was came in the form of "outposts" staffed by eight "health care teams," "community aides," and public health nurses. But their main duties consisted of routing patients to private physicians, who received direct reimbursements from OEO and Medicare and Medicaid. Not all of the work was a wash. There were other useful services like the distribution of vitamins and basic courses on narcotics addiction, personal hygiene, and nutrition. But overall, given the $1.3 million the program was receiving a year, its central functions—providing transportation to private facilities that already existed— were glaringly modest compared to typical OEO health initiatives. The closest the program came to bringing anything *new* was its hiring of a dentist. Viewed in the most critical light, it all amounted to a cynical mechanism for funneling OEO money and patients' fees into the coffers of the Floyd County medical profession.[26]

The money funnel didn't keep running unchecked. By 1969, the program received scrutiny from OEO operatives, prompted by agitation from the Eastern Kentucky Welfare Rights Organization. The eastern Kentucky node of the burgeoning national welfare rights movement was becoming one of its most active.[27] Its bylaws read: "We are tired of being affected by decisions that are made by people we never see and don't even know exist. We should have a voice in the decisions now made by medical review teams and administrators." Like its counterparts, EKWRO had taken on inefficient distribution of federal welfare funds, and it was starting to protest strip mining, too. But by the late

1960s, health care in Floyd County drew more and more of the organization's attention.[28]

A key leader in EKWRO's fight was Eula Hall, a single mother of four who had grown up in the Floyd County coalfields, joined a local War on Poverty program, and had led a successful protest of 100 people over the board of education's refusal to serve free school lunches to the county's indigent population.[29] Hall's ascendance in the organization was notable, given that the group's early founding rhetoric, as historian Jessica Wilkerson has noted, was imbued with masculinity and an economic critique that centered heavily on how poverty undermined normative gender roles.[30] But even though its nominal leadership was made up of men, the "organizing backbone" of day-to-day political spadework consisted of women, who "had the most to gain or lose from welfare policies."[31]

For Hall, when it came to health, lack of lay governance translated into lousy treatment. Decades later, Hall detailed how a typical patient fared in the Floyd County program. It was, in short, an experience lacking basic dignity. She recalled patients, including herself, stuffed into Ford Broncos for the ride to the private physicians' offices, many located far in the county from patients' homes, where there "would already be a waiting room full of patients." Some of the rooms were poorly maintained, especially in the summer months, when it became "so dusty I [Hall] wouldn't even go in to see the doctor even though I had an appointment, because I'd be too dirty and couldn't see him. It would settle in your eyes."[32] Yet the physical conditions of the waiting rooms themselves might have been better than the actual impersonal treatment toward patients. On arrival, the "community aide" often read people's names and their problems aloud. When physician visits were finally complete, patients were sometimes left and forgotten, especially in towns with commercial districts and other activities that distracted those in charge of return transportation. "I'd get a call about six o'clock and so and so was stranded in Prestonsburg and I'd have to go get 'em," Hall remembered.

It was enough to spur OEO inspections. The findings were damning and supported Hall's assertions. After a few years of operation, there was still no formal bookkeeping. A total of $130,000 worth of funds had gone entirely unused without comment. Staffers purchased equipment without any clearly defined approval process.[33] Many resources seemed to be flowing to administrators, with one report remarking on the generosity of the self-rewarded fringe benefits. And the program's director, a physician named Russell D. Hall, ran his own practice and was able to devote only 20 percent of his time to overseeing the Floyd County operation, even though he was supposed to supervise the main employees. "He has neither the time nor the propensity to provide the strong, clear direction which the project now needs," one assessment read. "There was almost no supervision of the personnel and no one to make day by day management decisions. . . . Lacking strong leadership, the staff had taken on program responsibilities on a nonchalant basis," stated another.[34]

When it came to program operations, the transportation network itself—its core feature—was "inefficient." The outposts where patients went for initial intake were oddly located, often a burdensome distance from where actual patients lived. This required patients to make double trips: one to an inconveniently sited outpost, then another to the physician, a journey that could take as much as forty miles for just the first leg. Part of the problem stemmed from a rule implemented by the county's board of health, which limited program participation of nonspecialist physicians to those within Floyd County only, even if more conveniently located physicians happened to operate outside county boundaries.[35] It effectively gave Floyd County's private medical profession a monopoly on the approximately 20,000 patients who used the new OEO program, and it created patient bottlenecks, with some county physicians "seeing up to 100 people per day." The program compounded the matter by regularly admitting patients who exceeded the income requirements and should have been ineligible—but whose inclusion generated additional revenue from more reimbursements. Like most other agencies, the board of health was stacked with Floyd County political power brokers and health professionals, including a county judge named Henry Stumbo, a surgeon, a dentist, two physicians, a nurse, the county attorney, and the wife of the area's state representative. As one OEO inspector put it: "The physicians are receiving fees for care of the program's consumers, while establishing policy for the program."[36]

Fiscal chicanery occurred alongside the flouting of OEO guidelines. Rather than hire low-income residents, the program had become an overt source of cronyism. Eighty percent of its approximately 100 hires in the first three years, OEO found, had come from "middle or upper income groups." There was no public advertising of positions, and residents claimed that political connections were necessary for most employment. Several job descriptions were vague, with no language detailing "experience prerequisites, area of responsibility, and level of performance expected."[37] An inspector speculated that some positions had gone unfulfilled because those who controlled the program feared the presence of "outsiders" who might see how things operated.[38]

## The Futility of Amelioration

Shocking as the OEO reports' findings were, the tone was another matter entirely. Federal operatives were cautious about coming off too critically, fearful of reprisals from politicians connected to the county. Politically disempowered as Floyd County's population was, its House representative, Carl Perkins, was one of the most powerful congressmen in the United States, chair of the Committee on Education and Labor, and he just happened to oversee OEO's programs. In addition to using circumspect and diplomatic language, OEO framed the program's problems as fundamentally bureaucratic, merely in need of a few administrative tweaks. After a 1970 meeting in Washington, D.C., moderate reforms followed.[39] To firewall the program from the Floyd County government, OEO operatives transferred control of funds from the local board of health to a newly created and incorporated agency, Floyd County Comprehensive Health Services Program, Inc. It hired a new physician as a program director who could devote full dedicated time. And it implemented a "delegate board" that included eight low-income members, though they'd have to work alongside a dozen businesspeople and professionals.[40]

Yet reforms were only as effective as their enforceability, and OEO's subsequent actions continued to be reactive, mainly after EKWRO's prodding. Problems kept arising. One registered nurse working at an outpost complained that Earl Compton, in charge of a health education program, persistently declined to give concrete answers to her questions about her exact duties and goals. "You are the Team Leader, do what you think is right," she quoted him. Compton then mentioned promoting a friend of his. The nurse concluded, "This is why our program is lacking in key personnel, it's not what you know, it's who you know. In the past year Mr. Compton did not do anything for our consumers, nor did he contribute anything to my health aides."[41] Clara Mays, a nurse stationed at an outpost in Martin, Kentucky, claimed that the last time she saw Compton, he was "totally unprepared to conduct any class," while Josephine Williamson, writing from another location, noted that he had not even visited her outpost in six months and "did little to obtain materials for us in the way of health education."[42]

At the same time, Floyd County figures who'd initially taken over the health program maneuvered to retain control. They folded the newly created Floyd County Comprehensive Health Services entity into the Big Sandy Community Action Program (CAP), a more general social service agency funded by War on Poverty dollars, named after a nearby river. Its chairman was none other than county judge Henry Stumbo, a dominant figure in county politics who sat on the board of health, which had controlled the health program before being given the OEO boot. Big Sandy CAP was hardly a model program to oversee the project and not just because county cronies ran it. Earlier in 1970, OEO had faulted it for problems big and small. All were familiar to those who'd seen the Floyd County health program: sloppy record keeping, questionable purchasing, and loose administration. Many of its programs existed on paper only. In one outreach initiative designed to enroll eligible people onto food stamp rolls,

OEO found that "very little actual outreach is done" and that the staff hired for the program "spend most of their time in the office," not out in the field.[43] Activists from EKWRO had confronted Big Sandy CAP publicly about several pork barrel projects, including construction of a superfluous bridge, plus the hiring of personal friends who were paid bloated salaries.[44]

Unsurprisingly, these features persisted in the supposedly revamped Floyd County health program, and EKWRO renewed efforts against its administrators. The organization had recently formed an ad hoc Mud Creek Health Rights Committee, a reference to where its most active members, including Eula Hall, lived. One of its first tasks was to fight the transfer of Helen Wells, a Floyd County administrator, to the Mud Creek health outpost, accusing her of delaying elections to choose the health program's citizen board. "Helen Wells is not wanted or liked by the poor people on Mud Creek," EKWRO wrote. "Her attitude toward the poor people is bad: she always has been opposed to the organization on Mud Creek—but when they have to talk to her, she talks hateful to them."[45] In the fall of 1970, Hall organized a public demonstration of 200 at the county's public library over Wells, persistent nepotism in hiring practices, and poor patient treatment. At one meeting, she took the floor and asked "why the aides had been permitted to pack people into the program's vehicles like dogs, and why simple courtesy had not been exhibited to the poor."[46]

A parallel fight occurred over who'd lead the new program. Arnold Schechter, a young Chicago physician, had arrived on a full-time basis as project director. But he soon clashed with Big Sandy CAP, which promptly fired him. The firing had been bound to happen. Schechter and his interim predecessor, Glen Hentschel, had both tried to bring more outside physicians, especially specialists, into Floyd County, all while implementing OEO's suggested reforms. They'd failed, and former project director Russell Hall characterized Schechter, Hentschel, and OEO as interlopers bent on sabotaging the program, complaining at one point that "the new director was a physician rather than an Eastern Kentucky Boy who wanted to come back home."[47] When Schechter wanted to hire nine physicians for the program, his bosses reacted disingenuously, claiming that the county's limited number of physicians could serve the entire county.[48]

Schechter's firing for alleged "insubordination" set off a chain of events with enormous consequences. The Eastern Kentucky Welfare Rights Organization staged a protest on the steps of the county courthouse, which garnered the attention of the muckraking *Louisville Courier-Journal*, the most visible of Kentucky's newspapers. Other detractors soon emerged. William Poole, a reverend in Prestonsburg, the county's largest town, discussed stymied attempts to employ new physicians: "Few doctors in East Kentucky are able to give patients the individual time they would like. One need only to visit the hollows to behold an ocean of rotting and rotten teeth." The retaliatory dismissal of Schechter for

# SICK AND TIRED?

## SO ARE WE!

HAVE YOU EVER GONE TO THE HOSPITAL AND BEEN TURNED AWAY BECAUSE YOU COULDN'T PAY CASH IN ADVANCE???

HAVE YOU EVER WAITED FOR HOURS TO SEE A DOCTOR??? AND AFTER WAITING HOURS YOU WERE SEEN ONLY BY THE NURSE AND SENT TO THE DRUGSTORE TO PICK UP PILLS AND DRUGS THAT NEVER SEEM TO HELP???

HAVE YOU EVER SEEN A SPECIALIST??? DID YOU HAVE TO TRAVEL 120 MILES EACH WAY TO LEXINGTON TO SEE ONE???

We are tired of waiting all day to see doctors and having to travel to Lexington to see specialists!

For the last three years millions of dollars in public money has been coming into Floyd County's Comprehensive Health Program to pay for health care for poor people. All over the country this kind of program has set up health clinics and hired doctors to serve the people. WHAT HAS HAPPENED TO $$$$$$ MILLIONS $$$$$$ HERE IN FLOYD COUNTY??? The local doctors, pharmacists and politicians have taken control of the Comprehensive Health Program and have kept THE POOR PEOPLE FROM SETTING UP CLINICS AND HIRING THEIR OWN DOCTORS. So far they have managed to keep all the money for themselves!!!!

Dr. Schecter, the director of the Comprehensive Health Program, tried to bring in more doctors and specialists to Floyd County. WHAT HAPPENED TO HIM??? He was fired by the county doctors, pharmacists and politicians who are afraid they will lose some of their money.

THIS IS OUR PROGRAM!!!! THE MONEY WAS GIVEN TO FLOYD COUNTY TO PROVIDE HEALTH SERVICES FOR POOR PEOPLE. WE THINK THE PROGRAM SHOULD BE CONTROLLED BY THE PEOPLE IT IS SUPPOSED TO SERVE.

WE WANT THE COMPREHENSIVE HEALTH PROGRAM CHANGED TO FIT THE NEEDS OF THE PEOPLE . . . SO THAT THE PEOPLE WHO USE IT WILL GET BETTER SERVICE AND THE PEOPLE WHO WORK IN IT WILL BE ABLE TO DO A BETTER JOB.

If you would like to know more about what Comprehensive Health is supposed to do for you ... And if you would like a chance to say what kinds of health services you need and want ...

COME TO A PUBLIC HEARING ON HEALTH CARE IN EASTERN KENTUCKY

Time:          Sunday, March 28, 1971, 1:00 p.m.
Place:         P.A.C.E. Community Center, Rt.23, Allen, Kentucky
Sponsored by:  Eastern Kentucky Welfare Rights Organization (EKWRO)
               c/o Eula Hall, Chairman, Health Committee
               Craynor, Kentucky    Phone: (606) 587-2246

Leaflet distributed in Floyd County on Comprehensive Health Services program, March 28, 1971.

*Source*: Box D-093, Folder 7, Carl Perkins Papers, Special Collections and Archives, Eastern Kentucky University, Richmond, Ky.

his efforts, the Reverend Poole suggested, only made the situation worse. It was "difficult to see how the people are benefitting from . . . rejection of staffing the Comp. Health program with 'outside' personnel as virtually every Comp. Health program in the nation does."[49]

The Office of Economic Opportunity, meanwhile, returned to inspect the program with an aggressiveness absent the first time round. The Eastern Kentucky Welfare Rights Organization had established a communication channel with Leon Cooper, a Black OEO administrator to whom Hall sent documents about the program, each time urging more investigations.[50] Cooper, who also had a hand in settling some of the New York City and Los Angeles OEO disputes, started visiting eastern Kentucky. He encountered hostility, not to mention race-baiting toward his presence, a welcome that did nothing to endear the Floyd County health program's administrators to swarming OEO auditors.[51] The federal office soon issued another damning review, writing that the recipients of OEO funds had "failed to develop a health care program which emphasizes comprehensive family-oriented health care for the low income residents of Floyd County" and that the transportation network operated "in a haphazard fashion." Its assessment this time, though, got to the exact roots of the problem. Program heads were blatantly gobbling OEO dollars for self-enrichment. One board member made purchases for his own private business, and several others hired family members as employees without regard to qualifications. A Prestonsburg physician, Douglas Adams, was a part-time owner in a local drug store where a large number of the programs' patients had been directed for prescriptions. The owners of the drug store, in turn, had financial stakes in a Prestonsburg nursing home owned by Eleanor Robinson, chairwoman of the Floyd County program's board.[52] Proposed mechanisms for participatory governance had yet to take off, with elections and meetings irregularly called, often at the last minute and in bad weather to deter attendance. Reprisals and threats were routine. The investigators found that Schechter's firing was just the first in a number of similar actions. "Patients who are actively involved in community affairs," they charged, "have been intimidated as to their employment and the employment of their relatives. These individuals have also been warned that they would experience difficulty in obtaining health, social and municipal services to which they are entitled." Vocally discontent employees received threatening phone calls and found that administrators tampered with their personnel files.

It was a disheartening situation, but it engendered a forceful reaction showcasing the power of a savvy grassroots activist response. Alongside OEO's formal work, EKWRO and another group called Mountain People's Rights held massive hearings, creating foment among residents. One gathering featured 250 witnesses who recounted experiences with the program. A participant, Maggie

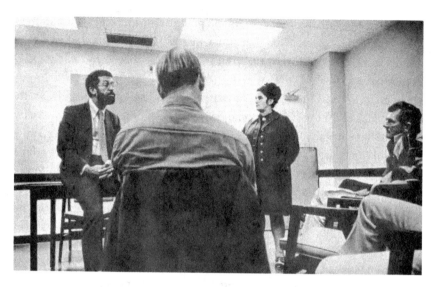

**Eula Hall (EKWRO) and Leon Cooper (OEO) meeting, ca. 1970–71.** Hall and Cooper lead a meeting at the height of the Floyd County health struggles. Cooper and OEO came to side with EKWRO, though meetings could sometimes become contentious because of EKWRO's perception that OEO's pace was insufficiently forceful.
*Source: Mountain Life and Work*, November 1971.

Hall, recalled being charged on a reimbursement card for "18 days of hospital care and 44 days in a nursing home," even though she'd only spent five days in a hospital and none at the nursing home. Another patient suspected that she was suffering from uterine bleeding but was never even examined by her physician.[53]

It was all enough for OEO to threaten termination of funds. Big Sandy CAP's defense was shrewd, if cynical, and turned on its head the communitarian foundations of the maximum feasible participation requirement. It invoked community defensively and cast OEO requirements as an invitation for interlopers to disrupt local life. "Why can the Office of Health Affairs [OEO's health division] in Washington, D.C., be permitted to plan and write a program for local people?" asked one administrator in protest.[54] This line of defense wasn't without some support among the larger Floyd County public, not all of which supported EKWRO's and other protestors' efforts. The writer of one letter to Judge Stumbo from a resident in Cliff, Kentucky, had heard about the conflicts around the program and concluded: "I think we have enough good people here in F.C. [Floyd County] to run this program without bringing other people in from other states to run it."[55] But mild dissents did little to reverse the traction of OEO or EKWRO. The latter had grown confident enough to challenge Representative Perkins himself, who had long avoided any direct intervention in the program's affairs. "Because you have not acted on your responsibilities as our Congressman," EKWRO activists wrote to him, "we can only assume that you are in collusion with the local doctors and politicians who control the Comprehensive Health Program. And that you, Congressman Perkins, are benefitting as they are for the political favoritism and the political pork barrel that the OEO money has provided."[56]

Because EKWRO had forged links between the hollows of Floyd County and the halls of OEO's Washington offices, rapid policy response followed. By May and June 1971, the program was on its last legs after OEO served Big Sandy CAP and the board of Floyd County Comprehensive Health Services a final warning notice. By then, the program's travails had gained national attention. A late turning point came with resignations from nurses. One of them, Veronica Click, was humiliated by her supervisor, Helen Wells, who posted a copy of the resignation on a public bulletin board. The most consequential and resonant of the resignations came from a Malvina Thomson, who identified herself as none other than Judge Henry Stumbo's own great-niece, before writing as well about Wells's conduct, lack of proper credentials for her position, and the loss of "time, energy, money," plus "mental and physical strain" caused by being "responsible to one that has no health education only a political tie." The resignations sapped the morale of many remaining employees, who in an anonymous note from "The Entire Staff of Incompetency" wrote: "We are losing two valuable, resourceful, capable, dependable, reliable, truthful, honest, lovable, energetic, knowledgeable, persevering[,] adaptable, commendable, compassionate, dedicated, experts, community minded, possessing great insight about the ability of fellow sub-professionals, and in general women with tremendous humanitarian instincts, honorable, humble, considerate, heroic, patriotic, revered."[57] A month later, OEO formally suspended the program's funds, bringing the five-year Floyd County health care experiment to a close.[58]

## The Ambiguities of Medical Governance Demands

At the end of her resignation letter, Thomson had asked: "Who does poor people look to when in need of Medical help?"[59] In the wake of a governance crisis—and one that went in favor of those who waged the battle—her question carried more profound implications than she probably realized at the time. The Eastern Kentucky Welfare Rights Organization and its supporters had broken the grip that an entrenched county political machine had held on a program that received almost $2 million to target medical maldistribution. But the victory raised larger questions about what governance victories meant in the grander scheme. After all, as Thomson's question noted, the challenge to corrupt local governance of the program had resulted in the parallel loss of the program, after OEO pulled funding. Thomson's question was even more important beyond eastern Kentucky, as President Nixon in his second term would soon signal his intention to wind down many of the programs it sponsored.

The Floyd County episode, more than any of the other neighborhood health projects in the country, illustrated the importance of the administrative mechanisms upholding the community governance imperative that swept through health planning during the War on Poverty years. Across the country, OEO functionaries played a crucial oversight function, intervening in response to locally reported disputes over ignorance of its guidelines. In New York and Los Angeles, that took the form of adjudicating between community health councils and the organization that had received its funds—the latter, in both cases, an academic medical center. In eastern Kentucky, where no such council had even been properly elected, intervention from the top eventually shut down rampant misuse of funds.

The federalist structure of War on Poverty programs was double-edged. In previous generations of federal legislation, state and local actors jockeyed for and often won more control of program administration. This was most notoriously the case with distribution of Aid to Families with Children and Social Security Act benefits in the South, part of a larger effort where "the South's representatives built ramparts within the policy initiatives of the New Deal and the Fair Deal to safeguard their region's social organization," in other words, Jim Crow, typically by providing administrators from below with huge discretion in how they allocated benefits and allowing them to do so in a racially discriminatory manner.[60]

Yet during the 1960s, in health care, many policy makers, including architects of the OEO neighborhood health centers program, believed that decentralization allowed for better provisioning of services, particularly through the hiring of local workers intimately familiar with local knowledge and trust networks. But these structures of decentralization opened the door to problems on frequent exhibit. Money typically flowed indirectly to an intermediary—an academic medical center, a university, a county—and placed the burden of realizing accountability mechanisms on users of the programs themselves and their advocates. This was emotionally taxing and time-consuming work, requiring concerted organizing efforts, both with Washington and on the ground at home. In Floyd County particularly, it was outright dangerous. The county health program, government agencies, and local businesses were one and the same and influenced residents' daily lives and well-being.

The problem had ramifications beyond any one local facility, whether Floyd County or otherwise. In 1972, a year after the height of the conflicts, the prestigious academic journal *Science* commissioned a lengthy story on the health care battles in eastern Kentucky. Its author explained the odd story choice by writing that "such facets of OEO health care as family-centered preventative medicine, salaried group practice, training of paramedicals, and consumer participation in decision making, have become elements in the debate over national health insurance. . . . And if Congress pours more money into the existing health care system on a national scale, the story of Floyd County could be repeated many times over."[61] The article highlighted the dilemma of queueing up abundant new health dollars alone without clearer planning over how to monitor where they ended up, a threat exacerbated by the enduring federalist impulse in U.S. health policy.

These were fairly abstract debates for the people of Floyd County. In the here and now, residents faced the prospect of a governance victory bearing no tangible fruits. After toppling the Floyd County machine, what now? The EKWRO organizers seemed to have anticipated the dilemma and had worked steadily on writing alternate proposals for a funded health program with a physician staff. In 1972, EKWRO's Health Committee launched an eight-week health program headed by a six-member team consisting of physicians and medical and nursing students. With a dozen teenagers who went door to door, they conducted 184 household visits and screened 711 people for anemia, low blood-sugar levels, and enteric diseases. The organizers hoped to lay prefiguratively a foundation for their own health program that would perform in all the ways that the prior initiative had failed, especially when it came to participatory governance and having its own physician staff. It planned to fund the program via third-party insurance payments and philanthropic donations.

Achieving local self-sufficiency without the fiscal muscle of OEO was, alas, an uphill task. The experience of seeing OEO funds in a boondoggle, combined with the refusal of surrounding private hospitals to accept indigent patients, resulted in an inward turn and suspicion of outsiders, but from a different angle. Several EKWRO members now wanted to pursue a self-sufficient route. "I'm looking forward for us to be working more alone to try to get doctors into our communities where the people can be served without going and being turned away with a snobby nose as we have right along in these hospitals," said George Tucker. In turn, this self-sufficiency, organizers argued, would actually allow for more effective realization of medical care run by people aware of how patients actually lived both inside and outside the clinic. "The reality of preventive medicine," read one proposal, required "changing the environment, changing working conditions," and other forms of "social change" to which EKWRO had been more broadly engaged. "Real preventive medicine" of the sort it hoped to practice "is not a light undertaking, but one that requires the full strength of a community. If it is seen as an attempt by aliens to change a community's way of life, it will be rejected. People will never change their way of life or fight political battles necessary to change their social condition because a stranger, separated by his professional and class status, tells them to. Ultimately, the process of preventive medicine must be carried out by we the people, who are the 'patients.'"[62]

Lofty ideals were one thing, actual operations another. A year later, during planning for the new facilities, program organizers admitted that "we have no idea what the success of our efforts will be, but we intend to try everything to keep our program going."[63] Despite the challenge of permanent sustainability, the group managed to raise enough funds, much of it from UMWA locals and $1,400 in seed money from the Appalachian Volunteers, which was folding, to open up the Mud Creek Clinic, staffed by two part-time physicians and a small team of nurses and paraprofessionals. Within a year, they moved into Eula Hall's thirty-dollars-a-month rental house, initially serving patients two days a week.[64]

But an independent clinic could go only so far, especially as UMWA donations became increasingly unreliable. In 1977, Hall and the clinic's staff agreed to merge with Big Sandy Health Care, Inc., an incorporated nonprofit that ran a cluster of clinics in the five-county Big Sandy area that the prior OEO program had served. Alarmingly, some holdovers from the Floyd County project, including its former chair, Eleanor Robinson, were involved in this new organization. But EKWRO's agitation had produced some important checks, including the presence of an EKRWO member on the board. And patients were no longer shuttled to private physicians and preexisting facilities. The Big Sandy operation instead employed its own staff and built its own infrastructure using funds allocated by the new Department of Health, Education, and Welfare's Health Services Development program, a successor to OEO's health program.

On paper, many features of the program reflected the influence of not just EKWRO but other neighborhood health initiatives nationwide. In contrast to the impersonal, even dehumanizing, prior initiative, Big Sandy formally declared that "health care should be administered with compassion and dignity." It employed "local people, not professional health educators," hired directly from the area. The clinical staff itself worked under a health team system, holding health conferences with patients and their families. "In a well-knit team, local people and professionals can become momentary peers in a common cause," read one statement of the program's philosophy.[65]

Yet things were hardly idyllic. Quentin Allen, the program's founder, accused the EKWRO-affiliated board member of fueling conflict, writing that "the tactic of confrontation and unfounded accusation continues as their most viable weapon in seeking relief for the assorted tensions affecting this polarized group," and relations with the Mud Creek Clinic were persistently antagonistic.[66] By March 1975, however, other board members had tired of Allen, after he hired a county judge's daughter-in-law for a job, and they ousted him. Other complaints centered on questionable administrative practices. A sliding scale had yet to be implemented, and orders for supplies often had gone unprocessed for weeks. Final decisions about new hires were also kept in the dark until employees already started working. Much of the opposition was led by Robert Young, a young new physician who had received death threats from anonymous physicians in the area after voicing his concerns.[67]

Allen's firing came at an opportune time, since Hall and the Mud Creek Clinic worked on a shoe-string budget with no centralized and reliable stream of financial support. And Hall contended with another source of stress as well, working on Mud Creek Clinic affairs while warding off a physically abusive ex-husband by regularly carrying a gun in self-defense each time she left the facility.[68] Sparse resources had resulted in an inability to recruit a stable physician force and diminished access to in-patient hospitalization services.[69] For the Mud Creek Clinic, incorporation into the five-county Big Sandy program solved its sustainability problem but compromised the autonomous vision to which at least some EKWRO organizers had aspired. As facilities elsewhere had learned—from small neighborhood facilities such as Gouverneur in New York to large county hospitals such as those in Los Angeles—the romance of the local, the autonomous, the participatory, and the communitarian was difficult to sustain given the budgetary scale required for infrastructural upkeep, personnel costs, and, in the case of outpatient clinics, hospitalization costs for patients requiring further inpatient care. Going it alone was doubly difficult in a region with historically severe medical maldistribution and few state and local sources of additional funds. Mud Creek's incorporation into Big Sandy was a compromise from total self-sufficiency but an ultimately tolerable one.

## Community Health in a Landscape of Hardship

Merging into a multicounty health care network put the Mud Creek Clinic on stable grounding. It also raised questions about Appalachian health projects writ large.

Several other similar clinics and networks existed in other parts of eastern Kentucky. All operated amid a landscape of hardship deleterious to the health and well-being of residents. The water supply around Mud Creek, for instance, had long been associated with enteric disease in the area. In 1958, a U.S. Public Health Service (USPHS) team of investigators had visited southeastern Kentucky and found that of eleven locations studied, Mud Creek was the only one where none of the households in the research sample contained a flush toilet or indoor hot and cold running water. Nearly all residents relied on dug wells for drinking water, 50 percent of which contained 100 or more coliforms per 100 milliliter water sample, the highest category measured. "In most instances, the water probably was contaminated both during drawing operations and by surface drainage" and other routine usage, wrote the study team. Rectal swabs for a number of parasitic worms and bacterial pathogens showed that a cluster of five small hollows that included Mud Creek reported the highest percentages of various *Shigella* species and *Ascaris* and *Trichuris* intestinal worms.[70]

In presenting the findings, the USPHS study explored connections between enteric diseases and living environments—namely, sanitary infrastructure and overcrowded housing. Although it ultimately assigned primary importance to sanitation, it didn't dismiss consideration of living conditions and economics, either, noting particularly that overcrowding—defined as more than 1.5 persons per room—was positively associated with a higher incidence of diarrheal disease and *Shigella* and *Ascaris*. The report stopped short of considering the larger reasons for the infrastructural deficits that it identified as the chief commonality among areas with higher enteric disease risks. Even if the researchers didn't draw direct links, there were hints, though, that they understood that more fundamental roots behind the problem existed. The authors, for instance, devoted extended sections of the report to discussing high unemployment in the region—35 percent in Mud Creek—and the effects of the coal industry's decline on people's ability to sustain themselves.[71]

A decade after the USPHS study, the EKWRO's health team found that these conditions had changed only slightly. During its door-to-door screening program in 1972, a little more than half of all stool samples taken contained at least one of four parasites (*Ascaris*, *Trichuris*, hookworm, *Strongyloides*), with stools taken from children aged six to fifteen exhibiting the highest prevalence, at 70 percent. Although use of a centralized water system and drilled wells had increased, water from dug wells was still common. A little under 80 percent of such wells contained "heavy contamination," defined as 500 coliform colonies per 100 cubic centimeters. Eighty percent of residents still used outdoor privies, resulting in "contamination of gardens and soil with human waste."[72] Successful earlier campaigns against hookworm in other parts of the South seemed to have bypassed Mud Creek entirely.[73]

The most dispiriting part of the EKWRO assessment, however, had nothing to do with sanitary infrastructure. It came when team members noted the high number of people taking pharmaceuticals to calm themselves. They wrote about feeling "struck by the large number of adults on 'nerve pills' and tranquilizers. Ninety-two people or slightly less than one-third of the adults reported that they were currently taking 'nerve pills.' Most commonly these were phenobarbital, but also included mellaril, thorazine, elavil, and other anti-depressants." But the conclusions were obvious: "This practice seems to be both a reflection of the economic and social pressures under which people live as well as the medical practice in the area," a reference to the Floyd County medical cronies.[74] Medical care—even when done the right way—was but one component in the health of the population. It was bound in a manifold of other health influences that EKWRO members were uncovering. This was an epiphany similar to the one Rodney Powell had when he'd testified about Watts's deeper and more fundamental inequities—beyond just lack of medicine—as he stood before Congress.

Then there was the problem of scale. Even a network such as Big Sandy Health Care was still just one part in a health care system that was fragmented and uneven, especially when it came to large hospital services that primary care clinics couldn't cover. The Eastern Kentucky Welfare Rights Organization had recently filed a lawsuit, one largely quixotic and symbolic, against the U.S. Treasury Department over charitable tax breaks given to private hospitals that refused to see indigent patients. The effort grew from the Mud Creek Clinic's battles with the frequent turning away of indigent patients by the surrounding network of Appalachian Regional Hospitals. At a 1975 public hearing, residents testified about trouble receiving hospital care. Among them was a woman from Marrowbone, Kentucky, who "took her father, suffering from pneumonia, to the Pikeville Methodist Hospital, where she claims he was denied treatment until she made arrangements to pay a 20-year-old bill. Later, when suffering from a stroke and heart attack, he was allegedly forced to wait two hours in the emergency room while the doctor on call traveled from Elkhorn City to Pikeville." Another patient from Melvin, Kentucky, "with asthma, arthritis, lung trouble and low blood" was told "she had to pay $15 before she could see a doctor. She was also unable to obtain medication until the next day 'because the pharmacy was closed at night,' even for the emergency room." A mother of two from Pike County reported that "it costs $40 to get an ambulance to come to her home and take her to Pikeville," the nearest town with a hospital. "You must pay before they take you. . . . I ain't got $40. I hope I never have to use one," she told the audience. Their comments showed that efforts like the OEO program, or other similar single-site projects, had not produced something resembling a coherent regional system.[75]

Others commented on the larger structures in which these patients were embedded. Robert Young, the physician who'd challenged and eventually forced Quentin Allen's resignation from Big Sandy Health Care, discussed the excessive concentration of specialists centered in urban Lexington, where the University of Kentucky's medical school was located, and openly wondered whether stricter "controls" over where physicians could practice would be required. Toward the end of the meeting, Eula Hall told the audience that they needed to be "putting pressure on facilities which will in turn force good service. People with a small amount of money get a small amount of service." But the battle would continue to be steep and unequally waged, especially considering how much effort had gone to keeping the Mud Creek Clinic alive—and just barely—during its first couple years. In 1976, the U.S. Supreme Court dismissed EKWRO's lawsuit on technical grounds, arguing that it lacked standing to bring the case on behalf of all indigent patients.[76]

A fractured nonsystem was easier to diagnose, in short, than to repair. In 1975, the Southeastern Kentucky Regional Health Demonstration Project ceased operation after dispersing grants to more than eighty projects. Its planners reflected on the difficulty of fusing decentralization with regional coordination, to say nothing of implementing participatory governance. One administrator wrote about different entities, each obeying distinct dictates: from individual projects to area development districts to the Appalachian Regional Commission. Others pointed to the obstinacy of local jurisdictions: "I know the people in this area well enough—their loyalty to their community, their suspiciousness—to doubt that we'd get anywhere." Still another pointed to naked self-interest: "Everybody wanted their little community hospital to be designated as a regional hospital because then they could get more equipment."[77]

Still, by the 1970s, medical maldistribution looked considerably different from how it did in the 1950s, when the high-profile reports about the problem had been published. In some places, philanthropic and governmental construction funds had created a favorable facilities-to-patient ratio. In Clay County, southwest of Floyd, the Frontier Nursing Service conducted a health survey and discovered that a surprisingly high 91 percent of residents had access, in theory, to a private physician and that 63 percent reported "more than one source of health care to use as a combination of services" if they needed it. Sixty percent reported access to three hospitals in the area, while others drew services from the Frontier Nursing Service's new station or the county health department. But an increase in medical care infrastructure masked class heterogeneity and ability to use it, as the local hearings demonstrated. In this respect, Appalachia wasn't that different from the East Side of Cleveland at its worst. Among those interviewed, many reported that the high cost of the care itself impeded more regular usage of services. "Although everyone could get out for acute care," the nursing service's field report read, "many people stated that because of the above problems they would have sought care more often if it had been more accessible." Some respondents reported, too, that limited resources meant that they were consigned to facilities featuring "long waits to see the doctor (and then only briefly), incomplete diagnostic work-ups, inconvenient clinic hours, and doctors more concerned with making money than with taking care of people."[78]

Another report by the Appalachian Regional Commission confirmed infrastructural improvements in Central Appalachia. The commission noted an overall rise in medical bed-to-patient ratios. But as had others, it then stressed that for a quarter of the population in medical indigency (and many others near it), strides made against maldistribution were themselves maldistributed. "The hospital system runs at or near capacity by apparently overserving those who can pay, while it is unable to cover much more than the bare emergency needs of the Medically Indigent," the commission's report concluded. Institutional trust funds supported some charity care at small private hospitals in the region, but they were "small, scattered, and produce little income."[79]

Moreover, the sustainability of any new infrastructure was precarious. Two common systems of insurance repayment—Medicaid and the UMWA's imperiled welfare and retirement funds—faced constant turbulence.[80] In the middle of the decade, the Appalachian Regional Hospitals system, itself a response to the sustainability crisis faced by the United Mine Workers' Miners Memorial Hospitals, found itself strapped for cash. It defaulted on some long-term loans, requiring state intervention and Appalachian Regional Commission funds to regain its footing. Compounding the problem were physicians and institutions who refused to accept Medicaid altogether because of dissatisfaction over reimbursement rates. This was a problem not exclusive to the region but one whose consequences were more pronounced, given the area's high rate of medical indigency. For the regional commission, the trouble of Central Appalachian medical care couldn't be analyzed in a vacuum. "Many of the medical problems in Central Appalachia," the commission concluded, "are a direct consequence of economic causes," such as troubling employment trends and industrial transformation.[81]

Medical care and Appalachian health, in other words, were embedded in a number of larger processes. The most dramatic was the advent of strip mining and the risks it posed to health, whether conceived more narrowly (water pollutants) or more broadly (forced displacement from one's home). Whether in Mud Creek, the Red Bird Valley, Floyd County, or Clay County, the strip mining of eastern Kentucky had proceeded apace since the mid-1960s. Projects similar in scale and mission to the Mud Creek Clinic and Big Sandy Health Care had opened in Harlan, Leslie, Knott, Letcher, and Perry Counties. But these were all places with conditions like those of Mud Creek in Floyd County and where residents were suffering, first from the loss of underground mining jobs resulting from the sharp rise in strip mining, then in turn from the environmental health effects of dual economic and technological change. Given the presence of these multiple influences on health, how much of a public health impact, many in the region asked, did these local single-site medical care experiments really have?

Eula Hall's daily itinerary reflected her and the EKWRO's acknowledgment of this fundamental dilemma of community health. Hall dealt with it by doing. Besides the Mud Creek Clinic, Hall's days were occupied protesting Floyd County strip mines, monitoring water pollution, and fighting the county's disbursements of food stamps. All carried major health implications. All were connected. And all grew out of processes including but also beyond the local.

Like many others working on medical care projects in the region, Hall had long understood that health included, but was more than, just local health care itself.

This reality was something that others like Hall around the country knew. In New York City, organizers with the Lower East Side Health Neighborhood Council–South had pointed out that poverty was the common link among those whom they surveyed door to door about their health problems. In Los Angeles, there was Rodney Powell, testifying before Congress, and Milton Roemer, assessing Watts for the official riot commission. They'd commented, respectively, on unpardonable levels of hunger in the area and wondered whether what were framed as "health problems" were really just the "final excrescence of malfunctions and failures in our whole society." In Cleveland, the Urban League argued that addressing health required understanding "the relation between low socio-economic status and social problems," while the Welfare Foundation of Cleveland's working definition of health came to include guarantees not just for medical care access but for food, housing, education, the end of racism, and remunerative work. Health wasn't just the doctor's office but something akin to Roosevelt's unfulfilled Second Bill of Rights. Whether in New York City, Los Angeles, Cleveland, or Central Appalachia, people who asked these questions came to wonder whether what they could do in their vicinity was enough. In other words: Whither localism?

This was the question that opened this book. And it was a question community health advocates would ask into the twenty-first century, just as a certain community organizer did when he entered his postcollegiate life.

# Conclusion

## Localism Is Dead—Long Live Localism!
## Or: All Health Politics Is Local*

This book spans the midcentury United States. The last events recounted in it occurred in the mid-1980s, right when the person whose story began this volume was just getting started.

When we last left Barack Obama, he'd thrown himself into work he found exhausting, fulfilling, and inspiring. Yet after a couple years of it, the community organizer began to wonder: a hard-fought victory against a negligent landlord here, a small grant secured for job training at a single school there, pockets of increased lay empowerment now and then, all against constant uphill battles for slim fiscal resources. What did it all mean when it came to larger social change? Perhaps not much; and so, community organizing began to feel something like the whack-a-mole carnival game, where for every beaver wacked with a foam mallet, three more just jumped right up. Likewise, for every community win, there were a dozen new exhausting battles to fight. And for all the laypersons whose political capacities were cultivated, realized, and activated, individuals were still constrained by entrenched political machines and obstinate, self-serving, sometimes cynical, elected officials at city hall. It all played out atop a shaky economic context: in this case, a rapidly disappearing decimated steel industry and, with it, jobs, pensions, and overall economic security.

In these circumstances, triumphs in local politics, Obama concluded, were bound to be pyrrhic. If one wanted to defy these limits, one had to transcend the intrinsic bounds of the local. That meant grabbing the formal levers of power at the highest levels possible. The block, the neighborhood, the city, and even the larger metropolitan area weren't it. So the organizer shifted his sights and astounded his friends by saying—with a straight face—that he had his eye on nothing less than the federal level and the executive office: yes, that one. It'd involve a sojourn in Cambridge (Harvard Law School) before a return to the Midwest, where he'd then plot his next steps (state senate, U.S. Senate, White House). Recollecting his thinking about local organizing at that time, he'd later recount that "the victories we achieved were extraordinarily modest" and that "the work that I did in those communities changed me much more than I changed the communities."[1] That was partly because they took place "in the armpit of the region, as far away from the center of power as you can get," recalled one of his close colleagues from those years.[2] To really effect change, you had to move from the "armpit" to the center, where the direct levers connected to the "center of power" were located.

## Localism at a Crossroads

Obama was attuned to dynamics and contradictions in local politics—its potential and its limits—that surfaced in the six cases you've read. In the four decades since this book's stories ended, the contradictions of localism have only sharpened. Consider two developments. In health care, Amazon, a multinational conglomerate then periodically flirting with a market capitalization of $1 trillion—which it's long since busted past—announced in 2018 that it was stepping into a new sector: health care. It'd embark, in partnership with J. P. Morgan Chase and billionaire investor Warren Buffett's Berkshire Hathaway firm, on a triple-titan entry into the American health care system, one with as yet nebulous goals that nonetheless prompted the *Wall Street Journal* to remark that the entity could pose "a potential threat to existing industries."[3] What that threat might entail was a mystery but could have included everything from operating its own primary care clinics to entering the insurance industry, acquiring distressed hospitals, getting into pharmaceutical purchasing, or replacing traditional health services delivery with online variants, among other possibilities. Alas, we never found out. The Big Three pulled the plug on the project in January 2021, having found the American health care system too labyrinthine and impermeable—at least for now—for even the most ambitious and well capitalized of entrants.[4]

But that hasn't stopped others. Venture capital and private equity–backed upstarts dot the landscape to the cool tune of $41.5 billion invested in so-called digital health between 2010 and 2017, an astonishing increase of 858 percent.[5] Special-purpose acquisition companies and initial public offerings for such firms regularly make the pages of the financial press. Then there's the recent wave of institutional consolidation—between 2007 and 2012, "432 merger and acquisition deals . . . involving 835 hospitals"—that analysts expect to continue into the coming decades, with economists David Cutler and Fiona Scott writing that "upcoming policy changes seem likely to further reinforce the pressure to consolidate."[6] Where it all heads is anybody's guess, but it signals a medical sector on the precipice of epoch-changing metamorphosis, even if it may come in fits, starts, and occasional abandonment. All these new developments and new players—Big Banks, Big Tech, Big Medicine, and whatever else—make local struggles over medicine seem bygone, modest, quaint.

That is even more the case when one turns to the biggest public health challenge of not just a generation but possibly humanity: climate change. By the end of the first decade of the twenty-first century, it became clear that rising temperatures were a problem that could not be solved at a single scale: city, county, state, province, or country. It was a global problem, and it required a global solution, coupled with radical changes in production and consumption patterns and the very way people lived. The world needed "treating an emergency like an emergency" so that "all our energies can go into action, rather than into screaming about the need for action," wrote the journalist and activist Naomi Klein.[7] Anything less—atomized, scattered, walled off—amounted to emptying the rapidly rising oceans with a teacup. As with analogs in the health care system, the graveness of climate change made local environmental politics of the past look, well, myopic.

And yet, despite its obvious limitations, the local impulse has powerfully persisted into twenty-first-century health politics. Medicine and public health in particular have seen a resurgence of interest in tackling problems not from 30,000 feet on high but from the ground up, where they begin and are ultimately experienced by everyday people. Two similar emerging frameworks, Health in All Policies (HiAP) and the Robert Wood Johnson Foundation's Culture of Health, are examples. Their adherents attempt to make health a society-wide "shared value." The hope is to unite those working in health with those outside the health sector—in housing, transportation, and community development, for example—for the common cause of population health improvement. This is achieved more effectively, so goes the thinking, than any efforts conducted by a single sector in isolation. It is at the level of municipalities, spearheaded by local health departments, where HiAP and the Culture of Health are being most rapidly implemented, with one group of writers highlighting the "pivotal role that multisector partnerships could play in transforming regional health and well-being."[8] Localism's persistence is also seen in the growing incorporation of community health workers "who can integrate knowledge of the local social service milieu with knowledge of patients' individual circumstances," acting as critical conduits between laypersons and the medical institutions that serve them: itself a legacy of War on Poverty–era health programs explored here.[9] This imperative has been even more pronounced in the field of global health, where organizations designing health interventions for developing countries have increasingly hired community health workers familiar with microlevel local context rather than deploying one-size-fits all programs from outside, with one eminence grise of the field recently declaring that doing so constitutes "the very highest standard of care available to the poor who live with chronic disease."[10] These trends mark a reversal from one identified by health policy expert Mark Schlesinger, datable to the mid-1990s, when interest from policy makers in such community-oriented approaches grew lukewarm after their heyday in the 1960s and 1970s.[11]

Localism has also played an unexpected role in climate change politics. It didn't look that way in 2015, when 196 countries, under United Nations auspices, entered the so-called Paris Agreement, pledging to curb carbon emissions with the goal of preventing global temperature increases beyond 2°C. Cautious optimism was the mood of the conference where the pact had been hashed out. Here was a global solution for a global problem—and now one with the commitment of the United States, long a holdout when it had come to previous attempts at addressing climate change as a global community. United Nations Secretary-General Ban Ki-moon declared: "I have listened to people—the young, the poor and the vulnerable, including indigenous peoples, from every corner of the globe. They have demanded that world leaders act to safeguard their well-being and that of generations to come. Here in Paris, we have heeded their voices—as was our duty."[12] The triumphant afterglow didn't last. A couple of years and one presidential election later, the United States announced that it intended to pull out of the accord, casting an ominous pall on the prospects of climate change mitigation. Ban, now having departed his office, wrote that he was "alarmed and disappointed at the inadequate pace of progress, especially by the major polluting economies."[13]

It all couldn't have come at a worse time. Twenty years into the twenty-first century, climate change activists could no longer be dismissed as kooky granola catastrophists crying wolf. Scenes of weeks-long forest fires in California and New South Wales looked outright apocalyptic and straight out of a Hollywood special-effects-laden scientific fiction film. But fiction it was not; rather, it was the new reality and the new normal: fires, flooding, polar vortexes, ever frequent hurricanes, record heat waves, melting ice sheaths the size of countries, and drought. And yet, with larger cracks in global governance more generally, a global response to climate change suddenly looked a lot less dependable.

Enter localism. If leadership wasn't going to come at the global and federal levels, then it would come from regions below them. American mayors who had been working together on climate change for more than a decade now felt an urgently renewed sense of purpose, whether they headed large metropolises or small towns. Now, in direct response to federal dereliction of duty, they pledged to work directly with the United Nations in achieving both the Paris climate goals and their own, spelled out in the U.S. Conference of Mayors' Climate Protection Agreement, whose participants vow to curb carbon emissions in their jurisdictions to 1990 levels.[14] It now contains more than 1,000 signatories. Looking at the larger cities on the list, it isn't hard to see why so many signed so rapidly: Los Angeles, New York City, Miami, and the first to commit, Seattle. All have already been hit—and will be hit even harder—by the effects of climate change. At the C40 World Mayors Summit, held in 2019, Los Angeles mayor Eric Garcetti asserted that "if cities are invited to be at the table, I believe they will help accelerate the work that needs to be done. Hopefully, we can do it in concert with our national governments, but [we can do it] even where there is conflict." He concluded by noting that "the United Nations works directly with cities all the time . . . so they shouldn't feel scared about jumping down to that local level."[15]

It wasn't surprising so much climate leadership was lurking, then activated, at the local level. As we have seen in this book, it was regional angst that gave rise to one of the most ambitious air pollution control schemes theretofore devised, and it was regional grievances about an ecological world turned upside down that gave rise to intense, if tragically futile, protest against strip mining. In the decades since, protest from below for environmental justice has burgeoned in predominantly minority and low-income areas that are a far more likely receptacle for a host of environmental health hazards, whether PCB waste, carcinogenic polyvinyl chloride production, diesel bus depots, garbage dumps, or whatever else.[16] And they had long been complemented by indigenous protestors, both in the United States and elsewhere, fighting the predations of extractive economies.[17]

The Green New Deal, the most ambitious framework for climate change legislation ever proposed in the United States, was shot through with undeniable localist impulses. Next to proposals for massive infrastructural conversion to renewable energy were references to "directing investments to spur economic development, deepen and diversify industry and business in local and regional economies," and "build[ing] wealth and community ownership." It reaffirmed a commitment to "justice and equity by stopping current, preventing future, and repairing historic oppression of indigenous peoples, communities of color, migrant communities, deindustrialized communities, depopulated rural communities, the poor, low-income workers, women, the elderly, the unhoused, people with disabilities, and youth"—the stuff of not just environmental justice but everyday local struggles.[18] The Green New Deal's public face and most ardent proponent was Alexandria Ocasio-Cortez, a first-term congresswoman representing parts of Queens and the Bronx, ground zero for generations of local political conflict over health, some analyzed in these very pages.

In late 2019, with the shock of the Covid-19 pandemic, the local dimension reasserted its importance, especially in the critical early months of the pandemic that entrenched its tragicomic and dystopian course a year before the arrival of highly effective vaccines. American observers initially viewed Covid-19 through the lens of SARS, MERS, and Ebola: something scary enough but also far away enough, too, and thereby subsumable to the category of "global." That complacency ended soon enough. As the virus spread into Iran, then Italy, then around the world, it gave rise to nation-to-nation comparisons. Why, three months since novel coronavirus's emergence, did some countries like New Zealand and South Korea seem to be effectively controlling spread while others, like the United States or Brazil, floundered? Explanations in the press ranged: cultures of mask wearing, the presence or absence of critical infrastructure for contact tracing, willingness on the part of the populace to accept centralized apparatuses for isolation, and the seriousness of political leadership, to name just some.[19]

Nation-to-nation comparisons were shortly followed by those plumbing lower units of analysis. In India, attention turned to the initial successes of Kerala state, which reported fewer cases than any other in the county. The "Kerala model of COVID-19 relief" was fueled by vigilance early in January, and it led to the quick establishment of contact tracers, readily available testing kiosks, and an early quarantine in March. What was as important, however, was the larger political milieu enabling these tools—namely, robust social welfare programs and persistent government commitment to public health infrastructure, including superior public hospitals. That commitment had been reinforced in recent years because of other outbreaks, like that of Nipah virus, which had allowed for the honing of techniques in "virus tracing, testing, and treatment" and the construction of an Institute of Advanced Virology that allowed for rapid testing within Kerala and no time delay for results. Even more important, in the view of social activists Aruna Roy and Saba Kohli Davé, was a "political culture of participatory governance" that led to widespread public trust and embrace of the disease control measures. "Kerala's preparedness for the pandemic was an offshoot of its historic governance tradition of using a combined social and political democratic framework, which included dialogue with its people before putting systems of social welfare in place," they wrote.[20]

Within the United States, states differed markedly in their response to the epidemic, particularly when it came to the timing of stay-at-home orders and, later, when to open up economies again. On one pole were those initially hit hardest: Washington, Michigan, Connecticut, New Jersey, Pennsylvania, and especially New York, along with California and Massachusetts, two states with robust public health traditions. Their stay-at-home orders were most stringent, lasted the longest, and were implemented the soonest. California's mandate ordered "all individuals . . . to stay home or at their place of residence" unless they were critical to the state's day-to-day functioning.[21] New York shut all nonessential businesses—with only a few exceptions—and banned "non-essential gatherings of individuals of any size for any reason."[22]

On the other end were such states as Texas, Florida, Iowa, and Georgia. In justifying his late April move to reopen Georgia even as coronavirus infections and deaths showed no signs of tapering off across the country, Governor Brian Kemp, who'd been one of the last governors to issue a stay-at-home order, declared, "I felt like the negative effects of not having our economy starting to open up was beginning to have the same weight as the virus itself, especially if you weren't in the medically fragile category or someone in a long-term care facility."[23] The move earned sharp rebuke from the usual suspects but skepticism from even South Carolina senator Lindsay Graham and President Donald Trump. It all unfolded as protests mounted over state-at-home orders in front of state capitols, most prominently in Michigan, whose governor, Gretchen Whitmer, was particularly singled out for attacks frequently laced with sexist venom and that culminated in a terrifying (and luckily thwarted) kidnapping plot.[24] These state-level controversies over divergent Covid-19 policy suggested that one's location might affect one's eventual Covid-19 risk.

But states revealed only so much. Within them, whatever their respective governors' policies, there was considerable variation at the local level from both politicos and everyday people. That was readily apparent in Georgia, where officials in a number of cities publicly repudiated Governor Kemp, with Atlanta mayor Keisha Lance Bottoms remarking: "I have searched my head and my heart on this and I am at a loss as to what the governor is basing this decision on."[25] It wasn't just politicians, either. Businesses and residents expressed concern, too, and did not initially throw themselves into Kemp's reopening. Storeowners who took a shot at opening doors reported extremely low foot traffic even a month afterward.[26] It was the resistance of local municipalities, however, that may well have insulated Georgia from taking a worse turn, such as was experienced in neighboring Florida, where Governor Ron DeSantis allowed, in September, counties to open restaurants and bars to full capacity and prohibited mask-wearing mandates.[27] By contrast, in Georgia, Kemp surprised observers in August when he allowed local mask ordinances, following months of legal wrangling with a number of municipalities, most prominently Atlanta and Mayor Bottoms. Kemp's move came with caveats; it would apply mainly to government buildings and to private businesses only "if the owner or occupant consents to enforcement."[28] But it was no doubt a reversal and an acknowledgment of local power. Mask wearing had by then turned into political theater, with President Trump mocking his challenger Joe Biden during a presidential debate for his advocating mask usage. But national spectacle masked the real terrain where the mask wars played out: the local.

In California, meanwhile, resistant localities showed that they could influence a state. There, despite an aggressive response by Governor Gavin Newsom, several localities saw a groundswell of resistance to public health measures.

In politically conservative Orange County, beaches were the site of protests against Newsom's closures, and in the town of Huntington Beach, 1,500 people gathered in a crowd to lash out.[29] Perhaps bowing to the pressure, Newsom allowed Orange County restaurants to open soon afterward, even as the sheriff's office there announced publicly that it wouldn't enforce mask-wearing guidelines.[30] Soon afterward, California diverged from New York as a success story, though pockets of it with early aggressive mitigation continued to boast relatively low infection rates. In the Midwest, state decisions were also very much felt locally. One early study analyzed the divergent fortunes of fifteen "border counties," half in Illinois (which issued a stay-at-home order in March), half in Iowa (which did not). Whereas both sets of counties initially had almost equal rates of Covid cases per 10,000 people, after the Illinois order, the Iowa ones reported 217 "excess cases," almost a third of the state's total count.[31] That early analysis of small numbers predicted later more consequential trends. By October, Iowa had the country's ninth highest positivity rate—the percentage of tests returned positive—fueled by local trends; half of its counties were in the federally defined "red zone," with a rate above 10 percent.[32]

By the end of the summer 2020, novel coronavirus moved from concentrated urban epicenters and into more diffuse nooks and crannies. Again, it would be local-level politics and behavioral compliance that shaped future spread, perhaps as much as edicts handed down from the state and federal government. Specialists in rural health were especially aware of the drift beyond the metropole, as early as April, with one study noting that Covid case prevalence in rural counties increased from 3.6 per 100,000 to 43.6 per 100,000 within just three weeks.[33] By fall, preliminary analyses of Covid's geographic spread indicated that large metropolitan areas no longer boasted the largest seven-day averages of new cases; rural areas did. Experts raised concerns over whether local rural capacity could meet the new demands of local rural spread, as they documented potential shortages in testing and bed capacity.[34] Even states with successful early mitigation, such as New York, later reported resurgence driven by local developments. In that state, the surge occurred in the rural western part, plus hotspot neighborhoods in the city, first Brooklyn, then Staten Island, where some residents resisted calls to wear masks and avoid large indoor social gatherings.[35]

But the local may only be so determinative. Throughout the early days of Covid-19, many Americans discovered a passion for the history of medicine and public health, particularly the 1918 flu pandemic. Much of the public interest centered on city-to-city variation in death rates, with the conclusion, confirmed since by medical historian Howard Markel and colleagues, that municipalities that implemented "nonpharmaceutical interventions" sooner and more comprehensively did much better than those who didn't or, worse, flouted the seriousness of the 1918 flu pandemic.[36] Just as all health politics was local in 1918, so it seemed the same might be true in 2020. The 1918 analogies had their limits, however. For one, the United States of 2020 was much more interconnected—by air travel, by extensive consumer rail, by automobiles—and many of its denizens regularly traversed from city to city and state to state. Thus roaring success in one locality was not necessarily a guarantee of anything in a tightly knit country and, for that matter, a world where a health injury to one could be a health injury to all. That was the lesson Kerala officials learned by the summer, when early success was checked by the return of migrant workers to local coastal towns, which brought the Kerala case numbers back up to levels of other states.[37]

## Toward a Multi-Scalar Health Politics

The Tip O'Neillian phrase "all health politics is local" is thus still accurate, but it must now be appended with an asterisk. That asterisk denotes local health politics' coexistence, sometimes uneasy, with larger parallel currents: recurrent economic turbulence, parasitic national energy infrastructure, and unforeseen new stakeholders in the health arena. Local health politics isn't dead but has morphed and been absorbed. And the current iteration of it has implications for readers of this book, whether scholars of health policy or those who enact it.

Chief among these is the need for what might be called a multiscalar health politics. Though preserving and prizing the value of localism, such a politics would also recognize and act on a multiplicity of vectors within and beyond it: formal institutions and informal formations; governmental and nongovernmental actors; individual clinics and health systems writ large; extractive sites next to one's home but also the larger energy infrastructure in which they are embedded; and spontaneous grassroots local activism alongside regional regulatory agencies and rarefied policy making.

Attempts to surpass the limits of single-site localism have certainly occurred in the past two decades. Following the 1999 protests against the World Trade Organization, neologisms and phrases like "glocal," "movement of movements," and "think globally, act locally" entered the political lingua franca, alongside real-world developments such as the World Social Forum, raucous meetings where activists from around the world gathered to swap tactics, share stories, and chart an alternative global future anchored in convergent radical localisms.[38] These impulses, though, carried more than a little antistatism and deep suspicion of traditional organizations. The limits of such a perspective were thrown into sharp relief with the 2008 financial crisis and the Covid-19 pandemic, which required nothing less than the full-bore proactive efforts of familiar institutions: nation-states, central banks, and economic consortiums. What is needed, rather, is an approach resembling what the political theorist Peter Funke has dubbed a "relay framework": a way of analyzing simultaneous but distinct modes of political engagement and thinking of them in a "more sequential, connected or capacious perspective, emphasizing the linkage and cooperation dynamics of multiple groups or networks."[39] A new local health politics must come with a wide-angle lens: embracing the virtues of those working on the ground at the most micro of levels but also looking up, left, right, and everywhere else at a multiplicity of developments, from the highly structured to the structureless. Likewise, a global or national policy or approach that fails to acknowledge local color is just as myopic as a hyperlocalism that ignores larger currents around it.

For all its flaws, the community health promise—undergirded by the "persistence of localism," in Thomas Sugrue's words—remains resounding for health politics, and it raises the question of why. It's an urgent one given the mounting supralocal forces that circumscribe localism's potential, and I have struggled with it. After all, when I started researching this book, I expected to dunk a huge bucket of ice-cold water on "community health," communitarianism's health-sector cousin, having dismissed it a priori as romantic fluff of the "small is beautiful" vein. And while there is certainly some of that critique in these pages, I found myself surprised at how much more respectful, if critically so, I felt toward community health as the research went on, particularly its most localist strands. I suspect that localism's enduring appeal—to me and others—stems from its fundamental accessibility and democratic promise. One's backyard and the institutions around it seem tangible, reachable, and most important, *changeable*, as opposed to elite institutions far away or large-scale processes that remain abstract. Here, the words of Frances Fox Piven and Richard Cloward, almost a half century ago, remain piercing, apt, and striking. On where people turn when they express discontent, the duo observed that "people experience deprivation and oppression within a concrete setting, not as the end product of large and abstract processes, and it is the concrete experience that molds their discontent into specific grievances against specific targets."[40] It is the immediate, the visceral, the everyday that most shapes people's worldviews and where they thus then seek modes of social change. In other words, the local. As Piven and Cloward elaborate, "Workers experience the factory, the speeding rhythm of the assembly line, the foreman, the spies and the guards, the owner and the paycheck. They do not experience monopoly capitalism." Similarly, "People on relief experience the shabby waiting rooms, the overseer or the caseworker, and the dole. They do not experience American social welfare policy."[41] It is the local lens that is far more likely to render one's surroundings in ways that are most tangible and meaningful.

In unequal societies where the levers of political power at the highest levels are foreclosed to most, it is the proximate where people often head when they first consider stretching the horizon of what is possible or are fending off impending threats to their welfare, whether in health or otherwise. It is what the subjects of this book did as they wrestled with the dilemmas that arose in the locales you have read about here. It has been my goal to excavate these local efforts—blood, sweat, struggles, triumphs, realization of limits and defeats— and to situate them as part of a larger national story and against a panoply of constricting influences.

It is only with this sober clarity of vision that we can evolve a multiscalar new health politics that can succeed, and one that still nonetheless remembers, in the end, that all health politics is local*.

# Acknowledgments

This book bears the name of only one author, but a lot of people commented on it, criticized it in draft, helped me think through analytic problems, funded the research, talked about things with me, or were just important people to have around in the process. I've been relishing the opportunity to show my appreciation here.

First, I want to thank my family, which is stationed in various parts of California and Thailand. I want to single out my two grandmothers, who've long passed age ninety, and my immensely talented sister, the mysterious Whitney Biennial–featured artist Milano Chow, who had the good sense—as her sibling didn't—to shrink her last name for professional purposes.

Next, I want to thank folks who shepherded the book to the finish line. I'd heard a lot of effusive chatter about one Brandon Proia as an editor, and I'm able to affirm the truth of it a thousand times over. He reads every word and line, sees the overall logic of a book, and then tells you the macro- and microlevel fixes you need to get to where you want to go. In an era where such close reading and editorial care are dwindling and the rubber stamp has increasingly been substituted for a strong editorial hand, Brandon is an exception. It's no surprise he has the reputation he does. Alongside Brandon was the careful attention to production detail—right down to figuring out the proper grayscale spectrums in my maps—by Cate Hodorowicz, Michelle Wallen, Kim Bryant, Lindsay Starr, Laura Jones Dooley, Andrew Winters, Elizabeth Orange, Mary Caviness, and Madge Duffey. A special thanks to Erin Granville for boundless patience toward the end of the process and her ability to explain the subtlest grammatical points with ease via horror movie examples.

Right up to the last minute of production, several archivists went out of their way to provide hard-to-find material or images: Harry Rice, Patty Tarter, Heather Dent, Chris Miller, and Jaime Bradley at Berea College; Matthew Smith at the University of Kentucky; Vicki Catozza at the Western Reserve Historical Society; Jennifer Nieves at the Dittrick Medical History Center; Cara Dellatte at the New York Public Library; Helen Conger at the Case Western Reserve University Archives; Steve Novak at the Columbia Health Sciences Library; Linnea Anderson at the University of Minnesota's Social Welfare History Archives; Doug DiCarlo at the LaGuardia and Wagner Archives; Bruce Crouchet at the daunting Los Angeles County Hall of Records; Jessica Becker at Yale University; and Caitlyn Rahschulte at Eastern Kentucky University. I also want to thank Terry Mizrahi, Robert Tranquada, and Rodney Powell for entrusting me with some of their personal papers. The New York City and Los Angeles chapters would have been greatly diminished without the material that they provided and that helped those cases come to life. Finally, thank you to Sarah Stoner-Duncan for help with some of the schematic illustrations and to Ashley Marshall for her expertise with digital elevation mapping.

It's not always fun to get a serious and thorough reading of your work, but the eventual repairs make it better. Connie Nathanson, James Colgrove, David Rosner, Ron Bayer, Jenny Leigh, Monica Gisolfi, and Lundy Braun gave careful readings of the full draft. A special thanks goes out to James for a particularly microscopic reading and for suggesting a set of organizational changes that greatly enhanced the overall coherence of the book. I am also grateful to Paul Kelleher, Kyle Nelson, Kavita Sivaramakrishnan, and Desiree Abu-Odeh, who read individual sections very closely. In the final stages, Henry Farrill read the penultimate version with his characteristic exacting eyes and intellectual energy. As usual, I can't thank the man enough.

Back in time a bit: I want to thank five undergraduate professors of mine at Columbia University who got me into the history racket in the first place. Betsy Blackmar taught me how to be a historian: everything from the drudgery of going through thirty boxes of documents and finding little to picking up the phone and calling people for archival leads and to learning how to situate oneself in various scholarly currents. Then there is Samuel Roberts. I wouldn't have even known that medicine and public health were things you could think about historically—and, frankly, what "public health" even was—without his class on African American public health history. His support has been unfailing through all these years. Barbara Fields taught generations of students to respect the craft of writing and to avoid looseness with concepts. Eric Foner's survey classes on American radicalism and Jacksonian democracy made me switch majors, and the senior thesis he advised jump-started some of the inquiries in this book. When I was a wayward college student, David Rosner took a chance on me for an important project on environmental health history; that led directly to some of the chapters on the topic here. He also set an example of how to write history accessible to public health professionals and with a broader purpose. Finally, she wasn't a historian or a professor at the time, but Jenn Lena was the first to teach me what sociology was, and in later years, she helped me stay out of trouble when she sensed I was getting into it. She has always been there for me.

At the University of Pennsylvania, I was lucky enough to study with Tom Sugrue. *Origins of the Urban Crisis* remains a clinic on how to historicize policy debates, ransack archives, and fuse social science and historical methods. Tom enthusiastically supported my work—both to me and, I later learned, to many others—and his writing remains a model of clarity and organization. He also fought for me at numerous administrative junctures through my doctoral program. The same goes for the late Michael B. Katz, whose books, essays, and polemics on the degrading treatment of the country's most marginalized made me want to study with him after I read *The Undeserving Poor*. Katz taught me how to traverse multiple academic quarters as a historian—including how to engage with those who think of history as background music or, worse, a complete waste of time—and how to negotiate the uncomfortable boundary between activism and academia. From David Barnes, I learned how to be a healthy skeptic of myths that the public health profession sometimes tells itself and how to root that skepticism in historical analysis. Besides cultivating a lifelong allergy—no, hostility—to John Snow and Edwin Chadwick hagiography, David also taught many people how to be an attentive and caring teacher. TAing for him was one of the highlights of my time at Penn. Stephanie McCurry taught one of the most brilliant classes I have ever taken on the Civil War, race, and nation; detects sophistry like nobody else; and underscored the importance of reading widely and outside of your field. Steven Hahn had zero obligation to spend as much time as he did talking to me. He took me through the classics of political economy, from Marx to Dobb to Wallerstein, and made sure I was well versed in the conceptual fundamentals. When I wondered why I couldn't get through more than five pages in an hour, he calmed me down and helped me ask the right questions to approach challenging material. On the MPH side, Carolyn Cannuscio was my advocate from the start, oversaw preliminary versions of work that ended up in this book, taught me how to present to audiences who weren't historians, and gave me important advice on self-confidence and not using self-effacement as an easy crutch. I am indebted to her for teaching me how to be more professional.

Finally, there is my friend, collaborator, and comrade Adolph L. Reed Jr. What can I say that can fit into this allotted space? I am one of hundreds whose fundamental way of thinking about politics, ideology, class, social movements, and race were matured and transformed by working with Adolph. He resists the fashionable and the platitudinal, interrogates unquestioned assumptions when others do not, and is a model of intellectual rigor. But people know less about him as a teacher: the seriousness and generosity he exhibits toward his students, both before and after they graduate. I am lucky to know him and glad we have continued to work together.

I also want to single out two people who were not on my committee or at Penn but were critical at keeping my morale and confidence high, especially when it flagged. Susan Reverby checked up regularly on how I was doing, put me in touch with a lot of people in the medical history field, gave me free lodging in Cambridge, and taught me a lot about how to navigate the public health and medical worlds as both an insider and an outsider. Susan introduced me to Lundy Braun, another brilliant scholar, who has also been a huge source of support, a model thorn in the side of ill-conceived racist medical science, and who has always treated me like an equal; I still feel honored and humbled when either of them asks me for my thoughts on their scholarship.

Then there are my fellow graduate students: Adam Goodman, Daniel Amsterdam, Jess Lautin, Sean Greene, Tshepo Chery, Hope McGrath, Clem Harris, Diana Burnett, Julie Davidow, and the absurdity from Rucker, Ricardo Howell. Karen Tani also was a critical sounding board at numerous fraught points and my regular intellectual interlocutor. Everyone in graduate school should be lucky to have a friend like her.

Elsewhere at Penn, I want to thank Sarah Igo, Rogers Smith, Charlie Branas, Christian Morssink, J. A. Grisso, Arnold Rosoff, Walter Tsou, Anthea Butler, and Barbara Savage for being supportive readers and teachers at various points. Joan Plonski, the late Deborah Broadnax, and Jackie McLaughlin helped me navigate administrative issues, especially between two degree programs. I miss the late Jean Whelan and her wit. Ditto Walter Lear, a legendary health activist and packrat who introduced me to the vast history of American health social movements.

For three years, I was a Graduate Fellow in the Center for Africana Studies' Summer Institute program. I want to thank Camille Charles, Gale Garrison, and Carol Davis for their exceptional vision and execution of the Institute and Rebbeca Tesfai, Yea Afolabi, and the aforementioned Ricardo character, who led the program and taught me about leadership and teamwork.

I received research funding from a few critical sources: the Penn Program on Democracy, Citizenship, and Constitutionalism; the national fellowship program, overseen by Brian Balogh, at the Miller Center of Public Affairs at the University of Virginia; and Penn's Institute of Education Sciences Predoctoral Training Program in Interdisciplinary Methods for Field-Based Research in Education, supervised by Rebecca Maynard and Laura Perna. This funding enabled me to hit a lot of archives I otherwise wouldn't have been able to visit, plus secured the entirety of my graduate education.

I didn't work on this book much—at least directly—in the two years that I was a Robert Wood Johnson Foundation Health & Society Scholar at the University of Wisconsin–Madison. But my time there was career altering and led me to overhaul and conceptually reframe the entire book. Under the structure that Stephanie Robert, John Mullahy, and David Kindig formulated, I regularly encountered major debates in health economics, population health, bioethics, demography, health policy, and other fields that helped me orient this book to a wider range of readers. Steph, John, and Dave have continued to help out whenever I've asked in the years since, and I'm grateful for what they set up. I am especially grateful to Dave for sharing his perspectives on many of the events recounted in this book that he lived through.

Our Madison program thrived because of the other fellows: Tova Walsh and Jayanti Owens (my years); above me, Fenaba Addo and Julie Maslowky; and below, Raj Mukkherjee, Daniel Hackman, and Christy Erving. A special thanks to Julie for the long talks on life and politics and Christy for the same, plus her willingness to see garbage films with me every now and then. Ashley Thompson provided assistance with numerous administrative issues, all with good humor and what can only be described as a lot of "energy." Jane Lambert was and is a recurring source of kindness, competence, intelligence, and curiosity who also can get anything done. Jenna Nobles and Joan Fujimura were my entrée into the school's storied sociology department and always hooked me up with new audiences and resources. On the other hand, there was Paul Kelleher, the philosopher-clown, who made up for his buffoonery by offering occasional insights on ethics, cooking amazing paella, and watching a lot of basketball with me (including a ridiculous trip to a Chicago Bulls game whose multiple detours somehow made us miss only one quarter). Last, I want to thank the staff at the Center for High-Throughput Computing, which introduced me to new methods and ways of doing things during my time that I hadn't even heard of.

At Columbia, I am fortunate to be part of the Center for the History and Ethics of Public Health at the Mailman School of Public Health, which navigates the space between historical scholarship and present-day public health concerns. David Rosner was instrumental in bringing me there and instantiating that vision alongside Ron Bayer and Amy Fairchild. James Colgrove has been a valuable guide on both teaching and scholarship. Kavita Sivraramakrishnan regularly stretches and challenges my intellectual assumptions and epistemic horizons in addition to just being a good friend. In the Department of Sociomedical Sciences, I want to thank Mark Hatzenbeuhler and Diana Hernandez for being welcoming faces when I first entered and Marilena Lekas, Karolynn Siegel, Connie Nathanson, Gerald Oppenheimer, Carly Hutchinson, Bob Fullilove, Raygine DiAquoi, Marni Sommer, Morgan Philbin, Marita Murrman, Gina Wingood, Rachel Shelton, WNBA superfan Angela Aidala, Kim Hopper, and my two chairs, Lisa Rosen-Metsch and Kathy Sikkema, and Dean Linda Fried for their support since. The Columbia Population Research Center also provided critical resources, and I thank Jennifer Hirsch for connecting me with it. Thanks also to my colleagues in the history department, particularly Mae Ngai, Betsy Blackmar, Sam Roberts, and Stephanie McCurry, for bringing me in on various initiatives or just being there to chat.

It's also awesome to have worked with truly brilliant MPH and doctoral students, many of whom helped me iron out my thinking on a number of political questions through conversations in and out of the classroom. They include Gabi Seplovich, Nora Landis-Shack, Nicole Mabry, Hongdeng Gao, Laura Nicole Sisson, Hannah Dowling, Jenn Wong, May Erouart, Carlos Gould, Matthew Lee, Ijeoma Eboh, Sadie Bergen, Lauren Broussard, Rachel Wolf, Brittney Cavaliere, Sarah Miller, Gray Lu, Matthew Kelly, Charles Halvorson, Winn Periyasamy, Nathan Albert, Sydney Giordano, Yoka Tomita, Desiree Abu-Odeh, Joanna Xing, Caitlin McMahon, Abbey Sussell, Dan Chong, Nina Paroff, Kristen Gardner, Sonia Mendoza-Grey, April Harrison, and Kristen Meister.

A lot of people at various academic gatherings contributed something to either this book or the larger thinking that went into it, people like fellow Los Angeles Lakers ideologue Selena Oritz, Lucia Trimbur, ace IHOP companion Julilly Kohler-Hausmann, Adam Biggs, Kelly Happe, Elizabeth Wrigley-Field, Robert Greene, Andrew Hartman (the saddest Nuggets fan in the world), Mike Yudell, Laura Weinrib, Laura Bothwell, Stephanie Woolhandler, David Himmelstein, Jacob Bor, Adam Gaffney, Amy Fairchild, Pallavi Podapati, the late Elizabeth Fee, Ted Brown, Oli Fein, Charlotte Phillips, Scott Podolsky, Susan Lederer, David Takeuchi, Nancy Tomes, Ansley Erickson, Alondra Nelson, Lindsey Leninger, Cynthia Connolly, Joanna Wuest, Mo Torres, Amy Offner, Tian Zheng, Tiffany Greene, Adam Kushner, Gina Greene, Kathleen Bachynski, Jess Nickrand, Jennifer Gunn, Megan Wolff, Dominique Tobbell, Jon Zelner, Terry Mizrahi, Seth Prins, Brianna Last, Ronda Kotelchuck, Robb Burlage, Jenny Stepp, Amy Zanoni, Barry Eidlin, Kelly O'Donnell, Sarah Cate, Daniel Moak, Andrew Highsmith, Arline Geronimus, Chris Sellers, Janet Golden, Joyce Chang, Sophia Lee, Gina Neff, Robert Pollin, Guian McKee, Harold Braswell, Kim Phillips-Fein, Sandro Galea, Keith Wailoo, Ben Howell, Kim Sue, Mary Marshall Clark, Roger Lancaster, Jenny Leigh, Walter Michaels, Daniel Immerwahr, Richard Clapp, Patricia D'Antonio, Annie Menzel, and Jimmy Casas Klausen.

Finally, I wouldn't have been able to navigate the occasional rough points of academic life without my friends: Carrie Babcock, Blair Mosner-Feltham, Shoshana Schwartz, Megan Rossi, Bill Bronston, Mick McGarvey, Susan Schnall, Madeline Gomez, Maya McKenzie, Albert Wu, Christine Karatnytsky, Zach Levenson, Andrew "Bruce" Liu, Abby Walthausen, Penelope Reilly, "Annteresting" McCall, Helen Wang, Bianca Segui, Eugene Puryear, Ali Clymer, Beth Sherouse, Chase Strangio, Kyle Nelson, Judd Schoenholtz, Becca Vanderwalde,

Victor Balta, Justin Sowa, Ben Becker, John Atkinson, Marcelo Davidow, Bret Nicely, Pat Taylor, Alexis Stephens, Anjoli Roy, Vern Liu, Kristin Harper, Tierney Yenreit, Samir Sonti, Eric Augenbraun, Hope McGrath, Joy McGrath, Yan Slobodkin, Deborah Dentler, and the world's most annoying pest-journalist, Sam "I need this in one hour" Bloch. Ben "Dr. Ben" Johnson and Brian Kwan helped counsel me through a scary health issue that surfaced unexpectedly at the end of this writing. Thanks also to the JW crew, especially Sara Noshari, Melissa McQueen, and Candace Cooper; my fantasy basketball league; and the Lakers Brain Trust (Tracy, Ryan, Leon, Mike, Mark, Scott, Meesh, and Garrett) for helping each other survive the Ryan Kelly and Robert Sacre "eras." I am grateful to have known Jessica Lambert and Courtney Szper for almost twenty years. Ditto John Alexander Farrill, Monica Gisolfi, and my Stanford-trained attack dog attorney, Jordan Segall!

I first met the person in my dedication when I took his class as a college sophomore and had no idea he was a titan of social science. He put up with a lot of callow braggadocio, and yet his support never wavered, both then and since. I owe him a lot.

My proceeds from this book will be donated to the Association of Flight Attendants–CWA, AFL-CIO Disaster Relief Fund.

# Notes

ABBREVIATIONS

*ARC Papers* Papers of the Appalachian Regional Commission, Special Collections Division, Margaret I. King Library, University of Kentucky, Lexington

*Beame Papers* Abraham Beame Papers, LaGuardia and Wagner Archives, LaGuardia Community College, City University of New York, Queens

*Celebrezze Papers* Anthony J. Celebrezze Papers, Western Reserve Historical Society, Cleveland, Ohio

*Cooper Papers* Papers of John Sherman Cooper, Special Collections Division, Margaret I. King Library, University of Kentucky, Lexington

*CSM (Part Two) Papers* Council of Southern Mountains (Part Two) Papers, Berea College Special Collections and Archives, Hutchins Library, Berea, Ky.

*CUMC Papers* Records of the Columbia University Medical Center, Office of the Vice President for Health Sciences, Dean of the Faculty of Medicine [semiprocessed], Archives and Special Collections, Augustus C. Long Health Sciences Library, New York

*Ford Papers* John Anson Ford Papers, Manuscripts Collection, Huntington Library, San Marino, Calif.

*Gottron Papers* Papers of Richard Gottron [semiprocessed], Cleveland Clinic Archives, Cleveland Clinic, Beachwood, Ohio

*Hahn Papers* Papers of Kenneth Hahn, Manuscripts Collection, Huntington Library, San Marino, Calif.

*Hall Papers* Papers of Helen Hall, Social Welfare History Archives, Elmer L. Andersen Library, University of Minnesota, Minneapolis

*Koch Papers* Edward Koch Papers, LaGuardia and Wagner Archives, LaGuardia Community College, City University of New York, Queens

*LAC Archives* Hall of Records, Kenneth Hahn Hall of Administration (Los Angeles County), Los Angeles

| Lindsay Papers | John Lindsay Papers (mayoral), LaGuardia and Wagner Archives, LaGuardia Community College, City University of New York, Queens |
| --- | --- |
| Perkins Papers | Carl Perkins Papers, Special Collections and Archives, Eastern Kentucky University, Richmond |
| Powell unpub. | Rodney Powell, unpublished essay on the South Central Multipurpose Health Center, in private collection |
| Stokes Papers | Papers of Carl Stokes, Western Reserve Historical Society, Cleveland, Ohio |
| Wagner Papers | Robert F. Wagner Papers, LaGuardia and Wagner Archives, LaGuardia Community College, City University of New York, Queens |
| Weinerman Papers | Edwin Richard Weinerman Papers, Manuscripts and Archives, Sterling Memorial Library, Yale University, New Haven, Conn. |
| Whitman Papers | Papers of Samuel Whitman, Case Western Reserve University (CWRU) Archives, Case Western Reserve University, Cleveland, Ohio |

## INTRODUCTION

1. This account is derived from David J. Garrow, *Rising Star: The Making of Barack Obama* (New York: William Morrow, 2017), 41, 189–325.

2. Garrow, 313.

3. Tip O'Neill, *All Politics Is Local and Other Rules of the Game* (New York: Random House, 1994).

4. Thomas Sugrue, "All Politics Is Local," in *The Democratic Experiment*, edited by Meg Jacobs, William J. Novak, and Julian E. Zelizer (Princeton, N.J.: Princeton University Press, 2003), 304.

5. Lily Geismer, *Don't Blame Us: Suburban Liberals and the Transformation of the Democratic Party* (Princeton, N.J.: Princeton University Press, 2014); Lisa McGirr, *Suburban Warriors: The Origins of the New American Right* (Princeton, N.J.: Princeton University Press, 2001).

6. Daniel Amsterdam, *The Roaring Metropolis: Businessmen's Campaign for a Civic Welfare State* (Philadelphia: University of Pennsylvania Press, 2016).

7. Robert Korstad and James Leloudis, *To Right These Wrongs: The North Carolina Fund and the Battle to End Poverty and Inequality in 1960s America* (Chapel Hill: University of North Carolina Press, 2010); Annelise Orleck and Lisa Gayle Hazirjian, eds., *The War on Poverty: A New Grassroots History, 1964–1980* (Athens: University of Georgia Press, 2011); Kent Germany, *New Orleans after the Promises: Poverty, Citizenship, and the Search for the Great Society* (Athens: University of Georgia Press, 2007); Annelise Orleck, *Storming Caesar's Palace: How Black Mothers Fought Their Own War on Poverty* (Boston: Beacon, 2006); and Crystal Sanders, *A Chance for Change: Head Start and Mississippi's Black Freedom Struggle* (Chapel Hill: University of North Carolina Press, 2016).

8. See Charles Payne, *I've Got the Light of Freedom: The Organizing Tradition and the Mississippi Freedom Struggle* (Berkeley: University of California Press, 1995); John Dittmer, *Local People: The Struggle for Civil Rights in Mississippi* (Urbana: University of Illinois Press, 1994); and Tomiko Brown-Nagin, *Courage to Dissent: Atlanta and the Long History of the Civil Rights Movement* (New York: Oxford University Press, 2012).

9. On the Democratic Congress under which most Great Society and War on Poverty legislation passed, see Julian Zelizer, *The Fierce Urgency of Now: Lyndon Johnson, Congress, and the Battle for the Great Society* (New York: Penguin Books, 2015); and Lyndon B. Johnson, Annual message to Congress on the State of the Union (speech, Washington, D.C., January 8, 1964), University of California, Santa Barbara, American Presidency Project, www.presidency.ucsb.edu/documents/annual-message-the-congress-the-state-the-union-25.

10. Peter Marris and Martin Rein, *Dilemmas of Social Reform: Poverty and Community Action*, 2nd ed. (Chicago: Aldine, 1973), 7.

11. Ira Katznelson, *City Trenches: Urban Politics and the Patterning of Class in the United States* (Chicago: University of Chicago Press, 1981), 104–5.

12. The absence of place is evident in otherwise outstanding works on health policy development. See Paul Starr, *The Social Transformation of Medicine: The Rise of a Sovereign Profession and the Making of a Vast Industry* (New York: Basic Books, 1984); Rosemary Stevens, *American Medicine and the Public Interest* (New Haven, Conn.: Yale University Press, 1971); Rosemary Stevens, *In Sickness and in Wealth: American Hospitals in the Twentieth Century* (New York: Basic Books, 1989); Colin Gordon, *Dead on Arrival: The Politics of Health Care in Twentieth-Century America* (Princeton, N.J.: Princeton University Press, 2003); Jill Quadagno, *One Nation, Uninsured: Why the U.S. Has No National Health Insurance* (New York: Oxford University, 2005); Jacob S. Hacker, *The Divided Welfare State: The Battle over Public and Private Benefits in the United States* (New York: Cambridge University Press, 2002); Jennifer Klein, *For All These Rights: Business, Labor, and the Shaping of America's Public-Private Welfare State* (Princeton, N.J.: Princeton University Press, 2003); Jonathan Oberlander, *The Political Life of Medicare* (Chicago: University of Chicago Press, 2003); Jonathan Engel, *Poor People's Medicine: Medicaid and American Charity Care since 1965* (Durham, N.C.: Duke University Press, 2006); Alice Sardell, *The U.S. Experiment in Social Medicine: The Community Health Center Program, 1965–1986* (Pittsburgh: University of Pittsburgh Press, 1989); Alan Derickson, *Health Security for All: Dreams of Universal Health Care in America* (Baltimore: Johns Hopkins University Press, 2005); and Robert Cunningham III and Robert M. Cunningham Jr., *Blues: A History of the Blue Cross and Blue Shield Systems* (DeKalb: Northern Illinois University Press, 1977). Ricky Hendricks, *A Model for National Health Care: The History of Kaiser Permanente* (New Brunswick, N.J.: Rutgers University Press, 1993), is not a national study per se, but centers almost entirely on the internal organizational dynamics of the respective programs the authors study. For a critique of national-level "grand narrative," see John Harley Warner, "Grand Narrative and Its Discontents: Medical History and the Social Transformation of American Medicine," *Journal of Health Politics, Policy and Law* 29, no. 4–5 (2004): 757–80.

Some recent exceptions include Evelyn Hammonds, *Childhood's Deadly Scourge: The Campaign to Control Diphtheria in New York City, 1880–1930* (Baltimore: Johns Hopkins University Press, 2002); Sandra Opdycke, *No One Was Turned Away: The Role of Public Hospitals in New York City since 1900* (New York: Oxford University Press, 2000); James Colgrove, *Epidemic City: The Politics of Public Health in New York* (New York: Russell Sage Foundation, 2011); Gabriel Winant, *The Next Shift: The Fall of Industry and the Rise of Health Care in Rust Belt America* (Cambridge, Mass.: Harvard University Press, 2021); Bonnie Lefkowitz, *Community Health Centers: A Movement and the People Who Made It Happen* (New Brunswick, N.J.: Rutgers University Press, 1997); Andrew Simpson, *The Medical Metropolis Health Care and Economic Transformation in Pittsburgh and Houston* (Philadelphia: University of Pennsylvania Press, 2019); and Judith Walzer Leavitt, *The Healthiest City: Milwaukee and the Politics of Health Reform* (Princeton, N.J.: Princeton University Press, 1982).

The history of environmental health remains a small field but exhibits the same orientation when it comes to non-place-based analysis, with national-level regulatory debates assuming central roles alongside environmental health scientists. See Christian Warren, *Brush with Death: A Social History of Lead Poisoning* (Baltimore: Johns Hopkins University Press, 2000); Nancy Langston, *Toxic Bodies: Hormone Disruptors and the Legacy of DES* (New Haven, Conn.: Yale University Press, 2011); and Naomi Oreskes and Erik M. M. Conway, *Merchants of Doubt: How a Handful of Scientists Obscured the Truth on Issues from Tobacco Smoke to Global Warming* (New York: Bloomsbury, 2011). For some exceptions, where the regional setting is integral to subsequent developments and the types of environmental health hazards produced, see Gregg Mittman, *Breathing Space: How Allergies Shape Our Lives and Landscapes* (New Haven, Conn.: Yale University Press, 2008), ch. 4; Alan Derickson, *Black Lung: Anatomy of a Public Health Disaster* (Ithaca, N.Y.: Cornell University Press, 1998); David Rosner and Gerald Markowitz, *Deceit and Denial: The Deadly Politics of Industrial Pollution* (Berkeley: University of California Press, 2003), chs. 8, 9. The bulk of *Deceit and Denial*, however, falls into the first category.

13. Robert Aronowitz, "The Social Construction of Coronary Heart Disease Risk Factors," in *Making Sense of Illness: Science, Society, and Disease* (New York: Cambridge University Press, 1998); Sejal Patel, "The Eclipse of the Community Study: The Roseto Study in Historical Context" (PhD diss., University of Pennsylvania, 2007).

14. Sugrue, "All Politics Is Local," 302.

15. My exploration of communitarian rhetoric is heavily influenced by Adolph Reed, "The Curse of Community," in *Class Notes: Posing as Politics and Other Thoughts on the American Scene* (New York: New Press, 2000); Reed, "Sources of De-Mobilization in the New Black Political Regime: Incorporation, Ideological Capitulation, and Radical Failure in the Post-Segregation Era," in *Stirrings in the Jug: Black Politics in the Post-Segregation Era* (Minneapolis: University of Minnesota Press, 1999); Rogers Brubaker, "Ethnicity without Groups," in *Ethnicity without Groups* (Cambridge, Mass.: Harvard University Press, 2004); Miranda Joseph, *Against the Romance of Community* (Minneapolis: University of Minnesota Press, 2002); and Daniel Immerwahr, *Thinking Small: The United States and the Lure of Community Development* (Cambridge, Mass.: Harvard University Press, 2015).

16. See David Kindig and Greg Stoddart, "What Is Population Health?," *American Journal of Public Health* 93, no. 3 (2003): 380–93; and Kindig, "Understanding Population Health Terminology," *Milbank Quarterly* 85, no. 1 (2007): 139–61.

17. On public and private factions of the welfare state, see Michael B. Katz, *In the Shadow of the Poorhouse: A Social History of Welfare in America* (New York: Basic Books, 1986); Katz, *Improving Poor People: The Welfare State, the "Underclass," and Urban Schools as History* (Princeton, N.J.: Princeton University Press, 1997), ch. 1; Hacker, *Divided Welfare State*; Klein, *For All These Rights*; and, from a cross-national perspective, Melani Cammet and Lauren M. MacLean, eds., *The Politics of Non-State Social Welfare* (Ithaca, N.Y.: Cornell University Press, 2014).

18. On the emergence of the "voluntary" ideology, see Stevens, *In Sickness and in Wealth*.

19. The literature on decision-making in the face of scientific uncertainty is vast, but for examples from health see Sara Vogel, *BPA and the Struggle to Define the Safety of Chemicals* (Berkeley: University of California Press, 2012); Rosner and Markowitz, *Deceit and Denial*; Langston, *Toxic Bodies*; Steven Epstein, *Impure Science: AIDS, Activism, and the Politics of Knowledge* (Berkeley: University of California Press, 1998); Ronald Bayer, *Private Acts, Social Consequences: AIDS and the Politics of Public Health* (New York: Free Press, 1989); Bayer, David Merritt Johns, and Sandro Galea, "Salt and Public Health: Contested Science and the

Challenge of Evidence-Based Decision Making," *Health Affairs* 31, no. 12 (2012): 2738–46; and Les Levidow, "Precautionary Uncertainty: Regulating GM Crops in Europe," *Social Studies of Science* 31, no. 6 (2001): 842–74.

20. On racism in medicine, see Gordon, *Dead on Arrival*, ch. 5; David Barton Smith, *Health Care Divided: Race and Healing a Nation* (Ann Arbor: University of Michigan Press, 1999); Alondra Nelson, *Body and Soul: The Black Panther Party and the Fight Against Medical Discrimination* (Minneapolis: University of Minnesota Press, 2011); Samuel K. Roberts, *Infectious Fear: Politics, Disease, and the Health Effects of Segregation* (Chapel Hill: University of North Carolina Press, 2009); Nayan Shah, *Contagious Divides Epidemics and Race in San Francisco's Chinatown* (Berkeley: University of California Press, 2001); Natalia Molina, *Fit to Be Citizens? Public Health and Race in Los Angeles, 1879–1939* (Berkeley: University of California Press, 2006); Karen Kruse Thomas, *Deluxe Jim Crow: Civil Rights and American Health Policy, 1935–1954* (Athens: University of Georgia Press, 2011); Vanessa Gamble, *Making a Place for Ourselves: The Black Hospital Movement, 1920–1945* (New York: Oxford University Press, 1995); David McBride, *Integrating the City of Medicine: Blacks in Philadelphia Health Care, 1910–1965* (Philadelphia: Temple University Press, 1989). On biomedical thinking specifically, see Michael Yudell, *Race Unmasked: Biology and Race in the 20th Century* (New York: Columbia University Press); Lundy Braun, *The Surprising Career of the Spirometer from Plantation to Genetics* (Minneapolis: University of Minnesota Press, 2014); Susan Reverby, *Examining Tuskegee: The Infamous Syphilis Study and Its Legacy* (Chapel Hill: University of North Carolina Press, 2009); Dorothy Roberts, *Fatal Invention: How Science, Politics, and Big Business Re-Create Race in the Twenty-First Century* (New York: New Press, 2011); and Troy Duster, *Backdoor to Eugenics* (New York: Routledge, 1990).

21. On the entry of lay participants into health and science, see Steven Epstein, "The Construction of Lay Expertise: AIDS Activism and the Forging of Credibility in the Reform of Clinical Trials," *Science, Technology, and Human Values* 20, no. 4 (1995): 408–37; Phil Brown, Rachel Morello-Frosch, and Stephen Zavestoski, eds., *Contested Illnesses: Citizens, Science, and Health Social Movements* (Berkeley: University of California Press, 2012); Kelly Moore, *Disrupting Science: Social Movements, American Scientists, and the Politics of the Military, 1945–1975* (Princeton, N.J.: Princeton University Press, 2008); Julie Sze, *Noxious New York: The Racial Politics of Urban Health And Environmental Justice* (Cambridge, Mass.: MIT Press, 2007; Rachel Kahn Best, *Common Enemies: Disease Campaigns in America* (New York: Oxford University Press, 2019). On the War on Poverty specifically, see Greta de Jong, "Plantation Politics: The Tufts-Delta Health Center and Intraracial Class Conflict in Mississippi, 1965–1972," and Laurie B. Green, "Saving Babies in Memphis: The Politics of Race, Health, and Hunger during the War on Poverty," both in Orleck and Hazirjian, *War on Poverty*.

22. On 1970s health planning and participatory initiatives specifically, see Louise Lander, "HSA: If at First You Don't Succeed," *Health/PAC Bulletin* no. 70 (May/June 1976); Barry Chackoway, ed., *Citizens and Health Care: Participation and Planning for Social Change* (New York: Pergamon, 1981). For critiques of community participation and elucidation of its limits more generally, including of the more substantive brand in the 1960s, see Alan Altshuler, *Community Control: The Black Demand for Participation in Large American Cities* (New York: Pegasus, 1970); and Michael Lipsky and Morris Lounds, "Citizen Participation and Health Care: Problems of Government Induced Participation," *Journal of Health Politics, Policy and Law* 1, no. 1 (1976): 85–111.

23. The literature on elite capture is dominated by studies of economic development programs. See, e.g., Jean-Phillippe Platteau, "Monitoring Elite Capture in Community-Driven Development," *Development and Change* 35, no. 2 (2004): 223–46; Platteau and Anita

Abraham, "Participatory Development in the Presence of Endogenous Community Imperfections," *Journal of Development Studies* 39, no. 2 (2002): 104–36; Ivor Chipkin and Mark Swilling, *Shadow State: The Politics of State Capture* (Johannesburg, South Africa: Wits University Press, 2018); and Aniruddha Dasgupta and Victoria A. Beard, "Community Driven Development, Collective Action and Elite Capture in Indonesia," *Development and Change* 38, no. 2 (2007): 229–49. For an important reminder of federalism's enduring importance, especially in the recent past, see Sara Mayeux and Karen Tani, "Federalism Anew," *American Journal of Legal History* 56 (2016): 128–38.

24. Mike Davis, *El Niño Famines and the Making of the Third World* (New York: Verso Books, 2000); Davis, *Ecology of Fear: Los Angeles and the Imagination of Disaster* (New York: Henry Holt, 1998); Vaclav Smil, *China's Environmental Crisis: An Inquiry into the Limits of National Development* (Armonk, N.Y.: M. E. Sharpe, 1993); James O'Connor, *Natural Causes: Essays in Ecological Marxism* (New York: Guilford Press, 1998); Susannah Hecht and Alexander Cockburn, *The Fate of the Forest: Developers, Destroyers, and Defenders of the Amazon*, 2nd ed. (Chicago: University of Chicago Press, 2010); Thomas Andrews, *Killing for Coal: America's Deadliest Labor War* (Cambridge, Mass.: Harvard University Press, 2008); and Philip Landrigan et al., "The *Lancet* Commission on Pollution and Health," *Lancet* 391, no. 10119 (2017): 462–512.

25. The work of medical demographer and physician Thomas McKeown catalyzed these debates in a series of articles captured by two works: *The Modern Rise of Population* (New York: Academic Press, 1976), and *The Role of Medicine: Dream, Mirage, or Nemesis* (Oxford: Blackwell, 1979). The debate still generates periodic cycles of debate. For overviews and a representative sampling of the subsequent debates' parameters, see James Colgrove, "The McKeown Thesis: A Historical Controversy and Its Enduring Influence," *American Journal of Public Health* 92, no. 5 (2002): 725–29; Bruce Link and Jo Phelan, "McKeown and the Idea That Social Conditions Are Fundamental Causes of Disease," *American Journal of Public Health* 92, no. 5 (2002): 730–32; Simon Szreter, "Rethinking McKeown: The Relationship between Public Health and Social Change," *American Journal of Public Health* 92, no. 5 (2002): 722–25; Simon Szreter, "The Importance of Social Intervention in Britain's Mortality Decline, c. 1850–1914: A Re-Interpretation of the Role of Public Health." *Social History of Medicine* 1, no. 1 (1988): 1–38; Allan Mitchell, "An Inexact Science: The Statistics of Tuberculosis in Late 19th-Century France," *Social History of Medicine* 3, no. 3 (1990): 387–403; David S. Barnes, "The Rise or Fall of Tuberculosis in Belle-Epoque France: A Reply to Allan Mitchell," *Social History of Medicine* 5, no. 2 (1992): 279–90; and Allan Mitchell, "Tuberculosis Statistics and the McKeown Thesis: A Rebuttal to David Barnes," *Social History of Medicine* 5, no. 2 (1992): 291–96. See also David Cutler, Allison Rosen, and Sandeep Vijan, "The Value of Medical Spending in the United States, 1960–2000," *New England Journal of Medicine* 355, no. 9 (2006): 920–27; Jo Phelan et al., "'Fundamental Causes' of Social Inequalities in Mortality: A Test of the Theory," *Journal of Health and Social Behavior* 45, no. 3 (2004): 265–85; and David R. Williams and Chiquita Collins, "US Socioeconomic and Racial Differences in Health: Patterns and Explanations," *Annual Review of Sociology* 21 (1995): 349–86.

26. Brandt and Gardner see some increasing "accommodation" between the two worlds in the postwar period, mainly in the form of epidemiologic methods making their way into biomedical research and practice. See Allan M. Brandt and Martha Gardner, "Antagonism and Accommodation: Interpreting the Relationship between Public Health and Medicine in the United States during the 20th Century," *American Journal of Public Health* 90, no. 5 (2000): 711–12. Elsewhere, however, they lament the hardening of the boundaries in other respects, including the incursion of biomedical hegemony into public health domains,

writing that "the rise of federal funding for medical research in the second half of the 20th century increasingly directed both medicine and public health research into a narrow biomedical paradigm."

27. A number of works address the boundaries of public health, many of them intellectual histories of major thinkers in the field. See Christopher Hamlin, *Public Health and Social Justice in the Age of Chadwick, Britain, 1800–1854* (New York: Cambridge University Press, 1998); William Coleman, *Death Is a Social Disease: Public Health and Political Economy in Early Industrial France* (Madison: University of Wisconsin Press, 1982); John Eyler, *Victorian Social Medicine: The Ideas and Methods of William Farr* (Baltimore: Johns Hopkins University Press, 1979); David S. Barnes, *The Making of a Social Disease Tuberculosis in Nineteenth-Century France* (Berkeley: University of California Press, 1995); and Richard J. Evans, *Death in Hamburg: Society and Politics in the Cholera Years, 1830–1910* (New York: Penguin Books, 1987). For a recent meditation on boundaries, see James Colgrove, Gerald Markowitz, and David Rosner, eds., *The Contested Boundaries of American Public Health* (New Brunswick, N.J.: Rutgers University Press, 2008); Amy L. Fairchild et al., "The Exodus of Public Health: What History Can Tell Us about the Future," *American Journal of Public Health* 100, no. 1 (2010), a provocative intervention that bemoans what the authors see as a narrow and technocratic orientation in late twentieth-century public health.

28. Howard J. Brown, "Urban Health Problems," November 30, 1969, Box 2, Folder "HJB Health Speeches 1967–1970," Papers of Howard J. Brown, Manuscripts and Archives Division, Humanities and Social Sciences Library, New York Public Library.

29. Jesse W. Tapp, Rena Gazaway, and Kurt Deuschle, "Community Health in a Mountain Neighborhood," *Archives of Environmental Health* 8 (1964): 516–17.

30. Major works in hospital historiography that analyze these features include Charles Rosenberg, *The Care of Strangers: The Rise of America's Hospital System* (New York: Basic Books, 1987); Sandra Opdycke, *No One Was Turned Away: The Role of Public Hospitals in New York City since 1900* (New York: Oxford University Press, 1999); David Rosner, *A Once Charitable Enterprise: Hospitals and Health Care in Brooklyn and New York, 1885–1915* (New York: Cambridge University Press, 1982); Stevens, *In Sickness and in Wealth*; and Joel Howell, *Technology in the Hospital: Transforming Patient Care in the Early Twentieth Century* (Baltimore: Johns Hopkins University Press, 1995). Their focus, however, tends to be on the Progressive Era to the late midcentury, before the period covered in this analysis.

31. The literature on health care costs—and increasing American uniqueness—is vast, but see Starr, *Social Transformation*, 381–419; Christy Chapin, *Ensuring America's Health: The Public Creation of the Corporate Health Care System* (New York: Oxford University Press, 2015), ch. 6; Walter J. McNerney, "Control of Health-Care Costs in the 1980's," *New England Journal of Medicine* 303, no. 19 (1980): 1088–95; and Victor Fuchs, "The Basic Forces Influencing Costs of Medical Care," in *Essays in the Economics of Health and Medical Care*, edited by Victor Fuchs (New York: National Bureau of Economic Research/Columbia University Press, 1972), 39–50.

32. Merlin Chowkwanyun, "Biocitizenship on the Ground: Health Activism and the Medical Governance Revolution," in *Biocitizenship: The Politics of Bodies, Governance, and Power* (New York: New York University Press, 2018), 178–99.

33. Constance Nathanson, *Disease Prevention as Social Change: The State, Society, and Public Health in the United States, France, Great Britain, and Canada* (New York: Russell Sage Foundation, 2007), 213.

34. On the social recognition of a health problem, see Robert Aronowitz, "Lyme Disease: the Social Construction of a Disease and Its Social Consequences," in *Making Sense of Illness:*

*Science, Society, and Disease* (New York: Cambridge University Press, 1998), 57–83; Nancy Krieger, "Does Racism Harm Health? Did Child Abuse Exist Before 1962? On Explicit Questions, Critical Science, and Current Controversies: An Ecosocial Perspective," *American Journal of Public Health* 93, no. 2 (2003): 194–99; Keith Wailoo, *Dying in the City of the Blues: Sickle Cell Anemia and the Politics of Race and Health* (Chapel Hill: University of North Carolina Press, 2000); Alan Derickson, *Black Lung*; David Rosner and Gerald Markowitz, *Deadly Dust: Silicosis and the Politics of Occupational Disease in Twentieth-Century America* (Princeton, N.J.: Princeton University Press, 1991). A leading progenitor of works in this vein is Charles Rosenberg and Janet Golden, eds., *Framing Disease: Studies in Cultural History* (New Brunswick, N.J.: Rutgers University Press, 1987). But from an earlier generation, see also Ludwik Fleck, *Genesis and Development of a Scientific Fact* (Chicago: University of Chicago Press, 1998).

CHAPTER ONE

1. Ray Trussell and Frank Van Dyke, *Prepayment for Hospital Care in New York State: A Report on the Eight Blue Cross Plans Serving New York Residents* (New York: School of Public Health and Administrative Medicine, Columbia University, 1961), 269–73.

2. Barbara Yuncker, "A Medical Dynamo Dedicated to Lifting Health Standards," *New York Post*, February 23, 1961; "Doctor of Many Hats: Ray Elbert Trussell," *New York Times*, February 24, 1961.

3. Sandra Opdycke, *No One Was Turned Away: The Role of Public Hospitals in New York City since 1900* (New York: Oxford University Press, 1999), 14, 55.

4. Commission on Health Services of the City of New York, organizational meeting, minutes, March 19, 1959, Box 504, Folder "Commission on Health Services Minutes 1959," CUMC Papers.

5. "Report of the Commission on Health Services of the City of New York," July 20, 1960, 5, Box 504, Folder "Commission on Health Services Gen. Corres. 1960," CUMC Papers.

6. Commission on Health Services of the City of New York, Executive Committee meeting, minutes, April 21, 1959, Box 504, Folder "Commission on Health Services Minutes 1959," CUMC Papers.

7. Commission on Health Services of the City of New York, organizational meeting, minutes, March 19, 1959; Ray Trussell to George Armstrong, memorandum on "interns and residents in municipal hospitals," November 16, 1959, Box 504, Folder "Commission on Health Services Gen. Corres. 1959," CUMC Papers. On foreign medical graduates, see Eram Alam, "Cold War Crises: Foreign Medical Graduates Respond to US Doctor Shortages, 1965–1975," *Social History of Medicine* 33, no. 1 (2020): 132–51.

8. Subcommittee on Coordination of the Medical Services, October 28, 1959, Box 504, Folder "Commission on Health Services Gen. Corres. 1959," CUMC Papers.

9. Committee of Interns and Residents of the New York City Municipal Hospitals, "The Crisis in the New York City Hospital System," October 1959, Box 504, Folder "Commission on Health Services Gen. Corres. 1959," CUMC Papers.

10. Commission on Health Services of the City of New York, organizational meeting, minutes, March 19, 1959.

11. Commission on Health Services of the City of New York, organizational meeting minutes, March 19, 1959, Box 504, Folder "Commission on Health Services Minutes 1959," CUMC Papers; Commission on Health Services of the City of New York, Technical

Advisory Committee memorandum, April 30, 1959, Box 504, Folder "Commission on Health Services Gen. Corres. 1959," CUMC Papers.

12. Commission on Health Services of the City of New York, special joint meeting of the Executive Committee and staff, minutes, October 6, 1959, Box 504, Folder "Commission on Health Services Minutes 1959," CUMC Papers.

13. Commission on Health Services of the City of New York, Executive Committee meeting, minutes, April 21, 1959. The origins of the affiliation are recounted in Nathan Smith, Peter Rogatz, and Martin Cherkasky, "The Case for Voluntary and Municipal Hospital Affiliation," *American Journal of Public Health* 53, no. 12 (1963): 1991. In the first year of the program, the two institutions shared one surgical resident, a figure that grew in following years.

14. "Report of the Commission on Health Services of the City of New York," 14; "Excerpts from the Opening Remarks of David M. Heyman at the final meeting of the Commission on Health Services," July 20, 1960, Box 504, Folder "Commission on Health Services Gen. Corres. 1960," CUMC Papers.

15. "Report of the Commission on Health Services of the City of New York," 8–9.

16. Commission on Health Services of the City of New York, Organizational Meeting of the Technical Advisory Committee on Coordination of Medical Services, minutes, July 16, 1959, Box 504, Folder "Commission on Health Services Minutes 1959," CUMC Papers.

17. Commission on Health Services of the City of New York, Organizational Meeting of the Technical Advisory Committee on Coordination of Medical Services, minutes, July 16, 1959.

18. The full membership list is in Commission on Health Services of the City of New York, organizational meeting, minutes, March 19, 1959.

19. On the impact of these scandals, beginning with Henry Beecher's 1966 *New England Journal of Medicine* article on ethics abuses in twenty-two cases, see David J. Rothman, *Strangers at the Bedside: A History of How Law and Bioethics Transformed Medical Decision Making* (New York: Basic Books, 1991).

20. Commission on Health Services of the City of New York, Executive Committee, minutes, October 27, 1959, Box 504, Folder "Commission on Health Services Minutes 1959," CUMC Papers; Commission on Health Services of the City of New York, special joint meeting of the Executive Committee and staff, minutes, October 6, 1959, Box 504, Folder "Commission on Health Services Minutes 1959," CUMC Papers. On the emergence of teaching hospitals—and different tiers of them—see Rosemary Stevens, *In Sickness and in Wealth: American Hospitals in the Twentieth Century* (New York: Basic Books, 1989), 137–38; Kenneth Ludmerer, *Time to Heal: American Medical Education from the Turn of the Century to the Era of Managed Care* (New York: Oxford University Press, 1999), ch. 9; and in New York City specifically, Opdycke, *No One Was Turned Away*, 58–60.

21. Commission on Health Services of the City of New York, Subcommittee for Coordination of Medical Services, minutes, October 28, 1959, Box 504, Folder "Commission on Health Services Minutes 1959," CUMC Papers.

22. Ray Trussell to Abraham Beame, August 10, 1961, Box 64, Folder 793, Departmental Files, Wagner Papers. The New York City Municipal Archives and the LaGuardia and Wagner Archives hold identical microfilmed copies of Departmental and Subject Files for most postwar New York City mayoral administrations.

23. Ray Trussell to Paul Screvane, September 19, 1961, Box 64, Folder 793, Departmental Files, Wagner Papers.

24. Henry Herman to Robert Wagner, September 5, 1962, Box 64, Folder 794, Departmental Files, Wagner Papers.

25. Gloria Clay to Robert Wagner, October 3, 1962, Box 64, Folder 794, Departmental Files, Wagner Papers.

26. Lillian Feigen to Robert Wagner, September 20, 1962, Box 64, Folder 794, Departmental Files, Wagner Papers.

27. "The Montefiore-Morrisania Affiliation July, 1962–December, 1963," ca. 1963–64, Box 65, Folder 797, Departmental Files, Wagner Papers.

28. Ray Trussell to Robert Wagner, October 18, 1963, memorandum on land offer, ca. fall 1963, Box 64, Folder 792, Departmental Files, Wagner Papers; Leo Larkin, "Board of Estimate Supplemental Report," November 1962, Box 64, Folder 792, Departmental Files, Wagner Papers.

29. "Proposal by the College of Physicians and Surgeons of Columbia University to Aid in the Improvement of the Care of Patients and to Increase the Education Opportunities for the Resident and Visiting Staffs of the Harlem Hospital in the City of New York," May 23, 1961, Box 322, Folder "Harlem Hospital 1932–1961," CUMC Papers.

30. On Columbia-Harlem relations at this time, see Stefan Bradley, *Harlem vs. Columbia University: Black Student Power in the Late 1960s* (Urbana: University of Illinois Press, 2009), 28–33.

31. Stanley Bradley to Houston Merritt, April 17, 1961, Box 322, Folder "Harlem Hospital 1932–1961," CUMC Papers.

32. For accounts of the 1968 protests, see Bradley, *Harlem vs. Columbia University*; and Robert McCaughhey, *Stand, Columbia: A History of Columbia University* (New York: Columbia University Press, 2003), ch. 15.

33. Grayson Kirk to Houston Merritt, March 28, 1961, Box 322, Folder "Harlem Hospital 1932–1961," CUMC Papers.

34. Ray Trussell, "The Municipal Hospital System in Transition," *Bulletin of the New York Academy of Medicine* 38, no. 4 (1962): 221–36. For a full list of initial affiliations, see "The Municipal and Other Health Care and Hospital Systems," in *Community Health Services for New York City: A Case Study in Urban Medical Delivery*, edited by Robert B. Parks (New York: Praeger, 1968), 302–10.

35. Dominique Tobbell, "Plow, Town, and Gown: The Politics of Family Practice in 1960s America," *Bulletin of the History of Medicine* 87, no. 4 (2013): 648–80.

36. See Robert Caro, *The Power Broker: Robert Moses and the Fall of New York* (New York: Vintage, 1975); and Samuel Zipp, *Manhattan Projects: The Rise and Fall of Urban Renewal in Cold War New York* (New York: Oxford University Press, 2010), chs. 4, 5.

37. Charles Scala, *Report on Status of Fordham Hospital and Hospital Situation in the Bronx* (New York: Fordham Hospital Alumni Association, 1961), 2, 3.

38. Scala, 4–7, 28.

39. Scala, 11–12, 14, 19.

40. Scala, 20, 22–23.

41. Scala, 30–31.

42. Lay Advisory Board, Fordham Hospital, "Your Hospital May Be Next to Close If the Mayor Closes Fordham July 1" (advertisement), *New York Times*, June 15, 1961; "Your Hospital May Be the Next to Close If the Mayor Closes Fordham July 1," *New York Times*, June 16, 1961.

43. Barbara Yuncker, "Trussell Yields, Won't Close Two City Hospitals," *New York Post*, June 26, 1961.

44. Trussell, "Municipal Hospital System."

45. City of New York, Office of the Mayor, press release on Fordham Hospital affiliation, July 28, 1963, Box 64, Folder 796, Departmental Files, Wagner Papers.

46. Mildred Loew vs. The City of New York, Dr. Ray E. Trussell, the Mount Sinai Hospital, 43 Misc.2d 1021 (N.Y. Sup. Ct. 1964).

47. Committee to Save City Hospital at Elmhurst, leaflet, February 18, 1964, Ray Trussell scrapbooks, Papers of Ray Trussell, LaGuardia and Wagner Archives, LaGuardia Community College, City University of New York, Queens.

48. Jane Jacobs, *Life and Death of Great American Cities* (New York: Random House, 1961); Herbert J. Gans, *The Urban Villagers: Group and Class in the Life of Italian-Americans* (New York: Free Press, 1962).

49. "Commissioner of Hospitals Acts to Affiliate All Municipal Hospitals: Authority with Disdain Causes Dissatisfaction," *Guild Bulletin* (Kings County Physicians Guild, Inc.) 14, no. 1 (March 1964).

50. Lester Tuchman, "Immediate and Long-Range Problems in the Municipal Hospitals of New York City," *Bulletin of the New York Academy of Medicine* 37, no. 8 (August 1961): 539–40.

51. Ray Trussell to Lester Tuchman, February 11, 1964, Papers of Ray Trussell, LaGuardia and Wagner Archives, LaGuardia Community College, City University of New York, Queens; Barbara Yuncker, "167 at Elmhurst OK Mt. Sinai Tie," *New York Post*, May 17, 1964; Ray Trussell, press release on City at Elmhurst, February 21, 1964, Box 65, Folder 797, Departmental Files, Wagner Papers; "Hospital Doctors Fight City Hall," *Medical World News*, March 27, 1964; "Matter of Lester R. Tuchman M.D. etc. VS. Ray E. Trussell, M.D.," May 25, 1964, Papers of Ray Trussell, LaGuardia and Wagner Archives, LaGuardia Community College, City University of New York, Queens.

52. Yuncker, "167 at Elmhurst"; Paul L. Montgomery, "130 Doctors Quit Merged Hospital," *New York Times*, July 2, 1964.

53. F. C. Fitts, "Recommendations and Comments: Gouverneur Hospital New York City, New York," August 23, 1955, Box 81, Folder 7, Hall Papers.

54. Fitts, "Recommendations and Comments."

55. George Freedman, New Era Club open letter, September 13, 1954, Box 81, Folder 6, Hall Papers.

56. "LENA to Conduct Drive to Obtain 20,000 Names on Hospital Petitions," *East Side (N.Y.) News*, June 2, 1956; George Freedman to Helen Hall, June 30, 1956, Box 81, Folder 8, Hall Papers; Health Committee of the Lower East Side Neighborhoods Association, petition, ca. 1956, Box 81, Folder 8, Hall Papers.

57. LENA Health Committee to Robert Wagner, June 28, 1956, Box 81, Folder 8, Hall Papers.

58. Hospital Council of Greater New York, "Report on Hospital Needs of Lower Manhattan," March 1956, Box 77, Folder 2, Papers of the Henry Street Settlement, Social Welfare History Archives, Elmer L. Andersen Library, University of Minnesota, Minneapolis.

59. Hulan E. Jack to Helen Hall, December 4, 1956, Box 81, Folder 8, Hall Papers; City of New York, Department of Hospitals, "Gouverneur Hospital, Manhattan Replacement, site and Planning," ca. late 1956, Box 81, Folder 8, Hall Papers; Winslow Carlton to Helen Hall, October 21, 1958, Box 81, Folder 9, Hall Papers.

60. George Freedman, "Is Gouverneur Hospital a Mirage?," *East Side News*, December 24, 1959.

61. Morris Kaplan, "Panel Urges City to Shut Hospital," *New York Times*, February 17, 1961.

62. Woody Klein, "Gouverneur Treating 300 Daily as Clinic's Fate Hangs in Doubt," *New York World-Telegram and Sun*, March 10, 1961.

63. Lower Eastside Neighborhoods Association (LENA) to Ray E. Trussell, March 10, 1961, Box 81, Folder 12, Hall Papers.

64. Lower Eastside Neighborhoods Association (LENA) to Ray E. Trussell, March 10, 1961.

65. "Howard J. Brown Curriculum Vitae," Box 6, Folder "Dr. Howard J. Brown—curriculum vitae," Papers of Howard J. Brown, Manuscripts and Archives Division, Humanities and Social Sciences Library, New York Public Library; Walter J. Lear, "A Tribute to Howard J. Brown," February 1975, Howard J. Brown Biographical File, Institute for Social Medicine and Community Health, Philadelphia.

66. Jennifer Klein, *For All These Rights: Business, Labor, and the Shaping of America's Public-Private Welfare State* (Princeton, N.J.: Princeton University Press, 2003), ch. 3.

67. "Demographic Characteristics of the Area," 1967, Box 15, Folder "Lower Manhattan Community Mental Health Center," Papers of Mobilization for Youth, Rare Books, Special Collections and Archives, Butler Library, Columbia University, New York.

68. Harold J. Brown and Raymond S. Alexander, "The Gouverneur Ambulatory Care Unit: A New Approach to Ambulatory Care," *American Journal of Public Health* 54, no. 10 (1944): 1663.

69. Harold L. Light and Harold J. Brown, "The Gouverneur Health Services Program: A Historical View," *Milbank Memorial Quarterly* 45, no. 4 (1967): 379–82.

70. Light and Brown, 388.

71. "WINS Radio 1010 NYC Hospital Commissioner (transcript)," June 6, 1965; Ray Trussell to Robert Wagner, June 28, 1965, Papers of Ray Trussell, LaGuardia and Wagner Archives, LaGuardia Community College, City University of New York, Queens.

72. "Lindsay: The Hospital Horror-Story," *New York Post*, October 15, 1965. On Lindsay, see Kim Philips-Fein, *New York's Fiscal Crisis and the Rise of Austerity Politics* (New York: Metropolitan Books, 2017), 34–38; Clarence Taylor, "Race, Rights, Empowerment," in *Summer in the City: John Lindsay, New York, and the American Dream*, edited by Joseph P. Viteritti (Baltimore: Johns Hopkins University Press, 2014), 61–78; and Ramón A. Gutiérrez, "Internal Colonialism: An American Theory of Race," *Du Bois Review* 1, no. 2 (2004): 286.

73. John Lindsay, "A 'White Paper' on New York City's Crisis in Hospital Facilities and Care: A Program of Positive Action and Progress (Part I)," October 15, 1965, Box 91, Folder 8, Papers of John Lindsay (personal), Sterling Memorial Library, Yale University, New Haven, Conn. This is a collection of Lindsay's personal papers, not those from his mayoral administration, which were deposited later with the city government.

74. "The New York City Municipal Hospitals: Interim Report to the Honorable Nelson A. Rockefeller Governor, State of New York," Box 506, Folder "New York City Dept. Hospitals Mar. 1966–Feb. 1967," CUMC Papers.

75. "New York City Municipal Hospitals."

76. "New York City Municipal Hospitals."

77. "New York City Municipal Hospitals."

78. Emergency rooms also found themselves becoming receptacles for unwanted patients. See, e.g., Beatrix Hoffman, "Emergency Rooms: The Reluctant Safety Net," in *History and Health Policy in the United States: Putting the Past Back*, edited by Rosemary A. Stevens, Charles E. Rosenberg, and Lawton R. Burns (New Brunswick, N.J.: Rutgers University Press, 2006), 250–72.

79. "New York City Municipal Hospitals."

80. *Report of the Blue Ribbon Panel to Governor Nelson A. Rockefeller on Municipal Hospitals of New York City* (Albany: New York State Department of Health, 1967), 2.

81. State of New York Commission of Investigation, *Recommendations of the New York State Commission of Investigation concerning New York City's Municipal Hospitals and the Affiliation Program* (New York: Community Council of Greater New York, 1968), 47–52.

82. Robb Burlage, *New York City's Municipal Hospitals: A Policy Review* (Washington, D. C.: Institute for Policy Studies, 1967), 224, 515–29.

83. "Medical Empires: Who Controls?," *Health/PAC Bulletin*, November–December 1968, 1–4; Merlin Chowkwanyun, "The New Left and Public Health: The Health Policy Advisory Center, Community Organizing, and the Big Business of Health, 1967–1975," *American Journal of Public Health* 101, no. 2 (2011): 238–49.

84. See "The Final Report of the Commission," in *Community Health Services for New York City: A Case Study in Urban Medical Delivery*, edited by Robert B. Parks (New York: Praeger, 1969), 14. The Parks volume contains the original report and supplementary studies written by the Piel Commission's staff.

85. "Problems, Causes, Solutions," 506–10, in Parks, *Community Health Services*.

86. "The Final Report of the Commission," 7, 19; "The Municipal and Other Health Care and Hospital Systems," 318–21, in Parks, *Community Health Services*.

87. "Community and Institutional Needs," 172, in Parks, *Community Health Services*.

88. "Community and Institutional Needs," 198–99.

89. "Community and Institutional Needs," 198–99.

90. For overviews of the Office of Economic Opportunity and Community Action Program, see James T. Patterson, *America's Struggle against Poverty 1900–1994* (Cambridge, Mass.: Harvard University Press, 1994), 142–54; Alice O'Connor, *Poverty Knowledge: Social Science, Social Policy, and the Poor in Twentieth-Century U.S. History* (Princeton, N.J.: Princeton University Press, 2001), 166–73; and Michael B. Katz, *The Undeserving Poor: America's Enduring Confrontation with Poverty*, 2nd ed. (New York: Oxford University Press, 2013), 119–35.

91. For examples of how War on Poverty–funded health initiatives commonly interpreted the phrase, see *The Comprehensive Neighborhood Health Services Program, Guidelines* (Washington, D.C.: Office of Economic Opportunity, 1968); and Robert Tranquada, "Participation of the Poverty Community in Health Planning," *Social Science and Medicine* 7, no. 9 (1973): 719–28.

92. "REVISED BY-LAWS—LESNHC-S," October 29, 1969, June 1970, private collection; "Incorporation Papers/Goals of LESNHC," May 1970, private collection. The by-laws appear to have hardly changed between 1969 and 1970 but are the earliest locatable versions. The organization's official mandate in these documents, however, matches the description of its original purpose, expressed in "Documented History of the Lower East Side Neighborhood Health Council–South Emphasizing the Relationship with the Beth Israel Medical Center under Dr. Trussell," ca. 1970, private collection. They also appear to match, almost word for word, the "Goals and Purposes of the Neighborhood Health Council" section of a summer 1967 council report: Frederick Warner, Robert Hawkins, Robert Farmer, and Terry Mizrahi, "Final Report of Lower Eastside Neighborhood Health Council Summer Project: Health Action and Survey Project by Older Youth," summer 1967, private collection.

93. "Antonin Flores-Action Leader for Action Group," *Gouverneur Reports: Community Health Bulletin* 2, no. 1 (1969), private collection.

94. On Saul Alinsky and his methods, see Sanford Horwitt, *Let Them Call Me Rebel: Saul Alinsky, His Life and Legacy* (New York: Vintage Books, 1992).

95. LESNHC-S, health survey, 1967, private collection.

96. For a broad overview of Medicaid, see Jonathan Engel, *Poor People's Medicine: Medicaid and American Charity Care since 1965* (Durham, N.C.: Duke University Press, 2006).

97. Warner et al., "Final Report of Lower Eastside Neighborhood Health Council Summer Project."

98. "Job Description for a Community Staff Person for the Health Council," 1967, private collection.

99. "Proposal for Additional Worker for the Lower East Side Neighborhood Health Council–South," ca. 1967, private collection; "Eight Months Struggle for a Health Council Staff," January 20, 1969, private collection; "A History of the Struggle for Staff for the Lower East Side Neighborhood Health Council-South with Some Conclusions Drawn and Some Questions Asked," ca. 1968–69, private collection; "Summary Minutes of the Meeting of Representatives of the Lower Eastside Neighborhood Health Council–South with the OEO Health Office in Washington, D.C.," May 31, 1968, private collection.

100. On the Young Lords, see Johanna Fernández, *The Young Lords: A Radical History* (Chapel Hill: University of North Carolina Press, 2020).

101. On HRUM's founding, see Fernández, 281–82.

102. "HRUM 10-Point Program," leaflet, ca. 1968–69, private collection.

103. "Eight Months Struggle for a Health Council Staff."

104. "Proposal for Additional Worker for the Lower East Side Neighborhood Health Council–South"; "Eight Months Struggle for a Health Council Staff"; "History of the Struggle for Staff for the Lower East Side Neighborhood Health Council–South"; "Summary Minutes of the Meeting of Representatives of the Lower Eastside Neighborhood Health Council–South."

105. "The Struggle for Partnership in the Planning and Delivery of Health Services: The Role of the Professional in Community Action," 1970, private collection; "Documented History of the Lower East Side Neighborhood Health Council–South Emphasizing the Relationship with the Beth Israel Medical Center under Dr. Trussell," ca. 1970, private collection.

106. Ray Trussell to Herbert Notkin, December 3, 1969, private collection.

107. "A Time for Health: A History of the Lower East Side Neighborhood Health Council–South," internal document, ca. early 1970s, private collection.

108. "Time for Health"; "Reinaldo Ferrer, MD New GHSP Director," *Gouverneur Reports: Community Health Bulletin* 3, no. 1 (1970), private collection.

109. Harvey Karkus to Antonin Flores, December 2, 1969, private collection; Health/PAC, "Health Rap," January 26, 1970, private collection; Mizrahi to Leonard Farbstein, February 5, 1970, private collection.

110. For a history of Local 1199, see Leon Fink and Brian Greenberg, *Upheaval in the Quiet Zone: A History of Hospital Workers' Union, Local 1199* (Urbana: University of Illinois Press, 1989).

111. Letter to Reinaldo Ferrer, Ray Trussell, Local 1199, Office of Economic Opportunity, March 2, 1970, private collection.

112. Local 1199's stance in part reflected tensions within its ranks at the time over whether the union's advocacy ought to extend beyond the welfare of union workers themselves and into quality-of-care issues in health facilities where they worked. See Fink and Greenberg, *Upheaval*, 198–208.

113. Ella Strother to Stephen C. Joseph, March 11, 1970, private collection.

114. "1199 and the Gouverneur Clinic Case," *1199 Drug and Hospital News*, February 1970, private collection.

115. Laura Ackerman, "Final Report and Evaluation of Activities with Gouverneur Health Services Program (GHSP) and the Lower East Side Health Council–South," April 14, 1970, private collection.

116. Frances L. Gesienice, "Breakdown of Patient's Complaints from the G.H.S.P. of the Beth Israel Medical Center," September 1969, private collection.

117. "Work Plan for Lower East Side Neighborhood Health Council–South 1970–1971," July 29, 1970, private collection.

118. Robert Alford, *Health Care Politics: Ideological and Interest Group Barriers to Reform* (Chicago: University of Chicago Press, 1975), 31; and Charles Brecher, "Historical Evolution of HHC," in *Public Hospital Systems in New York and Paris*, edited by Victor Rodwin et al. (New York: New York University Press, 1992), 59–83.

119. Antonin Flores to Joseph English, July 24, 1970, private collection.

120. "Notes for Meeting with Dr. English," fall 1971, private collection.

121. "Fact Sheet on the Crisis at the Gouverneur Health Services Program," November 29, 1971, private collection; "The Gouverneur Health Services Program of the New York City Health and Hospitals Corporation: Continuation Application," December 30, 1971, private collection.

122. Brief for Plaintiffs in Support of Their Motion for Leave to File a Second Amended and Supplemental Complaint and for a Preliminary Injunction, Lower East Side Neighborhood Health Council–South, Inc. et al. v. Elliot Richardson et al., 71 Civ. 5160 (1971); Terry Mizrahi, "Statement on the Affiliation Contracts with Specific Reference to the New Gouverneur Hospital," February 24, 1972, private collection.

123. For more on Mobilization for Youth, see Tamar Carroll, *Mobilizing New York: AIDS, Antipoverty, and Feminist Activism* (Chapel Hill: University of North Carolina Press, 2015), 22–78.

124. Roger Wetherington, "While Health Corps. Has Its Woes," *New York Daily News*, January 30, 1972.

125. The decision came on the heels of another similar case, *North City Area-Wide Council, Inc. vs. Romney*, just months before. In that case, a comparable neighborhood advisory board sued the Philadelphia Model Cities program, charging it with violating federal statutes that mandated a watchdog council's participation. Opinion of the Court, North City Area-Wide Council, Inc. et al. v. George Romney et al., 428 F. 2d 754 (1972).

126. Opinion of the Court, Lower East Side Neighborhood Health Council-South, Inc. et al. v. Elliot Richardson et al., 71 Civ. 5160 (1972).

127. "Inauguration," *Gouverneur Newsletter* 1, no. 2 (1972), private collection; "New Gouverneur Opens as the 19th City Hospital," *New York Times*, September 22, 1972.

128. Thomas Tam, "The Invisible Aides," *Gouverneur Newsletter* 1, no. 2 (1972), private collection.

129. "Voice of the People," *Gouverneur Newsletter* 1, no. 2 (1972), private collection.

130. "Voice of the People"; "Editorial: Our First Priority: Good Patient Care," *Gouverneur Newsletter* 1, no. 2 (1972), private collection.

131. Office of the State Comptroller, "Report on Review of Budget and Financial Operations, New York City Health and Hospitals Corporation," July 1, 1970–December 31, 1971, Box 43, Folder 568, Subject Files, "Health Servs. Admin—State Audit Report—Overpayment for Psychiatric 1972–1973," Lindsay Papers; Office of the State Comptroller, "Audit Report on a Review of Budget and Financial Operations of the New York City Health and Hospitals Corporation for the Period July 1, 1970 to December 31, 1971," Lindsay Papers.

132. Joseph T. English to David A. Grossman, memorandum on "Expense Budgets Fiscal Years 1971, 1972 and 1973 for the Health and Hospitals Corporation," ca. mid-1972 (from

context), Box 32, Folder 438, Subject Files, Lindsay Papers; Joseph T. English to John Lindsay, August 23, 1972, Box 32, Folder 438, Subject Files, Lindsay Papers.

133. Paul J. Kerz to Arthur Gordon, June 15, 1972, memorandum on interest-bearing accounts, Box 32, Folder 446, Subject Files, "H.H.C.—Audit—Central Processing Unit," Lindsay Papers; Office of the State Comptroller, "Audit Report on Review of Affiliation management of Cash Advances under Contracts with the New York City Health and Hospitals Corporation," July 1, 1970–December 31, 1971, Box 32, Folder 446, Subject Files, "H.H.C.-Audit-Central Processing Unit," Lindsay Papers.

134. Intergovernmental struggles over Medicaid burdens are discussed in Michael Sparer, *The Limits of State Health Reform* (Philadelphia: Temple University Press, 1996); and Jamila Michener, *Fragmented Democracy: Medicaid, Federalism and Unequal Politics* (New York: Cambridge University Press, 2012).

135. Commissioner of Health (New York City), staff meeting, February 8, March 14, 1968, Box 41, Folder 458, Subject Files, "Health Servs. Admin—Health, Department of (NYC)," Lindsay Papers.

136. Health and Hospital Planning Council of Southern New York, Inc., June 4, 1968, memorandum on "Notes on Progress and Problems in Neighborhood Health Center Planning and Development," Box 39, Folder 514, "Health Servs. Admin.—Comm.-Ambulatory Care Facilities," Lindsay Papers.

137. Kim Phillips-Fein, *Fear City: New York's Fiscal Crisis and the Rise of Austerity Politics* (New York: Metropolitan Books, 2017), 24–25.

138. Joseph T. English, memorandum on HHC activities, January 25, 1973, Box 43, Folder 566, Subject Files, "Health Servs. Admin—Reports, HHC," Lindsay Papers.

139. New York City Health Services Administration, "Special Analysis of National Legislative and Budgetary Developments and Their Implications for New York City," March 1973, Box 40, Folder 530, "Health Servs. Admin.—Correspondence," Lindsay Papers.

140. Author's calculations from U.S. Census data for 1950 and 1970, National Historical Geographical Information Systems database, Minnesota Population Center, University of Minnesota, Minneapolis.

141. New York City Health Services Administration, "Special Analysis of National Legislative and Budgetary Developments."

142. Joseph T. English, appendix, memorandum on miscellaneous HHC issues, February 10, 1972, Box 43, Folder 568, Subject Files, "Health Servs. Admin—State Audit Report—Overpayment for Psychiatric 1972–1973," Lindsay Papers.

143. Ester Fuchs, *Mayors and Money: Fiscal Policy in New York and Chicago* (Chicago: University of Chicago Press, 2010), 87; and Phillips-Fein, *Fear City*, 41–44.

144. Phillips-Fein, *Fear City*, 24–25.

145. Jonathan Soffer, *Ed Koch and the Rebuilding of New York City* (New York: Columbia University Press, 2012), 119; Fuchs, *Mayors and Money*, 86–93. On the crisis more generally, see Philips-Fein, *Fear City*; Joshua Freeman, *Working-Class New York: Life and Labor since World War II* (New York: New Press, 2000), ch. 15; Michael B. Katz, *In the Shadow of the Poorhouse: A Social History of Welfare in America* (New York: Basic Books, 1986), 290–92; William K. Tabb, *The Long Default: New York City and the Urban Fiscal Crisis* (New York: Monthly Review, 1982); Roger Alcaly and David Mermelstein, eds., *The Fiscal Crisis of American Cities: Essays on the Political Economy of Urban America with Special Reference to New York* (New York: Vintage Books, 1977); Jack Newfield and Paul DuBrul, *The Abuse of Power: The Permanent Government and the Fall of New York* (New York: Viking, 1977); and Robert W.

Bailey, *The Crisis Regime: The MAC, the EFCB, and the Political Impact of the Crisis Regime* (Albany: State University of New York Press, 1984).

146. Brecher, "Historical Evolution of HHC," 71.

147. James Colgrove, *Epidemic City: The Politics of Public Health in New York* (New York: Russell Sage Foundation, 2011), 91.

148. Memo to James A. Cavanagh, January 14, 1975, Box 9, Folder 133, Subject Files "Health and Hospitals Corporation—Report (1)," Beame Papers; Melvin Lechner to John L. S. Holloman, September 22, 1975, Box 9, Folder 131, Subject Files, "Health and Hospitals (1)," Beame Papers; John L. S. Holloman to Marvin Brecher, December 10, 1975, Box 9, Folder 131, Subject Files, "Health and Hospitals (1)," Beame Papers.

149. On Bellin more generally, see Colgrove, *Epidemic City*, 82–100.

150. Lowell Bellin to Edward Koch, June 13, 1975; Edward Koch to Lowell Bellin, June 9, 1975, Box 9, Folder 137, Subject Files, "Health Department," Beame Papers.

151. Lowell Bellin to Abraham Beame, September 24, 1975, Box 9, Folder 137, Subject Files, "Health Department," Beame Papers.

152. On the Koch, Bellin, and hospital closures, see also Colgrove, *Epidemic City*, 95, 99.

153. Stevens, *In Sickness and in Wealth*, 291.

154. Samuel Wolfe, "The Hospitals of the City of New York: A Policy Overview of the Municipal Hospitals in Relation to the City's Other Hospitals," 31–32, January 1976, Box 504, Folder "Health and Hospitals Corp. Nov. 1976–Dec. 1976," CUMC Papers.

155. Wolfe, 35.

156. Wolfe, 34.

157. "Harlem Community Health Survey: Utilization of Harlem Hospital," August 13, 1975, Box 323, Folder "Harlem Hospital 1975," CUMC Papers; "Sydenham Fact Sheet," March 6, 1979, Box 32, Folder 1, Departmental Correspondence, Koch Papers; Bernard Challenor to Donald F. Tapley, memorandum on Sydenham Hospital closure, May 19, 1976, Box 323, Folder "Harlem Hospital," CUMC Papers.

158. Basil A. Paterson, Martin Horwitz, and Walter L. Eisenberg, "Report and Recommendations of the Ad Hoc Panel on the Threatened Strike over Proposed Layoffs at Four Municipal Hospitals," June 17, 1976, Box 504, Folder "Health and Hospitals Corp. Nov. 1976–Dec. 1976," CUMC Papers.

159. "Pres. Nixon's Cut and Gouverneur," *Gouverneur Newsletter* 2, no. 1 (1973); Hanson Chan, "Community Demonstration against H.E.W. 13% Budget Cut," *Gouverneur Newsletter* 2, no. 1 (1973), private collection.

160. "Struggle for Health," *Gouverneur Newsletter* 2, no. 3 (1973), private collection.

161. Allen G. Schwartz to Edward Koch, May 11, 1979, Box 32, Folder 1, Departmental Files, Koch Papers.

162. Victor Botnick to Edward Koch, memorandum on "Montefiore Hospital Expansion," January 2, 1979, Box 45, Folder 17, Departmental Files, Koch Papers; Robert J. O'Connor to Edward I. Koch, January 22, 1979, Box 45, Folder 18, Departmental Files, Koch Papers.

163. New York City Health and Hospitals Corporation, "Closing of Cumberland Hospital Testimony," March 7, 1983, Box 33, Folder 6, Departmental Files, Koch Papers; Edward Koch to Stanley Brezenoff, memorandum on Greenpoint and Cumberland Hospitals, August 12, 1983, Box 67, Folder 29, Departmental Files, Koch Papers.

164. Adele Oltman, "Liberalism and the Crisis of Health Care in Harlem in the 1960s," *Social History of Medicine* 29, no. 1 (2015): 65. And for an analysis along these lines from the

time, see Barbara Ehrenreich and John Ehrenreich, eds., *American Health Empire: Power, Profits, and Politics* (New York: Random House, 1970).

165. On the multiplicity of late twentieth-century conservatism or "neoliberalism's" sources, see Kim Phillips-Fein, "The Roots of American Conservatism," *Nation*, May 4, 2016; Suleiman Osman, "'We're Doing It Ourselves': The Unexpected Origins of New York City's Public-Private Parks during the 1970s Fiscal Crisis," *Journal of Planning History* 16, no. 2 (2017): 162–74; and Timothy P. R. Weaver, *Blazing the Neoliberal Trail Urban Political Development in the United States and the United Kingdom* (Philadelphia: University of Pennsylvania Press, 2016).

## CHAPTER TWO

1. "Mayors' Conference on Control of Smoke and Fumes: Reporter's Transcript of Proceedings," May 8, 1946, Box 25, Folder B III 5 a aa (5), Ford Papers.

2. "Butadiene Smoke Again Blankets City in Haze," *Los Angeles Times*, September 9, 1943.

3. "City Hunting for Source of 'Gas Attack,'" *Los Angeles Times*, July 27, 1943.

4. L. S. Adams to Los Angeles County Board of Supervisors, December 2, 1949, Box 20-5014-210 (3260 APBP0008), Folder "April 19," LAC Archives. Los Angeles County records are unprocessed and organized by box numbers that do not consistently match subjects. I have included all numerical information that appears on the boxes.

5. Miriam Yergin to Los Angeles County Board of Supervisors, November 21, Box 20-5014-210 (3260 APBP0008), Folder "April 19," LAC Archives.

6. Raymond W. Berg to Los Angeles County Board of Supervisors, December 2, 1949, Box 25, Folder B III 5a aa (8), Ford Papers.

7. Fred Mayer to Los Angeles County Board of Supervisors, July 5, 1950, Box 20-5014-210 (3260 APBP0008), Folder "April 19," LAC Archives.

8. William C. Ring to Ed Ainsworth, December 27, 1949, Box 25, Folder B III 5a aa (8), Ford Papers; F. N. Doty, October 2, 1949, Box 20-5014-210 (3260 APBP0008), Folder "April 19," LAC Archives.

9. Berg to Los Angeles County Board of Supervisors, December 2, 1949.

10. Adams to Los Angeles County Board of Supervisors, December 2, 1949.

11. Lynne Swaim to Fletcher Bowron, August 30, 1949, Box 20-5014-210 (3260 APBP0008), Folder "April 19," LAC Archives.

12. On the initial reception of the work, see Linda Lear, "Rachel Carson's 'Silent Spring,'" *Environmental History Review* 17, no. 2 (1993): 23–48.

13. Dean Beckwith to Board of Supervisors, December 3, 1951, Box 20-5014-210 (3260 APBP0008), Folder "April 19," LAC Archives; Gordon Larson [from context] to Mignon P. Zallee, December 9, 1949, Box 20-5014-210 (3260 APBP0008), Folder "April 19," LAC Archives.

14. F. E. Mills to Office of Air Pollution Control, October 2, 1948, Box 20-5014-210 (3260 APBP0008), Folder "April 19," LAC Archives.

15. C. F. Harvey to Board of Supervisors, October 24, 1950, Box 20-5014-210 (3260 APBP0008), Folder "April 19," LAC Archives.

16. Florence D. Aberle to Board of Supervisors, undated [filed by county, September 30, 1949], Box 20-5014-210 (3260 APBP0008), Folder "April 19," LAC Archives.

17. Ford Sammis to Board of Supervisors, September 14, 1953, Box 20-5014-210 (3260 APBP0008), Folder "April 19," LAC Archives.

18. William B. [illegible] to Mayor's Office, ca. 1949, Box 20-5014-210 (3260 APBP0008), Folder "April 19," LAC Archives.

19. John M. Allswang, "Tom Bradley of Los Angeles," *Southern California Quarterly 74*, no. 1 (1992): 57; and Mike Davis, *City of Quartz: Excavating the Future in Los Angeles* (New York: Verso, 1990), 133.

20. "Chronological Record of Decisions and Activities by Supervisor John Anson Ford on the Problem of Smog Control," ca. 1955, Box 25, Folder B III 5a aa, Ford Papers.

21. Los Angeles County Department of Health, Discussion of Ordinance No. 4460, June 18, 1946, Box 25, Folder B III 5a aa (4), Ford Papers.

22. Mayors' Conference on Control of Smoke and Fumes: Reporter's Transcript of Proceedings," May 8, 1946, Box 25, Folder B III 5 a aa (5), Ford Papers.

23. On the police power generally, see Lawrence O. Gostin, *Public Health Law: Power, Duty, Restraint* (Berkeley: University of California Press, 2008), 92–94; and Gostin, "*Jacobson v. Massachusetts* at 100 Years: Police Power and Civil Liberties in Tension," *American Journal of Public Health* 95, no. 4 (2005): 576–81.

24. In a retrospective essay, Howard W. Kennedy describes this in detail. See Howard W. Kennedy, "Legislative and Regulatory Action in Air Pollution Control," *Public Health Reports* 78, no. 9 (1963): 799–806. Most scholarship on the development of public nuisance law is centered on the nineteenth century, not on more recent developments. On this longer history, see Christine Meisner Rosen, "'Knowing' Industrial Pollution: Nuisance Law and the Power of Tradition in a Time of Rapid Economic Change, 1840–1865," *Environmental History* 8, no. 4 (2003): 565–97; and Elizabeth Blackmar, "Accountability for Public Health: Regulating the Housing Market in New York City," in *Hives of Sickness: Public Health and Epidemics in New York City*, edited by David Rosner (New Brunswick, N.J.: Rutgers University Press, 1995), 42–64.

25. "Mayors' Conference on Control of Smoke and Fumes: Reporter's Transcript of Proceedings," May 8, 1946, Box 25, Folder B III 5 a aa (5), Ford Papers.

26. Christopher Sellers, *Crabgrass Crucible: Suburban Nature and the Rise of Environmentalism in Twentieth-Century America* (Chapel Hill: University of North Carolina Press, 2012), 211, 226.

27. I. A. Deutsch, "Various Aspects of Air Pollution Control," May 8, 1946, Box 25, Folder B III 5 a aa (5), Ford Papers.

28. On these tensions, see Paul Sabin, *Crude Politics: The California Oil Market, 1900–1940* (Berkeley: University of California Press, 2005), esp. ch. 3.

29. "Mayors' Conference on Control of Smoke and Fumes."

30. John Anson Ford, "Statement for Mr. Daugherty's Conference," January 1950, Box 20-052140-419, Folder "Thursday-Aug. 8 (1)," LAC Archives.

31. An essay that analyzes the early days of the American film industry's westward move and touches on the centrality of the Los Angeles landscape is Steven J. Ross, "How Hollywood Became Hollywood: Money, Politics, and Movies," in *Metropolis in the Making: Los Angeles in the 1920s*, edited by Tom Sitton and William Deverell (Berkeley: University of California Press, 2001), 255–76; Sabin, *Crude Politics*, ch. 3.

32. H. O. Swartout, "The 'Smog' Problem," September 1945, Box 25, Folder B III 5a bb (1), Ford Papers.

33. Swartout.

34. Annual Report of Los Angeles County Office of Air Pollution Control, 1946–1947, in Box 20-05214-411, 3260 APBP0001, Folder "Nov. 3 (4)," LAC Archives.

35. Annual Report of Los Angeles County Air Pollution Control District, 1947–1948, Box 20-5014-210 (3260 APBP0008), Folder "April 19," LAC Archives.

36. Annual Report of Los Angeles County Air Pollution Control District, 1947–1948.

37. Louis McCabe to W. S. Simpson, April 15, 1948, Box 25, Folder B III 5a aa (7), Ford Papers.

38. Annual Report of Los Angeles County Air Pollution Control District, 1947–1948. On the chamber of commerce's acquiescence to pollution control, see Sarah Elkind, *How Local Politics Shape Federal Policy: Business, Power, and the Environment in Twentieth-Century Los Angeles* (Chapel Hill: University of North Carolina Press, 2011), ch. 2.

39. A complete list of the early rules is in John A. Danielson, *Air Pollution Engineering Manual: Air Pollution Control District of Los Angeles* (Research Triangle Park, N.C.: Environmental Protection Agency, 1973).

40. George C. Murray to Board of Directors, Los Angeles County Air Pollution Control District, February 9, 1948, Box 20-05214-411 (3260 APBP0001), Folder "Nov. 3 (4)," LAC Archives.

41. Murray to Board of Directors, Los Angeles County Air Pollution Control District.

42. Frank H. Eichler to Los Angeles County Board of Supervisors (and "Smoke Control"), February 9, 1948, Box 20-05214-411 (3260 APBP0001), Folder "Nov. 3 (4)," LAC Archives.

43. "Report of Los Angeles County 1948 Grand Jury, Special Committee on Smog, Recommendations in Regard to Smog Abatement Proceedings within Los Angeles County," December 14, 1948, Box 20-05014-210 (APBP0008), Folder "April 19," LAC Archives.

44. Los Angeles County Air Pollution Control District, "Statement on Smog," December 8, 1948, Box 25, Folder B III 5a aa (7), Ford Papers.

45. Geo. P. Taubman Jr. to Board of Supervisors, March 10, 1948, Box 20-05014-210 (3260 APBP0008), Folder "April [illegible]," LAC Archives.

46. Summary of meeting between Citizens Smog Advisory Committee, Los Angeles, and St. Louis Smoke Abatement Campaign, September 29, 1947, Box 25, Folder B III 5a aa(6), Ford Papers; "Mayors' Conference on Control of Smoke and Fumes: Reporter's Transcript of Proceedings," May 8, 1946, Box 25, Folder B III 5 a aa(5), Ford Papers. On Donora, Pennsylvania, see Lynne Page Snyder, "'The Death-Dealing Smog over Donora, Pennsylvania': Industrial Air Pollution, Public Health Policy, and the Politics of Expertise, 1948–1949," *Environmental History Review* 18, no. 1 (1994): 117–39.

47. Morris Neiburger and James Edinger, "Meteorological Aspects of Air Pollution in the Los Angeles Area," October 1947, 3–4, Box 20-05214-411 (3260 APBP0001), unlabeled folder, LAC Archives. The authors researched the paper from September 1946 to May 1947.

48. Neiburger and Edinger, 11.

49. Neiburger and Edinger, 14.

50. Helman P. Roth and Engelbrekt A. Swenson, "Physiological Studies of Irritant Aspects of Atmospheric Pollution," October 15, 1947, 5, Box 20-05214-411 (3260 APBP0001), unlabeled folder, LAC Archives.

51. Roth and Swenson, 10–11.

52. Roth and Swenson, 31–42.

53. Roth and Swenson, 33.

54. H. F. Johnstone, "Technical Aspects of the Los Angeles Smog Problem: A Report Prepared for the Los Angeles County Air Pollution Control District," May 15, 1948, 6, Box 20-05014-210 (APBP0008), Folder "April [illegible]," LAC Archives.

55. Johnstone, 5–6.

56. Johnstone, 9, 12–13.

57. Johnstone, 13.

58. Johnstone, 16–20, 22–26.

59. "Average Daily Cycle of Sulfur Dioxide Concentration Showing Comparison Between September 1949 and September 1952 in Refinery Area," ca. 1952, Box 20-05214-311 (APBP0010), Folder "July 17 (3)," LAC Archives.

60. Johnstone, "Technical Aspects," 21.

61. "Table I. Sulfur Balance Charts," in Johnstone (no page).

62. Gordon Larson, "Estimated Daily Sulfur Dioxide," December 20, 1949, in Box 20-05214-410, Folder "Thursday-Aug. 8 (1)," LAC Archives.

63. Johnston, "Technical Aspects," 28.

64. Fletcher Bowron to Robert Millikan, October 2, 1945, Box 25, Folder B III 5a aa (4), Ford Papers; John Anson Ford to Fletcher Bowron, October 5, 1945, Box 25, Folder B III 5a aa (4), Ford Papers.

65. Louis McCabe, statement to Board of Supervisors, September 13, 1948, Box 20-5014-210 (3260 APBP0008), Folder "April 19," LAC Archives.

66. George L. Schuler to Los Angeles County Grand Jury, November 22, 1948, Box 25, Folder B III 5a aa (7), Ford Papers; George L. Schuler, "Conclusions," March 23, 1948, Box 20-5014-210 (3260 APBP0008), Folder "April," LAC Archives.

67. Mrs. J. G. Schutte to Raymond Darby, October 20, 1948, Box 25, Folder B III 5a aa (7), Ford Papers.

68. "ES" to John Anson Ford, November 1, 1948, Box 25, Folder B III 5a aa (7), Ford Papers.

69. Louis McCabe to Board of Supervisors, April 23, 1948, Box 20-5014-210 (3260 APBP0008), Folder "April," LAC Archives.

70. John Anson Ford to Mrs. A. W. Urquhart, November 15, 1948, Box 25, Folder B III 5a aa (7), Ford Papers.

71. Annual Report of the Los Angeles County Air Pollution Control District, 1949–1950, 37, 40, Box 20-05015-211 (APBP0012), LAC Archives; Annual Report of Los Angeles County Air Pollution Control District, 1947–1948, 15, Box 20-05014-210 (3260 APBP0008), Folder "April 19," LAC Archives; Annual Report of Los Angeles County Office of Air Pollution Control, 1946–1947, 5, Box 20-05214-411 (3260 APBP0001), Folder "Nov. 3 (4)," LAC Archives.

72. These are summarized in "Second Technical and Administrative Report on Air Pollution Control in Los Angeles County, 1950–1951," Box 20-05015-211 (APBP0012) (no folder), LAC Archives.

73. "Report Digest," November 24, 1950, Box 20-05015-211 (APBP0012) (no folder); "Second Technical and Administrative Report on Air Pollution Control in Los Angeles County, 1950–1951," 43–44.

74. Annual Report of the Los Angeles County Air Pollution Control District, 1949–1950, 10–11.

75. Annual Report, 8–9.

76. Annual Report, 27.

77. Annual Report, 19.

78. "Second Technical and Administrative Report on Air Pollution Control in Los Angeles County, 1950–1951."

79. "Excerpt Transcript of Proceedings of the Board of Supervisors, Consisting of Report Made by Gordon P. Larson," October 7, 1952, Box 20-05214-311 (APBP0010), Folder "July 17," LAC Archives.

80. Petition to Gordon Larson and Roy O. Gilbert, July 11, 1951, Box 20-05015-211 (3260 APBP0012) (no folder), LAC Archives.

81. A list of each violation and variance granted from 1948 to 1951 is in "Memorandum," December 31, 1952, Box 20-05214-311 (APBP0010), Folder "July 17," LAC Archives; Gordon Larson to Kenneth Hahn, ca. January 1953, Box 20-05214-311 (APBP0010), Folder "July 17," LAC Archives.

82. Harold W. Kennedy to Board of Supervisors, February 7, 1952, Box 20-05015-211 (APBP0012) (no folder), LAC Archives.

83. Gordon Larson to Kenneth Hahn, January 6, 1953, Box 20-05015-211 (APBP0012) (no folder), LAC Archives; Gordon Larson to Board of Supervisors, February 25, 1953, Box 20-05015-211 (APBP0012) (no folder), LAC Archives.

84. "ES" to John Anson Ford, March 16, 1953, Box 26, Folder B III 5a ff (4), Ford Papers.

85. Mike Davis, City of Quartz: Excavating the Future in Los Angeles (New York: Verso, 1990), 180–86.

86. R. L. Daugherty to Kenneth Hahn, ca. January–February 1953, Box 20-05015-211 (APBP0012) (no folder), LAC Archives.

87. "Second Technical and Administrative Report on Air Pollution Control in Los Angeles County, 1950–1951," 28–32; A. J. Haagen-Smit et al., "Investigation on Injury to Plants from Air Pollution in the Los Angeles Area," Plant Physiology 27, no. 1 (1952): 18–19.

88. A. J. Haagen-Smit, "The Air Pollution Problem in Los Angeles," Engineering and Science 14 (December 1950): 13.

89. A. J. Haagen-Smit, "Chemistry and Physiology of Los Angeles Smog," Industrial and Engineering Chemistry 44, no. 6 (1952): 1343. A more detailed account of the actual experimental procedure and apparatus appeared in an article published a year earlier. See Haagen-Smit et al., "Investigation on Injury to Plants," 21–24.

90. The researchers began with "straight-chain" olefins, $C_2$ to $C_{14}$, identifying "olefins with 5 and 6 carbon atoms with the double bond in the end position" as those resulting in maximum effects. Haagen-Smit, "Chemistry and Physiology of Los Angeles Smog," 1343.

91. Haagen-Smit et al., "Investigation on Injury to Plants," 30.

92. The experiments identified 3-methylheptane and diethyl acetic acid undergoing this process. See Haagen-Smit, "Chemistry and Physiology of Los Angeles Smog," 1346.

93. Haagen-Smit, 1346.

94. Haagen-Smit, 1344–45.

95. Haagen-Smit, 1346.

96. Haagen-Smit, 1346.

97. Haagen-Smit, 1345.

98. "Second Technical and Administrative Report on Air Pollution Control in Los Angeles County, 1950–1951," 38.

99. "Second Technical and Administrative Report on Air Pollution Control in Los Angeles County, 1950–1951," 37–44. The ACPD also calculated figures for 1940 for a baseline measure but through an estimation technique.

100. "Report of Special Committee on Air Pollution: Made to Governor Goodwin J. Knight's Air Pollution Control Conference," December 5, 1953, 14, Box 20-05214-311 (3260 APBP0010), Folder "Nov. 14 (5)," LAC Archives.

101. "Report of Special Committee on Air Pollution," 13.

102. "Report of Special Committee on Air Pollution," 13.

103. "Report of Special Committee on Air Pollution," 14.

104. "Report of Special Committee on Air Pollution," 14.

105. "Report of Special Committee on Air Pollution," 15–16.

106. John Anson Ford, "Statement for Mr. Daugherty's Conference," January 1950, Box 20-052140419, Folder "Thursday-Aug. 8 (1)," LAC Archives.

107. "Report of Special Committee on Air Pollution," 15.

108. Frederick G. Hehr to Los Angeles County Board of Supervisors, December [23], 1954, Box 20-5014-210 (3260 APBP0008), Folder "April 19," LAC Archives.

109. "Warning: The Death Fog Is Coming," November 19, 1955, Box 25, Folder B III 5a ee, Ford Papers.

110. "Warning: The Death Fog Is Coming."

111. S. C. Glassman to Kenneth Hahn, October 10, 1953, Box-Folder 3.6.1.1, Hahn Papers.

112. Robert Hope to Kenneth Hahn, October 9, 1953, Box-Folder 3.6.1.1, Hahn Papers.

113. S. S. Brown to Kenneth Hahn, October 16, 1953, Box-Folder 3.6.1.1, Hahn Papers.

114. Paul Reed to Kenneth Hahn, October 14, 1953, Box-Folder 3.6.1.1, Hahn Papers.

115. L. O. Burwell to Kenneth Hahn, October 12, 1953, Box-Folder 3.6.1.1, Hahn Papers; Harold Lincoln Thompson to Kenneth Hahn, October 16, 1953, Box-Folder 3.6.1.1, Hahn Papers.

116. These campaigns are documented in Colin Gordon, *Dead on Arrival: The Politics of Health Care in Twentieth-Century America* (Princeton, N.J.: Princeton University Press, 2003), 221–23; and Jill Quadagno, *One Nation, Uninsured: Why the U.S. Has No National Health Insurance* (New York: Oxford University Press, 2005), ch. 1. On the impact of McCarthyism on medical Los Angeles, see Merlin Chowkwanyun, "'The Neurosis That Has Possessed Us': Political Repression in the Cold War Medical Profession," *Journal of the History of Medicine and Allied Sciences* 73, no. 3 (2018): 255–73.

117. "Medical Research on Effects of Smog on Health to Begin at Once," *Bulletin of the Los Angeles County Medical Association* 82, no. 4 (March 15, 1951), 268.

118. "Working Outlines for Proposed Smog Research Health Program," ca. late 1953–1954, Box 20-05211-301 (3260 APBP0011), LAC Archives; K. C. Young to Los Angeles County Board of Supervisors, March 11, 1954, Box 26, Folder B III 5a gg, Ford Papers.

119. Los Angeles County Medical Association (LACMA), trustee minutes, October 14, 1954, Los Angeles County Medical Association Papers, Manuscripts Collection, Huntington Library, San Marino, Calif.

120. Gordon Larson to Los Angeles County Board of Supervisors, December 3, 1954, Box-Folder 3.6.1.1, Hahn Papers; Gordon Larson, open letter, January 1954, Box 26, Folder BIII 5a, Ford Papers.

121. Arthur A. Atkisson, "Air Contaminants as Factors in Industrial Land Use Planning and Zoning," July 21, 1956, Box 26, Folder B III 5a hh (2), Ford Papers.

122. "Report of Air Pollution Control District on Accomplishment of Recommendations of Governor's Report on Air Pollution Control (Beckman Report) of December 5, 1953," July 14, 1955, Box 20-05015-211 (3260 APBP0012) (no folder label), LAC Archives.

123. Gordon Larson, "Report to the Board of Supervisors," February 23, 1954, Box 26, Folder B III 5a, Ford Papers.

124. *Transportation in the Los Angeles Area* (Los Angeles: Citizens Traffic and Transportation Committee for the Extended Los Angeles Area, 1957), 6.

125. R. L. Daugherty, "The Problem of Automobile Exhaust," ca. 1955, Box 59, Folder "Pollution," Fletcher Bowron Papers, Manuscripts Collection, Huntington Library, San Marino, Calif.

126. *First Technical Progress Report Covering Work Done in 1954* (Los Angeles: Air Pollution Foundation, 1955), 70.

127. R. L. Daugherty to Kenneth Hahn, January 18, 1954, Hahn 3.6.1.1, Hahn Papers.

128. Herbert C. Legg, press release, December 15, 1953, Box 20-05214-311 (3260 APBP0010), Folder "NOV 14," LAC Archives.

129. "Round Table Discussion," April 29, 1954, Huntington Hotel, Pasadena, Calif., Box 25, Folder B a CC, Ford Papers.

130. "Round Table Discussion," 3.

131. "Round Table Discussion," 4.

132. "Round Table Discussion," 3.

133. "Round Table Discussion," 8, 10.

134. U.S. Census data for 1940, 1950, and 1960 taken from "Total Population" tables, National Historical Geographical Information Systems database, Minnesota Population Center, University of Minnesota, Minneapolis.

135. "Round Table Discussion," 8, 10.

136. "Round Table Discussion," 14.

137. "Round Table Discussion," 30.

138. "Round Table Discussion," 7–8.

139. "Round Table Discussion," 15.

140. "Round Table Discussion," 11.

141. Peter Thorsheim, "Interpreting the London Fog Disaster of 1952," in *The Politics and Culture of Air Pollution*, edited by E. Melanie DuPuis (New York: New York University Press, 2004), 162–64.

142. "Meeting of the Supervisors' Special Advisory Committee on Smog," December 15, 1954, Box 25, Folder BIII 5a cc (5), Ford Papers.

143. These surveys are discussed in John Goldsmith and Lester Breslow, "Epidemiological Aspects of Air Pollution," *Journal of the Air Pollution Control Association* 9, no. 3 (1959): 129–32.

144. Paul Kotin and W. C. Hueper, "Relationship of Industrial Carcinogens to Cancer in the General Population," *Public Health Reports* 80, no. 3 (1955): 332–33.

145. More than half of the initial seventy-one-mouse sample had died before a tumor. The authors calculated the 42 percent figure from the total number of mice alive. See Paul Kotin et al., "Aromatic Hydrocarbons: I. Presence in the Los Angeles Atmosphere and the Carcinogenicity of Atmospheric Extracts," *A.M.A. Archives of Industrial Hygiene and Occupational Medicine* 9, no. 2 (1954): 160.

146. Kotin et al., 160.

147. Paul Kotin, Hans L. Falk, and Marilyn Thomas, "Aromatic Hydrocarbons: II. Presence in the Particulate Phase of Gasoline-Engine Exhausts and the Carcinogenicity of Exhaust Extracts," *A.M.A. Archives of Industrial Hygiene and Occupational Medicine* 9, no. 2 (1954): 176; Paul Kotin, Hans L. Falk, and Marilyn Thomas, "Aromatic Hydrocarbons: III. Presence in the Particulate Phase of Diesel-Engine Exhausts and the Carcinogenicity of Exhaust Extracts," *A.M.A. Archives of Industrial Hygiene and Occupational Medicine* 11, no. 2 (1955): 119. The diesel results followed two unsuccessful previous attempts wherein mice died due to overly potent solution or failed to show any results due to an overly diluted solution intended to keep them alive long enough to survive the experiment.

148. Kotin, Falk, and Thomas, "Aromatic Hydrocarbons: III," 119.

149. "Smog Is Blamed for Lung Cancer," *New York World-Telegram and Sun*, April 20, 1955.

150. Kotin et al., "Aromatic Hydrocarbons: I," 161–62.

151. *Proceedings of the Second Southern California Conference on Elimination of Air Pollution, Ambassador Hotel, Los Angeles, November 14, 1956: Twelve Months' Progress—and the Year Ahead* (California State Chamber of Commerce, 1956), 147.

152. *Proceedings of the Second Southern California Conference*, 154.

153. For an intriguing exploration of mice studies, see Nicole C. Nelson, *Model Behavior: Animal Experiments, Complexity, and the Genetics of Psychiatric Disorders* (Chicago: University of Chicago Press, 2018).

154. *Proceedings of the Second Southern California Conference*, 153.

155. The participants focused particularly on the work of Clarence Mills, a University of Cincinnati environmental health researcher who had conducted the studies based on Chicago mortality records. See Clarence A. Mills, "Air Pollution and Community Health," *American Journal of the Medical Sciences* 224, no. 4 (October 1952).

156. *Proceedings of the Second Southern California Conference*, 166–71.

157. Lester Breslow and John Goldsmith, "Health Effects of Air Pollution," *American Journal of Public Health* 48, no. 7 (1958): 916.

158. Danielson, *Air Pollution Engineering Manual*, 3.

159. The Apartment Association of Los Angeles County, for example, wrote that the ban was "an ill-considered experimental program" that lacked scientific grounding. "Statement by C. A. Owen, President Apartment Association of Los Angeles County," ca. 1955, Box 20-05214-411 (3260 APBP0001), Folder "August 26 (2)," LAC Archives.

160. "Activities of the Automobile Industry on the Control of Hydrocarbon Losses from Automobile Exhaust," August 8, 1955, Box-Folder 3.6.1.4, Hahn Papers. The association had also visited Los Angeles a year earlier outlining its idea about reducing emissions. See J. M. Campbell, "What Are We Doing about Combustion?," August 16–18, 1954, Box-Folder 3.6.1.2, Hahn Papers; and Charles Chayne, "Motor Vehicles and the Air We Breathe," November 4, 1954, Box-Folder 3.6.1.2, Hahn Papers.

161. "Summary Report of Air Pollution Control District Auto Exhaust Research," August 9, 1957, Box-Folder 3.6.1.6, Hahn Papers.

162. *Transportation in the Los Angeles Area* (Los Angeles: Citizens Traffic and Transportation Committee for the Extended Los Angeles Area, 1957), 6.

163. Paul Mader et al., "Effects of Present-Day Fuels on Air Pollution," *Industrial and Engineering Chemistry* 48, no. 9 (1956): 1508–11; and Mader et al., "Photochemical Formation of Air Contaminants from Automobile Exhaust Vapors: Effects of Different Motor Fuels," *Industrial and Engineering Chemistry* 50, no. 8 (1958): 1173–74.

164. Mader et al., "Photochemical Formation," 1174.

165. This is a point made by Christopher Sellers, who writes: "Addressing only those pollutants detectable by sight and sting, whose bodily impact could be so direct and dire, it helped ensure that whatever else emanated from our collective bonfire lay beyond the perception of ordinary citizens." Sellers, *Crabgrass Crucible*, 234.

166. A compendium of this research is in *Health Consequences of Sulfur Oxides: A Report from CHESS, 1970–1971* (Research Triangle Park, N.C.: Environmental Protection Agency, 1974), which contains studies conducted in Idaho and Montana, Chicago, Cincinnati, Ohio, New York, and the Salt Lake City, Utah, area, some of which contained smelter activity similar to that in Los Angeles. See also *Air Quality Criteria for Sulfur Oxides* (Washington, D.C.: United States Government Printing Office, 1969), a Department of Health, Education, and Welfare compendium of similar research. On the Clean Air Act and the transition from regional to national regulation (and tensions therein), see Richard N. L. Andrews, *Managing the Environment, Managing Ourselves: A History of American Environmental Policy* (New Haven: Yale University Press, 1999), ch. 12. The development was somewhat ironic given the influence APCD rule making exerted on federal environmental protection.

167. Paul Kotin, "The Role of Atmospheric Pollution in the Pathogenesis of Pulmonary Cancer: A Review," *Cancer Research* 16, no. 5 (1956): 390. An exemplary article repeating Kotin's claim is Robert C. Toth, "Experts Blame Air Pollution for More Lung Cancer in Cities," *New York Times*, December 12, 1962. Robert Proctor, *Cancer Wars: How Politics Shapes What We Know and Don't Know about Cancer* (New York: Basic Books, 1995), 136, discusses the tobacco industry's appropriation of air pollution research. Far from falling into disrepute, Kotin later became the inaugural head of the National Institute of Environmental Health Sciences.

168. Campbell, "What Are We Doing about Combustion?"; and Daugherty, "Problem of Automobile Exhaust."

169. "Summary Report of Air Pollution Control District Auto Exhaust Research."

170. Robert Kehoe quoted in David Rosner and Gerald Markowitz, *Deceit and Denial: The Deadly Politics of Industrial Pollution* (Berkeley: University of California Press, 2003), 109. Two comprehensive accounts of the controversy over Kehoe and leaded gasoline are in Rosner and Markowitz, *Deceit and Denial*, ch. 4; and Christian Warren, *Brush with Death: A Social History of Lead Poisoning* (Baltimore: Johns Hopkins University Press, 2000), ch. 11.

171. Robert Kehoe to Gordon P. Larson, March 22, 1950, in M. Chowkwanyun, G. Markowitz, and D. Rosner, *Toxic Docs: Version 1.0* (database) (New York: Columbia University and City University of New York, 2020), www.toxicdocs.org/d /4akOXXqgkVzvovo3w3aK91OY1?lightbox=1.

172. H. A. Beatty to Robert Kehoe, August 6, 1954, in Chowkwanyun, Markowitz, and Rosner, *Toxic Docs: Version 1.0*, https://www.toxicdocs.org/d/jy5kvGqvo52w1x88 MRDbZBkk5?lightbox=1.

173. Joseph C. Aub, "Comparison of Organic and Inorganic Lead Poisoning," in *Proceedings of the Third Day of the Fourth Air Pollution Medical Conference* (Berkeley: California State Department of Health, 1960), 52–61, 71. Aub's career is detailed throughout Warren, *Brush with Death*; and in Christopher C. Sellers, *Hazards of the Job: From Industrial Disease to Environmental Health Science* (Chapel Hill: University of North Carolina Press, 1997), ch. 6, with Sellers noting subtle tensions between Aub's fidelity to both lead companies and his own academic inquiry, some of which surfaced at this Harvard conference.

174. Rosner and Markowitz, *Deceit and Denial*, 117.

175. Much of the regulatory debate around airborne lead centered around filtration and its efficacy (or lack thereof). See Carole R. Sawicki, *Seminar Summary: Sampling and Analysis of the Various Forms of Atmospheric Lead* (Research Triangle, N.C.: United States Environmental Protection Agency, 1975).

176. "Peoples Lobby Anti Pollution Initiatives; APCD expenditures," December 22, 1969, Box 3260-20-5011-207 (no folder), LAC Archives.

177. On the People's Lobby, see David Schmidt, *Citizen Lawmakers: The Ballot Initiative Revolution* (Philadelphia: Temple University Press, 1991), ch. 3.

178. Elkind, *How Local Politics Shape Federal Policy*, 82.

179. Christopher Boone, "Zoning and Environmental Inequity in the Industrial East Side," in *Land of Sunshine: An Environmental History of Metropolitan Los Angeles*, edited by William Deverell and Greg Hise (Pittsburgh: University of Pittsburgh Press, 2006), 167–78.

180. Eric Avila, *Popular Culture in the Age of White Flight: Fear and Fantasy in Suburban Los Angeles* (Berkeley: University of California Press, 2004), 195–215. On automobile registrations, see Scott Bottles, *Los Angeles and the Automobile: The Making of the Modern City* (Berkeley: University of California Press, 1987), 269; and Traffic Survey Committee, *Street*

*Traffic Management for Los Angeles: Appraisal and Recommendations Prepared for the City of Los Angeles* (Los Angeles: Traffic Survey Committee, 1948), 13–15.

181. On CARB, see Ellyn Adrienne Hershman, "California Legislation on Air Contaminant Emissions from Stationary Sources," *California Law Review* 58, no. 6 (1970): 1474–98; and Arie Haagen-Smit, "A Lesson from the Smog Capital of the World," *PNAS* 67, no. 2 (1970): 887–97.

182. Andrews, *Managing the Environment, Managing Ourselves*, 233–34.

183. Dwight Eisenhower quoted in Andrews, 227.

CHAPTER THREE

1. On domestic counterinsurgency, see Stuart Schrader, *Badges without Borders: How Global Counterinsurgency Transformed American Policing* (Berkeley: University of California Press, 2019).

2. Los Angeles County Board of Supervisors, transcript on "County Hospital in Watts-Willowbrook Area," March 8, 1966, Box 20-05113-202 (HOBP0025), Folder "October 29, 1968," LAC Archives.

3. On the 1960s rioting, see Thomas Sugrue, *Sweet Land of Liberty: The Forgotten Struggle for Civil Rights in the North* (New York: Random House, 2008), ch. 10. Throughout this chapter, I mostly use "riot" to discuss this event (and that in Cleveland), though I realize the term is imperfect. On connotations attached to riots, see Jonathan Metzl, *The Protest Psychosis: How Schizophrenia Became a Black Disease* (Boston: Beacon, 2010).

4. An account of the relationship between the county general hospital and surrounding institutions, along with a reproduction of the first contract, is in Helen Eastman Martin, *The History of the Los Angeles County Hospital (1878–1968) and the Los Angeles County–University of Southern California Medical Center (1968–1978)* (Los Angeles: University of Southern California Press, 1979), 90, ch. 36, 517–20; Charlie Barnett, "S-County Contract May Face Court Test," *Daily Trojan*, February 26, 1953, provides an account of Ford's brief challenge.

5. Arthur J. Will to War Assets Administration, August 20, 1946, Box 20-05112-207, Folder 40.10/1786 (Harbor Gen. Hosp.), LAC Archives; Arthur J. Will to Los Angeles County Board of Supervisors, memorandum on "Negotiations with U.C.L.A. Medical School," August 19, 1948, Box 20-05112-207, Folder 40.10/1786 (Harbor Gen. Hosp.), LAC Archives.

6. Harry Lee Hufford, "City-County Health Department Mergers in Los Angeles County, July 1, 1964: A Case Study" (MSc thesis, University of Southern California, 1966). The mergers were part of a nationwide trend of consolidation between city-county health departments. See A. James Thomas and R. L. Peterson, "City-County Health Department Mergers," *Public Health Reports* 77, no. 4 (1962): 341–48; William Shonick and Walter Price, "Reorganizations of Health Agencies by Local Government in American Urban Centers: What Do They Portend for 'Public Health'?," *Milbank Memorial Fund Quarterly: Health and Society* 55, no. 2 (1977): 233–71.

7. A. L. Thomas to County Board of Supervisors, memorandum on County-UCLA-Harbor agreements, May 21, 1958, Box 20-05112-207, Folder 40.10/1786 (Harbor Gen. Hosp.), LAC Archives.

8. Los Angeles County Board of Supervisors, motion, March 16, 1948, Box 20-05112-208 (HOBP0019) (no folder label), LAC Archives; Arthur J. Will to Los Angeles County Board of Supervisors, memorandum on additional beds needed, September 12, 1946, Box 20-05112-208 (HOBP0019) (no folder label), LAC Archives.

9. Arthur J. Will to Los Angeles County Board of Supervisors, March 1, 1948, Box 20-05112-208 (HOBP0019) (no folder label), LAC Archives.

10. William A. Barr, question and answer session, April 23, 1956, Box 20-05112-211 (HOBP0022), Folder "Jan 11 (2)," LAC Archives; Harold Kennedy to Los Angeles County Board of Supervisors, April 16, 1956, Box 20-05112-211 (HOBP0022), Folder "Jan 11 (2)," LAC Archives; Los Angeles County Department of Charities, "John Wesley County Hospital General Test Check Audit, Fiscal Year 1956–1957," October 7, 1958, Box 20-05112-211 (HOBP0022), Folder "Jan 11 (2)," LAC Archives; Isaac Pacht to Los Angeles County Board of Supervisors, memorandum on "purchase option for county acquisition of John Wesley County Hospital (Methodist Hospital)," September 1, 1960, Box 20-05112-211 (HOBP0022), Folder "Jan 11 (2)," LAC Archives; "County Will Buy Wesley Hospital," Los Angeles Times, September 5, 1965.

11. James A. Hamilton, "Report of Preliminary Hospital Survey," April 22, 1946, Box 20-05112-208 (HOBP0019) (no folder label), LAC Archives.

12. Los Angeles County Board of Supervisors, transcript of hearing on Los Angeles County General Hospital, August 27, 1957, Box 002219653 (3-K-0045-3-04-06, HOBP-15) (no folder label), LAC Archives.

13. Albert H. Gilpin to Los Angeles County Board of Supervisors, September 30, 1954, Box 20-05112-211 (HOBP0022), Folder "April 14," LAC Archives.

14. "Los Angeles County Patients Deserve Good Nursing Care: A Statement on Behalf of the Nursing Personnel Employed by the County of Los Angeles Submitted to the Board of Supervisors," September 24, 1957, Box 002219653 (3-K-0045-3-04-06, HOBP-15) (no folder label), LAC Archives.

15. Los Angeles County Board of Supervisors, transcript of hearing on nursing shortages, September 24, 1957, Box 002219653 (3-K-0045-3-04-06, HOBP-15) (no folder label), LAC Archives.

16. Los Angeles County Board of Supervisors, transcript of hearing on Los Angeles County General Hospital, August 27, 1957, Box 002219653 (3-K-0045-3-04-06, HOBP-15) (no folder label), LAC Archives.

17. John Anson Ford to William A. Barr et al., September 25, 1957, Box 002219653 (3-K-0045-3-04-06, HOBP-15) (no folder label), LAC Archives.

18. Los Angeles County Board of Supervisors, "Summary of the 10 Calendar Years of the Los Angeles County Hospital Advisory Commission's Activities," November 9, 1966, Box 20-05112-212 (HOBP0023), Folder 1-23-68 (4), LAC Archives.

19. L. S. Hollinger to Los Angeles County Board of Supervisors, memorandum on County General Hospital, June 5, 1959, Box 002219653 (3-K-0045-3-04-06, HOBP-15) (no folder label), LAC Archives.

20. Karen Kruse Thomas, Deluxe Jim Crow: Civil Rights and American Health Policy, 1935–1954 (Athens: University of Georgia Press, 2011), 179.

21. James A. Hamilton, "Report of Preliminary Hospital Survey," April 22, 1946, Box 20-05112-208 (HOBP0019) (no folder label), LAC Archives.

22. For conventional accounts of the Great Migration's various waves that do not focus on the westward stream, see William Cohen, At Freedom's Edge: Black Mobility and the Southern White Quest for Racial Control, 1861–1915 (Baton Rouge: Louisiana State University Press, 1991); and James Grossman, Land of Hope: Chicago, Black Southerners, and the Great Migration (Chicago: University of Chicago Press, 1991). An excellent quantitative analysis of mid-century African American migration is in Leah Bouston, Competition in the Promised Land (Princeton, N.J.: Princeton University Press, 2017).

23. On migration and neighborhood conditions of the South Central area, see Josh Sides, *L.A. City Limits: African American Los Angeles from the Great Depression to the Present* (Berkeley: University of California Press, 2003), esp. 112–20; and Gerald Horne, *The Fire This Time: The Watts Uprising and the 1960s* (Charlottesville: University of Virginia Press, 1995), 31–42.

24. Roy O. Gilbert to Arthur J. Will, October 6, 1953, Box-Folder 1.24.2, Hahn Papers.

25. "Medical Plan Membership Agreement," ca. early 1950s, Box 79, Folder 06.243, Weinerman Papers; Cyril C. Shepro, Irwin Cole, and Robert M. Peck to Stephen H. Fritchman, June 5, 1955, Box 79, Folder 06.243, Weinerman Papers; "Notes on Discussions with Dr. Weinerman," November 12–13, 1954, Box 79, Folder 06.243, Weinerman Papers; "Newsletter Issued by the Community Medical Foundation," December 1951, Box 79, Folder 06.243, Weinerman Papers; Lafe Thorne-Thomson to K. Hartford, March 2, 1955, Box 79, Folder 06.243, Weinerman Papers.

26. Author's calculations using standard isolation index P*= $\Sigma$ $(b_i / B)(b_i / t_i)$, with b = Black population and t = Black and white population, and U.S. Census data for 1960, in National Historical Geographical Information Systems database, Minnesota Population Center, University of Minnesota, Minneapolis.

27. Sol White to Los Angeles County Board of Supervisors, February 23, 1965, Box-Folder 1.24.2.6.5.1, Hahn Papers.

28. Kenneth Hahn, memorandum on Sol White proposal, March 16, 1965, Box-Folder 1.24.2.6.5.1, Hahn Papers. Some additional biographical information on White and his previous initiatives comes from Arthur Viseltear, Arnold I. Kisch, and Milton Roemer, *The Watts Hospital: A Health Facility Is Planned for a Metropolitan Slum Area* (Arlington, Va.: United States Department of Health, Education, and Welfare, 1967), 18–19; and Simeon Booker, "Watts Report: Doctor with 10,000 Patients," *Jet*, April 14, 1966.

29. The most detailed account of the Watts uprising is in Horne, *Fire This Time*.

30. California Governor's Commission on the Los Angeles Riots, *Violence in the City: An End or a Beginning? A Report* (1965), 74.

31. Milton Roemer, "Health Services in the Los Angeles Riot Area," in *Transcripts, Depositions, Consultants' Reports, and Selected Documents of the Governor's Commission on the Los Angeles Riots* [microfilm] (California: Governor's Commission on the Los Angeles Riots, 1966), 5–6, 17, California State Library, Sacramento.

32. Roemer, 9.

33. Roemer, 11–12.

34. Roemer, 14–16.

35. Roemer, 1.

36. Roemer, 18, 42, 49–50.

37. Biographical details about Roemer's background and politics are taken from: Milton Roemer, oral history with Ann C. Boyer, 1988, Special Collections, Charles E. Young Research Library, UCLA; Milton Roemer, oral history with Lewis Weeks, 1985, in Center for Hospital and Healthcare Administration History, American Hospital Association, Chicago; and Emily Abel, Elizabeth Fee, and Theodore Brown, "Milton I. Roemer: Advocate of Social Medicine, International Health, and National Health Insurance," *American Journal of Public Health* 98, no. 9 (2008): 1596–97.

38. Viseltear, Kisch, and Roemer, *Watts Hospital*, 21–22; "HM" to Kenneth Hahn, lettergram on various hospital proposals, December 16, 1965, Box-Folder 1.24.2.6.5.1, Hahn Papers; Hospital Planning Association of Southern California, "Review: Completion of First Phase of Special Study of South and Southeast Los Angeles Metropolitan Area Relating to Existing General Acute Hospital Facilities and Proposals for Acute Facilities," December 14, 1965, Box

20-05113-202 (HOBP0025), Folder "October 29, 1968," LAC Archives; L. S. Hollinger and William A. Barr to Los Angeles County Board of Supervisors, February 10, 1966, memorandum on "A Hospital in the Southeast Area," Box 20-05113-202 (HOBP0025), Folder "October 29, 1968," LAC Archives.

39. Watts Health Advisory Committee to Los Angeles County Board of Supervisors, ca. March 1966 (from context), Box 20-05113-202 (HOBP0025), Folder "October 29, 1968," LAC Archives.

40. Los Angeles County Board of Supervisors, transcript on "County Hospital in Watts-Willowbrook Area."

41. Los Angeles County Board of Supervisors, transcript on "County Hospital in Watts-Willowbrook Area."

42. Kenneth Hahn, Los Angeles County Board of Supervisors motion, February 15, 1966, Box 20-05113-202 (HOBP0025), Folder "October 29, 1968," LAC Archives.

43. Los Angeles County Board of Supervisors, transcript on "County Hospital in Watts-Willowbrook Area."

44. Susan D. Adams to Los Angeles County Board of Supervisors, March 7, 1966, Box 20-05113-202 (HOBP0025), Folder "October 29, 1968," LAC Archives.

45. A discussion of various algorithms used to calculate these ranges is Milton Roemer, "The New Watts General Hospital: What Size Should It Be?," in Viseltear, Kisch, and Roemer, *Watts Hospital*, 52–60.

46. Watts Health Advisory Committee to State Advisory Hospital Council, February 23, 1966, Box-Folder 1.24.2.6.5.8, Hahn Papers.

47. Watts Health Advisory Committee to State Advisory Hospital Council.

48. Watts Health Advisory Committee to Los Angeles County Board of Supervisors, ca. March 1966 (from context), Box 20-05113-202 (HOBP0025), Folder "October 29, 1968," LAC Archives.

49. "Statement by Supervisor Kenneth Hahn," March 8, 1966, Box-Folder 1.24.2.6.5.31, Hahn Papers.

50. Meeting with Winter, O'Dell, and Smith on "Hospital Bond Issue," ca. spring 1966 (from context), Box-Folder 1.24.2.6.5.8, Hahn Papers.

51. "Better Health for Everyone: Yes on A Hospital Bonds," ca. spring 1966 (from context), Box-Folder 1.24.2.6.5.17, Hahn Papers.

52. Callie Dixon, "Appendix E: Socio-Economic and Health Characteristics of Population South Health District," March 7, 1966, Box-Folder 1.24.2.6.5.8, Hahn Papers; Richard Bergholz, "Watts Hospital: A Touchy Issue," *Los Angeles Times*, May 31, 1966. Avoiding explicitly racial framing may also have been grounded in an interpretation of the problem as one of place and geography as much as racial marginalization. Milton Roemer, in his analysis of Watts health, had also primarily framed the problem by comparing place, not race.

53. Los Angeles County Board of Supervisors, transcript on Watts hospital, June 14, 1966, Box 20-05113-202 (HOBP0025), Folder "October 29, 1968," LAC Archives.

54. "Preliminary Financing Analysis: Los Angeles County Southeast General Hospital," September 21, 1966.

55. Los Angeles County Board of Supervisors, transcript on Watts hospital.

56. At a county hearing, E. P. Alexander of the *Los Angeles Herald-Dispatch* was the only person who raised the question, asking: "The hospital you propose putting in the Palm Lane district, what do you propose, gentleman, to do with the people that are living in this area now? I would like to know where they are going and where are they to live?" See "Few Former Palm Lane Residents in Public Housing," *Los Angeles Sentinel*, November 3,

1966; Los Angeles County Board of Supervisors, transcript on "County Hospital in Watts-Willowbrook Area."

57. Office of Economic Opportunity, press release on Watts OEO center, July 3, 1968, Box-Folder 1.24.2.5.4, Hahn Papers; for an account of the center with a different take and disciplinary perspective, see Jenna Loyd, *Health Rights Are Civil Rights: Peace and Justice Activism in Los Angeles, 1963–1978* (Minneapolis: University of Minnesota Press, 2014), 70–74.

58. "Announcement," *South End Bee*, November 16, 1966, private collection.

59. "Neighborhood Family Health Service Center," grant proposal, ca. 1966, Box-Folder 1.24.2.5.4, Hahn Papers. On paraprofessionals in education, see Nick Juravich, "'Harlem Sophistication': Community-Based Paraprofessional Educators in Harlem and East Harlem," in *Harlem: A Century of Schooling and Resistance in a Black Community*, edited by Ansley T. Erickson and Ernest Morrell (New York: Columbia University Press, 2019), 234–56.

60. "Statement by Councilman Billy G. Mills Re: Watts Health Services Center," ca. 1966 (from context), Box-Folder 1.24.2.5.4, Hahn Papers.

61. "Neighborhood Family Health Service Center."

62. Roger Egeberg, Robert Tranquada, and Elsie Giorgi, "A University of Southern California Proposal for Development and Operation of the Family Neighborhood Health Services Center," in Powell unpub.

This document is an analysis of the Watts center's early years by Rodney Powell, who later serves as its director. Written shortly after the events he describes, the Powell piece is a mix of his own prose and large quotations from documents, some reproduced in their entirety. It is all the more invaluable given the thin accessible paper trail the center left. I have triangulated Powell's interpretation of several events with other sources and have cited a number of the reproduced documents inside of it.

63. Biographical information on Bates comes from Robert Tranquada, unpublished memoir, private collection; James Bates, "South Central Multipurpose Health Center," ca. late 1960s (from context), Powell unpub.

64. Tranquada, memoir.

65. "Neighborhood Family Health Service Center," grant proposal.

66. Jim Bates, document on Community Health Council formation, ca. 1966–67 (from context), Powell unpub.; on antiracism and radicalism in Los Angeles during this era, see Scott Kurashige, *The Shifting Grounds of Race: Black and Japanese Americans in the Making of Multiethnic Los Angeles* (Princeton, N.J.: Princeton University Press, 2008); and Laura Pulido, *Black, Brown, Yellow, and Left: Radical Activism in Los Angeles* (Berkeley: University of California Press, 2006).

67. Augustus Hawkins to South Central Multi-Purpose Health Services Center, October 10, 1966, Powell unpub.

68. Tranquada to Hawkins, ca. October 1966 (from context), Powell unpub.

69. Robert Tranquada, "Historical Notes," October 25, 1966, private collection.

70. Robert Tranquada and Elsie Giorgi, "A Report on the Relationship between the Grantee Institution and the Community Health Council of a Neighborhood Health Center; With Specific and General Recommendations for the Solution of Some Problem Encountered," August 1966, private collection. On controversies around hiring and contracting, see David Goldberg and Trevor Griffey, eds., *Black Power at Work Community Control, Affirmative Action, and the Construction Industry* (Ithaca, N.Y.: Cornell University Press, 2011).

71. Robert Tranquada and Elsie Giorgi, "Suggested Policy Guidelines for CAP 207 (211) Councils," ca. August 1966 (from context), private collection.

72. The authoritative source on Drew is Spencie Love, *One Blood: The Death and Resurrection of Charles R. Drew* (Chapel Hill: University of North Carolina Press, 1997); Michael G. Kenny, "A Question of Blood, Race, and Politics," *Journal of the History of Medicine and Allied Sciences* (October 2006).

73. Charles R. Drew Medical Society, meeting minutes, June 6, 1966, Powell unpub.

74. Charles R. Drew Medical Society, meeting minutes.

75. Charles R. Drew Medical Society, meeting minutes.

76. "Miracle in Charcoal Alley," *Time*, November 17, 1967.

77. "Why We Oppose the USC Health Center," *Star Review*, October 20, 1966.

78. "Why We Oppose the USC Health Center."

79. "Watts Doctors Oppose U.S.C. Clinic," *Star Review*, October 20, 1966.

80. Jim Bates, document on Community Health Council formation, ca. 1966–67 (from context), Powell unpub.

81. Tranquada, unpublished memoir.

82. "Where Were You, Doctor?," ca. 1966–67 (from context), private collection.

83. Jim Bates, document on Community Health Council formation, ca. 1966–1967 (from context), Powell unpub.

84. Tranquada, unpublished memoir.

85. "Slide Titles for South Central Multipurpose Health Services Center Dedication," ca. October–September 1967 (from context), private collection; "Watts Medical Center Has Opening," *Los Angeles Sentinel*, September 14, 1967; William McPhillips, "Shriver Dedicates Watts Health Center," *Los Angeles Times*, September 17, 1967.

86. Tranquada to Roger Egeberg, confidential memo on Elsie Giorgi, June 3, 1967, private collection; Tranquada, unpublished memoir.

87. Elsie Giorgi to Tranquada, memo on Sol White, ca. early 1967 (from context), private collection.

88. Tranquada to Professional Advisory Board, memorandum "Concerning the Status of Dr. Sol White," October 1967 (from context); Tranquada to Egeberg, October 12, 1967, private collection.

89. Julian Zelizer, *The Fierce Urgency of Now: Lyndon Johnson, Congress, and the Battle for the Great Society* (New York: Penguin Books, 2015), 257.

90. Tranquada to Community Health Council, January 17, 1968, memorandum on OEO budget situation, Powell unpub.

91. Powell discusses this background briefly in Rodney Powell, "What Has Happened in the Watts-Willowbrook Program," in *Medicine in the Ghetto*, edited by John C. Norman (New York: Appleton-Century-Crofts, 1969), 73–85.

92. Harry Nelson, "New Watts Clinic Fights to Survive Many Problems," *Los Angeles Times*, July 8, 1968.

93. Powell unpub., 47–48.

94. Powell unpub., 47–48.

95. Powell unpub., 49.

96. Powell unpub., 52–53.

97. See Amy Offner, *Sorting Out the Mixed Economy: The Rise and Fall of Welfare and Developmental States in the Americas* (Princeton, N.J.: Princeton University Press, 2019), esp. ch. 3 and 7.

98. Powell unpub., 67.

99. Alice O'Connor, *Poverty Knowledge: Social Science, Social Policy, and the Poor in Twentieth-Century U.S. History* (Princeton, N.J.: Princeton University Press, 2001), 140–43;

Robert Self, *American Babylon: Race and the Struggle for Postwar Oakland* (Princeton, N.J.: Princeton University Press, 2003), 201.

100. On local-level job creation during the War on Poverty, see Guian McKee, *The Problem of Jobs: Liberalism, Race, and Deindustrialization in Philadelphia* (Chicago: University of Chicago Press, 2008).

101. Powell, "What Has Happened," 82.

102. Powell, 85.

103. *Hearings before the Select Committee on Nutrition and Human Needs of the United States Senate: Second Session and Ninety-First Congress (First Session on Nutrition and Human Needs Part 9—California)*, 2737–44.

104. *Hearings before the Select Committee*, 2738, 2741.

105. *Hearings before the Select Committee*, 2739.

106. The most trenchant observation of this contradiction is Anne-Emanuelle Birn, *Marriage of Convenience: Rockefeller International Health and Revolutionary Mexico* (Rochester, N.Y.: University of Rochester Press, 2006); and see Birn, "Gates's Grandest Challenge: Transcending Technology as Public Health Ideology," *Lancet* 366, no. 9484 (2005): 514–19.

107. Los Angeles County Hospital Advisory Commission, "Report on So-Called 'Heal-In'" at General Hospital, July 13, 1965; Los Angeles County Hospital Advisory Commission, "Progress Report, 1965–1966," July 7, 1966, Box 20-05112-212 (HOBP0023), Folder "1-1-23–68 (4)," LAC Archives.

108. Los Angeles County Hospital Advisory Commission, "Progress Report, 1965–1966."

109. Bunnie Berry to Los Angeles County Board of Supervisors, April 24, 1966, Box 20-05112-212 (HOBP0023) (no folder title), LAC Archives.

110. Joseph Spinazzola, spring 1966 (from context), Box 20-05112-212 (HOBP0023) (no folder title), LAC Archives.

111. Mary E. McShane to Ishmael Corona, April 24, 1966, Box 20-05112-212 (HOBP0023) (no folder title), LAC Archives.

112. Alex A. Roger to Los Angeles County Board of Supervisors, May 13, 1966, Box 20-05112-212 (HOBP0023) (no folder title), LAC Archives.

113. L. S. Hollinger to Los Angeles County Board of Supervisors, memorandum on Medi-Cal and appropriations increase, December 17, 1968, Box 20-05115-211 (HOBP0058) (no folder), LAC Archives.

114. Spencer Williams to Lynne Frantz, June 28, 1967, Box 20-05115-211 (HOBP0058) (no folder), LAC Archives.

115. L. S. Hollinger to Los Angeles County Board of Supervisors, memorandum on "Recommendations concerning Medi-Cal Financing," December 14, 1966, Box 20-05115-211 (HOBP0058) (no folder), LAC Archives.

116. L. S. Hollinger to George A. Carter, memorandum to Los Angeles County Grand Jury on "Medicare and Medi-Cal Programs in Los Angeles County," June 26, 1967, Box 20-05115-211 (HOBP0058) (no folder), LAC Archives; Los Angeles County Grand Jury (1967) Audit Committee to William Barr, L. S. Hollinger, Roscoe Hollinger, and Alvin Karp, May 18, 1967, Box 20-05115-211 (HOBP0058) (no folder), LAC Archives; Casper Weinberger, "With the Current Ruckus—Just What Is Medi-Cal?," *Los Angeles Times*, September 29, 1967.

117. Graduate Social Work Students' Association, Sacramento State College, resolution on Medi-Cal cuts, November 9, 1967, Box 20-05115-211 (HOBP0058) (no folder), LAC Archives.

118. James Mize to Ronald Reagan, November 22, 1967, Box 20-05115-211 (HOBP0058) (no folder), LAC Archives; Los Angeles County Board of Supervisors, statement on Reagan Medi-Cal proposal, November 1967 (from context), Box 20-05115-211 (HOBP0058) (no

folder), LAC Archives; Los Angeles County Board of Supervisors, "Special Item: Chief Administrative Officer," November 1967 (from context), Box 20-05115-211 (HOBP0058) (no folder), LAC Archives.

119. "Medi-Cal: It Seems to Be Solvent for Now," *Los Angeles Times*, January 7, 1968; Robert Fairbanks, "After 'Deficit Flurry: Medi-Cal "Numbers Game' in New Phase," *Los Angeles Times*, January 14, 1968.

120. "Appendix" in Los Angeles County Committee on Emergency Medical Care, "Subcommittee Report to the Board of Supervisors: Investigation of Charges Made by the Interns and Residents Regarding the Quality of Patient Care at the Los Angeles County/USC Medical Center," April 1971, 18, Box 3260 40.2, "County-USC Medical Center 1-6-70 to 5-28-74," Folder "#2 County-USC Medical Center-Outside Medical Relief [unintelligible] 40.2 From: 10-6-70 To: 1-18-72," LAC Archives.

121. "Five Year Analysis" in Los Angeles County Committee on Emergency Medical Care, "Subcommittee Report," 22.

122. "Report of Los Angeles County Hospital Commission on Los Angeles County/University of Southern California Medical Center," April 13, 1971, Box 3260 40.2 "County-USC Medical Center 10-6-70 to 5-28-74," Folder "#2 County-USC Medical Center-Outside Medical Relief [unintelligible] 40.2 From: 10-6-70 To: 1-18-72," LAC Archives; George Getze, "Hospital Criticism Labeled 'Hogwash,'" *Los Angeles Times*, December 17, 1970.

123. "Report of Los Angeles County Hospital Commission," 13, 17–18.

124. "Report of Los Angeles County Hospital Commission," 14.

125. "Report of Los Angeles County Hospital Commission," 14–15.

126. "Report of Los Angeles County Hospital Commission," 15–16; "Subcommittee Conclusions and Recommendations" in Los Angeles County Committee on Emergency Medical Care, "Subcommittee Report," 3–4.

127. "Report of Los Angeles County Hospital Commission," 18–19; Ray Zeman, "County Spending Slashes Ordered," *Los Angeles Times*, January 6, 1971.

128. "Report of Los Angeles County Hospital Commission," 18–19; Zeman, "County Spending Slashes Ordered."

129. "Recommendations for LAC/USC Medical Center" in "Report of Los Angeles County Hospital Commission."

130. Los Angeles County Health Services Planning Committee, *Report on the Study of Health Services of the County of Los Angeles*, February 24, 1970, 12, 18–19, in Los Angeles County Department of Public Health, Public Health Library, Los Angeles; Malcolm Merrill, *Future Directions for Health Services: Review of the Program of the Los Angeles County Health Department*, undertaken at the request of the Los Angeles County Board of Supervisors (1970), in Los Angeles County Department of Health Services Library, Los Angeles.

131. Elmer A. Anderson, "The Watts Health Miracle," *California Medicine* 115, no. 5 (1971): 65.

132. Harry E. Douglas, "Proposal for Hospital Occupations Training Center, Martin Luther King, Jr. General Hospital," ca. 1972 (from context), Box-Folder 1.24.2.6.5.64, Hahn Papers; L. A. Witherill, "Statement before the Senate Committee on Health and Welfare, Subcommittee on Medical Education," October 30, 1972, Box-Folder 1.24.2.6.5.68, Hahn Papers.

133. Mitchell W. Spellman to Sherman M. Mellinkoff, memorandum on UCLA affiliation with Drew Postgraduate Medical School, August 1, 1969; "Drew Postgraduate Medical School Maintains Close Ties with UCLA, USC," *UCLA Weekly*, April 19, 1971, Series 255,

Box 3, Folder "Drew Postgraduate Medical School 1978," UCLA School of Medicine, UCLA Archives, Charles E. Young Research Library, University of California, Los Angeles.

134. C. O. McCorkle Jr. to Charles Young, memorandum on UCLA dispersal of state funds, September 26, 1974, Series 226, Box 3, Folder "Drew Postgraduate Medical School 1974," UCLA School of Medicine, UCLA Archives, Charles E. Young Research Library, University of California, Los Angeles.

135. Joseph Graves, "Fact and Fiction: High Blood Pressure: Point of View," *Grapevine* (June 1975), Box 66, Augustus Hawkins Papers, Library Special Collections, Charles E. Young Research Library, UCLA, Los Angeles; Los Angeles County Department of Health Services, "Martin Luther King, Jr. General Hospital, Report No. 11," July 30, 1974, Box "Hospitals County-USC Med. Ctr. 40 40-1 40-2," Folder "Hospitals 40.0 From: 1-9-73 To: 1-23-75 #3," LAC Archives.

136. Los Angeles County Department of Health Services, "Ten-Year Capital Project Report," March 25, 1974, Box 3260-20-5218, Folder "185 Misc. #1," LAC Archives.

137. Los Angeles County Department of Health Services, "Ten-Year Capital Project Report."

138. Los Angeles County Department of Health Services, Biennial Report 1974–1976, Box 3260 20-5218- [illegible], Folder "185 Misc. #2," Location ID: X16-03202-0104, LAC Archives.

139. On national health insurance in this time period, see Starr, "Rebounding with Medicare: Reform and Counterreform in American Health Policy," *Journal of Health Politics, Policy and Law* 43, no. 4 (2018): 707–30; and Flint J. Wainess, "The Ways and Means of National Health Care Reform, 1974 and Beyond," *Journal of Health Politics, Policy and Law* 24, no. 2 (1991): 305–33.

140. Unfortunately, county trend summaries do not disaggregate between inpatient and outpatient admissions, though the sharp one-year increases for LAC–USC were likely the partial result of mid-decade patient pressures on the institutions.

141. Los Angeles County Department of Health Services, Biennial Report 1974.

142. Interns and Residents of Martin Luther King, Jr. General Hospital, statement on resolution of action, ca. late May 1975 (from context); "House Staff Manifesto," May 1975 (from context); "We, the Community Need—Quality Patient Care," May 1975; Interns and Residents of Martin Luther King, Jr. General Hospital, press statement, June 11, 1975, all in Box-Folder 1.24.2.6.5.81, Hahn Papers.

143. Los Angeles County, Department of Health Services, "Report on Task Forces to Review Intern and Resident Demands at Martin Luther King, Jr. General Hospital, LAC-USC Medical Center and Harbor General Hospital," May 30, 1975, in Box-Folder 1.24.35, Hahn Papers.

144. California Nurses' Association, *Proceedings: Community Nursing Service in Poverty and Ghetto Areas, November 6 & 7, 1970* (San Francisco: California Nurses Association, 1970), 112; "Black Grassroots Caucus Proves 'Highly Successful,'" *Los Angeles Sentinel*, March 23, 1972; Wendell Green, "Southeast Residents Seek Voice in New Hospital," *Los Angeles Sentinel*, February 27, 1972.

145. Black Grassroots Caucus, "Informational Bulletin," May 27, 1975, Box-Folder 1.24.35, Hahn Papers.

146. "A Long-Term Relationship between the University of California and the Charles R. Drew Postgraduate Medical School," January 3, 1978, Series 255, Box 3, Folder "Drew Postgraduate Medical School 1978," UCLA School of Medicine, UCLA Archives, Charles E. Young Research Library, University of California, Los Angeles.

147. On Arthur Jensen, see Michael Yudell, *Race Unmasked: Biology and Race in the 20th Century* (New York: Columbia University Press), 175–76.

148. The episode is recounted in Alondra Nelson, *Body and Soul: The Black Panther Party and the Fight against Medical Discrimination* (Minneapolis: University of Minnesota Press, 2011), 159–80. Nelson is careful to note that the UCLA professor chiefly responsible for the center, Louis West, was less overtly racialist and heavy-handedly biologistic than *Violence and the Brain*'s authors even as he accepted most of their core assumptions.

149. Coalition of Organizations to Leroy Weekes, ca. 1978 (from context), Box-Folder 1.24.35, Hahn Papers.

150. Los Angeles County Hospital Commission, "Site Inspection to Martin Luther King, Jr., General Hospital," November 5, 1980, Box-Folder 2.35.2, Hahn Papers.

151. On Proposition 13, see Peter Schrag, *Paradise Lost: California's Experience, America's Future* (Berkeley: University of California Press, 1998), 129–87; Robert Self, *American Babylon: Race and the Struggle for Postwar Oakland* (Princeton, N.J.: Princeton University Press, 2003), 316–27; Clarence Y. Lo, *Small Property versus Big Government: Social Origins of the Property Tax Revolt* (Berkeley: University of California Press, 1990); and Mike Davis, *City of Quartz: Excavating the Future in Los Angeles* (New York: Verso, 1990), 180–86.

152. Edmund Edelman, motion before Los Angeles County Board of Supervisors, August 1, 1978, Box 3260-20-5019-207, Folder "185-10 Closures," LAC Archives.

153. The initial cuts for these two districts (Central and Southeastern) were initially much higher, at 22 percent and 26 percent, respectively, prompting an inquiry that led to a more even distribution of cuts across the county. See Robert W. White to Art Torres, memorandum on 1981–82 health services budget appropriation, August 5, 1981, Box 3260-20-5218, Folder "185 Misc. #2," LAC Archives.

154. Harry L. Hufford to Art Torres, memorandum on 1981–82 health services budget appropriation, August 10, 1981, 1, Box 3260-20-5218, Folder "185 Misc. #2," LAC Archives.

155. South Central Multipurpose Health Services Corporation, "Refunding Proposal: Comprehensive Health Services," 1973, Library for International and Public Affairs, University of Southern California, Los Angeles.

156. Clifton A. Cole to Augustus Hawkins, February 23, March 9, 1973, Box 93, Augustus Hawkins Papers, Library Special Collections, Charles E. Young Research Library, UCLA, Los Angeles.

157. "Watts Health Foundation Will Lay Off 100 Workers," *Los Angeles Sentinel*, August 18, 1994; "Watts Health Agency to Lay Off 200 Staff," *Los Angeles Sentinel*, March 5, 1987; F. Finley McRae, "Watts Health Foundation Closes Doors," *Los Angeles Sentinel*, March 12, 1987; Denise Gellene, "Regulators Seize Control of Watts Health Foundation," *Los Angeles Times*, August 9, 2001.

158. Los Angeles County Auditor-Controller, "Department of Health Services—Martin Luther King, Jr. General Hospital—Fiscal Year 1973–1974 Audit," March 22, 1976, Box 3260-20-5219-310, Folder "Jan. 1976 through Oct. 1979," LAC Archives.

159. "Conditions of Martin L. King Hospital," ca. 1977 (from context), Box-Folder 1.24.2.6.5.84, Hahn Papers.

160. Darnell Hunt and Ana-Christina Ramon, "Killing 'Killer King': The Los Angeles Times and a 'Troubled' Hospital in the 'Hood,'" in *Black Los Angeles: American Dreams and Racial Realities*, edited by Hunt and Ramon (New York: New York University Press, 2010), 283–320.

161. Jube Shiver Jr., "Hospital Closings Called Evidence of Health Care Crisis for Blacks, Poor," *Los Angeles Times*, May 20, 1984; Geraldine Dalleck and Stan Dorn, "Same Old Story for Public Health," *Los Angeles Times*, August 19, 1986.

162. Stanley G. Robertson, "L.A. Confidential," *Los Angeles Sentinel*, February 4, 1988.

163. Claire Spiegel, "Angry Crowd Defends King Hospital," *Los Angeles Times*, September 28, 1989.

164. Larry Aubry, "King-Drew: Another View," *Los Angeles Sentinel*, October 5, 1989.


CHAPTER FOUR

1. Thomas H. Reed and Doris H. Reed, *The Organization of the Cleveland City Hospital: A Report to the Cleveland Bureau of Governmental Research* (New York: National Municipal League, 1949), 1, 27.

2. Reed and Reed, 11–12; Charles Rosenberg, *The Care of Strangers: The Rise of America's Hospital System* (New York: Basic Books, 1987); David Rosner, *A Once Charitable Enterprise: Hospitals and Health Care in Brooklyn and New York, 1885–1915* (New York: Cambridge University Press, 1982).

3. Reed and Reed, *Organization of the Cleveland City Hospital*, 17–18.

4. Reed and Reed, 20–23.

5. Reed and Reed, 36–44.

6. Author's calculations from U.S. Census for 1950 and 1960 in *Census of Population: 1950*, vol. 2, *Characteristics of the Population, Part 35, Ohio* (Washington, D.C.: U.S. Government Printing Office, 1952) and *Census of Population: 1960*, vol. 1, *Characteristics of the Population, Part 37, Ohio* (Washington, D.C.: U.S. Government Printing Office, 1961).

7. *A Study of Community Health Services in Cleveland and Cuyahoga County, Ohio: Report of Study Team to Public Health Study Group of Cleveland Metropolitan Services Commission* (Cleveland: Cleveland Metropolitan Services Corporation [METRO], 1957), 63, 70, in Public Administration Library, Cleveland Public Library, Cleveland, Ohio; A. Harmon to Bell Grave, memorandum on "Daily Rates for Patient Care—City Hospital," March 6, 1956; A. Harmon to Bell Grave, memorandum on "Daily Rates for Patient Care—City Hospital," March 1, 1956, Container 1, Celebrezze Papers.

8. *Study of Community Health Services*, 64; *Plan and Policies for Future Development of Western Reserve University School of Medicine and University Hospitals of Cleveland* (Cleveland: Committee on Plans and Development, 1954), 103–4, in Cleveland Health Sciences Library, Allen Memorial Library, Case Western Reserve University.

9. Anthony Celebrezze to Thomas Kinney, March 19, 1956, Container 1, Folder 18, Celebrezze Papers.

10. Arthur Cieslak to Celebrezze, November 9, 1956, Container 1, Folder 18, Celebrezze Papers.

11. Charles Rammelkamp to Celebrezze, September 15, 1957, Container 1, Folder 19, Celebrezze Papers.

12. "A Financial Formula for Transfer of City Hospital, Cleveland Boys' School and Blossom Hill School for Girls from the City of Cleveland to the County of Cuyahoga," June 5, 1957, Container 1, Folder 32, Celebrezze Papers.

13. A. Harmon to Lewis Cutrer, June 19, 1958, Container 1, Folder 20, Celebrezze Papers.

14. On right-to-work, see Elizabeth Tandy Shermer, "'Is Freedom of the Individual Un-American?' Right-to-Work Campaigns and Anti-Union Conservatism, 1943–1958," in *The Right and Labor in America: Politics, Ideology, and Imagination*, edited by Nelson Lichtestein and Shermer (Philadelphia: University of Pennsylvania Press, 2012), 114–36.

15. Mike Curtin, "The O'Neill-DiSalle Years, 1957–1963," in *Ohio Politics*, edited by Alexander P. Lamis and Mary Anne Sharkey (Kent, Ohio: Kent State University Press, 1958),

49–50; "Pattern for a Medical Care Program: Climate for a New Organization of Health Care," September 1964, Box 40, Folder 245, Weinerman Papers.

16. "Section V: Financing Medical Care," ca. 1961, Box 38, Folder 239, Weinerman Papers; "Summary of Preliminary Cleveland Report," September 21, 1961, Box 38, Folder 240, Weinerman Papers. On the 1950s rise in health care costs, see Christy Chapin, *Ensuring America's Health: The Public Creation of the Corporate Health Care System* (New York: Oxford University Press, 2015), ch. 6.

17. Biographical information on Richard Weinerman is taken from the author's canvas of his personal papers; and "E. Richard Weinerman, M.D.," *American Journal of Public Health* 60, no. 5 (1970): 797–99, two obituaries written after his death in a plane crash. For Yedidia, see Ora Huth, interview with Avram Yedidia, Kaiser Permanente Medical Care Program Oral History Project in Bancroft Library, University of California, Berkeley, CA. For Wilson, see "Health Report," July 1963, Box 40, Folder 261, Weinerman Papers.

18. "Pattern for a Medical Care Program."

19. "Statement of Principles: Cleveland Health Foundation / Western Reserve University School of Medicine / University Hospital," March 20, 1962, Box 38, Folder 241, Weinerman Papers.

20. "A Proposal to Plan an Integrated Comprehensive Health Service," ca. 1964–65 (from context), Box 38, Folder 241, Weinerman Papers.

21. "Filling in the Financial Picture," ca. 1962 (from context), Box 38, Folder 241, Weinerman Papers.

22. The best account of McCarthyist attacks on prepaid group practice is Rickey Hendricks, "Medical Practice Embattled: Kaiser Permanente, the American Medical Association, and Henry J. Kaiser on the West Coast, 1945–1955," *Pacific Historical Review* 60, no. 4 (1991): 439–73.

23. "Schedule of Anticipated Sources of Cash and Budgeted Capital Requirements During the Pre-Operating Period," October 8, 1962, Box 40, Folder 254, Weinerman Papers.

24. "A Program to Recruit Subscribers for the Cleveland Health Foundation," February 25, 1962, Box 38, Folder 241, Weinerman Papers.

25. Glenn Wilson, "Some Observations on Prepaid Group Practice and the Enrollment of Subscribers," presentation before Group Health Association of America (GHAA), 1966, Box 40, Folder 261, Weinerman Papers.

26. "The Community Health Foundation as a Demonstration in Comprehensive Health Planning," ca. 1966–68 (from context), Box 40, Folder 264, Weinerman Papers.

27. "CHF Takes New Health View," *Cleveland Plain Dealer*, December 14, 1966.

28. "Basic Health Record," March 23, 1964, Box 41, Folder 271, Weinerman Papers.

29. Community Health Foundation, "Health Maintenance Project," August 12, 1964, Box 41, Folder 270, Weinerman Papers.

30. Community Health Foundation, "Health Maintenance Project."

31. See Nancy Tomes, *Remaking the American Patient: How Madison Avenue and Modern Medicine Turned Patients into Consumers* (Chapel Hill: University of North Carolina Press, 2016), 262–63, 270–76.

32. See Marie Gottschalk, "The Elusive Goal of Universal Health Care: Organized Labor and the Institutional Straightjacket of the Private Welfare State," *Journal of Policy History* 11, no. 4 (1999): 367–98; Jacob S. Hacker, *The Divided Welfare State: The Battle over Public and Private Social Benefits in the United States* (New York: Cambridge University Press, 2002).

33. Todd Swanstrom, *The Crisis of Growth Politics: Cleveland, Kucinich, and the Challenge of Urban Populism* (Philadelphia: Temple University Press, 1985), ch. 7. In this regard, the

CHF kept well within the bounds of midcentury American welfare state logic when it came to health provision and the role of labor in abetting (sometimes not entirely wittingly) it. See Jennifer Klein, *For All These Rights: Business, Labor, and the Shaping of America's Public-Private Welfare State* (Princeton, N.J.: Princeton University Press, 2003), ch. 6, on the limits of group practice; and, more generally, Hacker, *Divided Welfare State*. Critiques of group practice from the left, however, can underappreciate their nonfiduciary upside on matters such as patient experience.

34. Eugene Vayda, "Changing Patterns of Medical Care," *Bulletin of the Academy of Medicine of Cleveland* 50, no. 6 (1965): 10–12.

35. The hardening of racial segregation in the area began during the first Great Migration. See Kenneth Kusmer, *A Ghetto Takes Shape: Black Cleveland, 1870–1930* (Urbana: University of Illinois Press, 1978), ch. 7.

36. "Public Education Program: In Support of the Community Health Foundation Hospital Independence, Ohio," ca. late 1967 (from context), Box 39, Folder 252, Weinerman Papers; Thomas Sugrue, "Crabgrass-Roots Politics: Race, Rights, and the Reaction against Liberalism in the Urban North, 1940–1964," *Journal of American History* 82, no. 2 (1995): 551–78.

37. William F. Miller, "Kaiser-CHF Hospital Plans New Element Here," *Cleveland Plain-Dealer*, December 20, 1968.

38. Leonard Moore, *Carl B. Stokes and the Rise of Black Political Power* (Urbana: University of Illinois Press, 2002), 23, 42.

39. "Special Grand Jury Report Relating to Hough Riots," 3–9, August 9, 1966, Box 23, Folder 6, Gottron Papers.

40. "Special Grand Jury Report Relating to Hough Riots," 3–9.

41. "Special Grand Jury Report Relating to Hough Riots," 13–14.

42. "Mayor's Emergency Committee: Final Report," 13, August 23, 1966, Box 23, Folder 6, Gottron Papers.

43. On Cleveland radicalism and activism, see Nishani Frazier, *Harambee City: The Congress of Racial Equality in Cleveland and the Rise of Black Power Populism* (Fayetteville: University of Arkansas Press, 2017); and Kimberley Phillips, *Alabama North: African-American Migrants, Community, and Working-Class Activism in Cleveland, 1915–45* (Urbana: University of Illinois Press, 1999).

44. "Cleveland Citizens Committee on Hough Disturbances" (Exhibit 106), October 13, 1966, in *Federal Role in Urban Affairs: Hearings before the Subcommittee on Executive Reorganization of the Committee on Government Operations, United States Senate, Eighty-Ninth Congress, Second Session, Part 4* (Washington, D.C.: U.S. Government Printing Office, 1966), 1039–46.

45. On urban renewal, see Herbert J. Gans, *The Urban Villagers: Group and Class in the Life of Italian-Americans* (New York: Free Press, 1962), esp. chs. 13, 14; Martin Anderson, *The Federal Bulldozer: A Critical Analysis of Urban Renewal, 1942–1962* (New York: McGraw-Hill, 1967); and, more recently, Arnold Hirsch, *Making the Second Ghetto: Race and Housing in Chicago, 1940–1960* (New York: Cambridge University Press, 1983); Samuel Zipp, *Manhattan Projects: The Rise and Fall of Urban Renewal in Cold War New York* (New York: Oxford University Press, 2010); Andrew Highsmith, *Demolition Means Progress: Flint, Michigan, and the Fate of the American Metropolis* (Chicago: University of Chicago Press, 2015); and Francesca Ammon, *Bulldozer: Demolition and Clearance of the Postwar Landscape* (New Haven, Conn.: Yale University Press, 2016).

46. "Cleveland Citizens Committee on Hough Disturbances" (transcripts; microfilm), 75–86, August 23, 1966, Social Sciences Department, Cleveland Public Library, Cleveland, Ohio.

47. *Plan and Policy for Future Development*, 46–48, 71–72.

48. The school had gained national attention among medical schools for innovative (and controversial) curricular reform in the mid-1950s that, among other things, eliminated many disciplinary walls in Western Reserve students' four-year-programs; more clinical immersion, including at City Hospital; and increased emphasis on the sociological dimensions of medicine. See Greer Williams, *Western Reserve's Experiment in Medical Education and Its Outcome* (New York: Oxford University Press, 1980), esp. chs. 21–23.

49. John D. Clough, ed., *To Act as a Unit: The Story of the Cleveland Clinic*, 4th ed. (Cleveland, Ohio: Cleveland Clinic Foundation, 2004), 221.

50. Thomas Hatch to Richard DeChant, memorandum on "Phase II of the University-Euclid Urban Renewal Program," January 5, 1966, Box 3, Office Files, Clipping Files, 1965–1966, Papers of Thomas Hatch [semiprocessed], Cleveland Clinic Archives, Cleveland Clinic, Beachwood, Ohio.

51. Terry Demchak, Barbara Ehrenreich, and the Cleveland Women's Liberation, Health Task Force, "People's Guide to Health Care: The Politics of Health Care," January 1972, Ms Coll. 641, Box 46, Folder 522, Medical Committee for Human Rights Papers, Kislak Center for Special Collections, Rare Books and Manuscripts, Van Pelt Library, University of Pennsylvania, Philadelphia.

52. For background on Hough, see J. Mark Souther, *Believing in Cleveland: Managing Decline in "The Best Location in the Nation"* (Philadelphia: Temple University Press, 2017), 45–70; David Stradling and Richard Stradling, *Where the River Burned: Carl Stokes and the Struggle to Save Cleveland* (Ithaca, N.Y.: Cornell University Press, 2017), 49–54. On deindustrialization more generally, see Thomas Sugrue, *The Origins of the Urban Crisis: Race and Inequality in Postwar Detroit* (Princeton, N.J.: Princeton University Press, 1996); Robert Self, *American Babylon: Race and the Struggle for Postwar Oakland* (Princeton, N.J.: Princeton University Press, 2003); Judith Stein, *Running Steel, Running America: Race, Economic Policy, and the Decline of American Liberalism* (Chapel Hill: University of North Carolina Press, 1998); and Jefferson Cowie, *Capital Moves: RCA's 70-Year Quest for Cheap Labor* (Ithaca, N.Y.: Cornell University Press, 1999).

53. "A Note on Sources and Methods," in Digital Scholarship Lab, "Renewing Inequality," *American Panorama*, ed. Robert K. Nelson and Edward L. Ayers, https://dsl.richmond.edu/panorama/renewal/#view=0/0/1&viz=cartogram; Housing and Home Finance Agency, *Urban Renewal Project Characteristics* (Washington, D.C.: Urban Renewal Administration, 1964), 44.

54. An earlier version of the project, originally proposed in 1956, extended as far as East Sixty-Fifth Street. For general background on the project and developmental trends in the neighborhood not specifically anchored to the clinic, see Daniel R. Kerr, *Derelict Paradise: Homelessness and Urban Development in Cleveland, Ohio* (Amherst: University of Massachusetts Press, 2011), 148–54; Thomas Hatch to Richard DeChant, memorandum on "Phase II of the University-Euclid Urban Renewal Program," January 5, 1966, Box 3, Office Files, Clipping Files, 1965–1966, Papers of Thomas Hatch [semiprocessed], Cleveland Clinic Archives, Cleveland Clinic, Beachwood, Ohio; and Thomas Hatch, "University-Euclid Urban Renewal Program Phase II" (second draft), February 2, 1965; Thomas Hatch, daily journal entries, February 8, 10, 1965; Thomas Hatch to Richard A. Gottron, March 4, 1965, all in Box 23, Folder 3, Gottron Papers.

55. Hatch, "University-Euclid Urban Renewal Program Phase II" (second draft).

56. On the public health enterprise's complicity in different waves of urban renewal efforts, see Samuel K. Roberts, *Infectious Fear: Politics, Disease, and the Health Effects of*

*Segregation* (Chapel Hill: University of North Carolina Press, 2009), 201–21; Russ Lopez, "Public Health, the APHA, and Urban Renewal," *American Journal of Public Health* 99, no. 9 (2009): 1603–11.

57. Cleveland Clinic meeting with Ralph Locher and Cleveland City Council, January 11, 1965, Box 23, Folder 3, Gottron Papers.

58. Thomas Hatch, daily journal entries, May 26, 1965, Box 23, Folder 4, Gottron Papers.

59. Richard Gottron, memorandum on Hough riots, July 20, 1966, Box 23, Folder 6, Gottron Papers.

60. Thomas Hatch, "Notes on Urban Renewal," December 28, 1966, Folder 23, Folder 4, Gottron Papers.

61. Thomas Hatch to Richard A. Gottron, memorandum on "Possible riots in 1967, and proposals to meet them," February 24, 1967; and "For Discussion with Tom Hatch," February 1967, both in Box 23, Folder 6, Gottron Papers.

62. Thomas Sugrue, *Sweet Land of Liberty: The Forgotten Struggle for Civil Rights in the North* (New York: Random House, 2008), 326.

63. Thomas Hatch to Richard A. Gottron, memorandum on "Possible riots in 1967, and proposals to meet them," February 24, 1967, Box 23, Folder 6, Gottron Papers.

64. Thomas Hatch to J. H. Nichols, memorandum on "Policies in re Community Development," September 6, 1968, Box 23, Folder 13, Gottron Papers.

65. "Elections: The Real Black Power," *Time*, November 17, 1967.

66. Swanstrom, *Crisis of Growth Politics*, 100–107; Moore, *Carl B. Stokes and the Rise of Black Political Power*, 23, 42; Carl Stokes, *Promises of Power: A Political Autobiography* (New York: Simon and Schuster, 1973), 53.

67. "Support Cleveland: NOW!," ca. 1968 (from context); and Richard Gottron to Cleveland Clinic employees, May 24, 1968, both in Box 23, Folder 8, Gottron Papers; Moore, *Carl B. Stokes*, 73–76; Swanstrom, *Crisis of Growth Politics*, 105. The program fizzled after one of its grants was linked to weapons purchases by a Black nationalist named Ahmed Evans that were later used in the Glenville incident.

68. Moore, *Carl B. Stokes*, 68–70, 73.

69. Richard Gottron, "Plan for a Community Health Facility," ca. 1968 (from context), Box 23, Folder 9, Gottron Papers; Moore, *Carl B. Stokes*, 83–91.

70. Gottron, "Plan for a Community Health Facility"; Fay A. Lefevre to Glenn Wilson, August 12, 1968, Folder "Mayor Stokes' Plan," Cleveland Clinic Archives.

71. Gottron, "Plan for a Community Health Facility."

72. Thomas Hatch, "The Fairfax Community" (second draft), June 5, 1969, Folder "Mayor Stokes' Plan," Cleveland Clinic Archives. This intraracial distinction made by planners at a predominantly white and elite institution calls to mind Arnold Hirsch's account of University of Chicago and its administrators' resigned acceptance of a Black middle-class population in the Hyde Park area. See Arnold Hirsch, *Making the Second Ghetto: Race and Housing in Chicago, 1940–1960* (Chicago: University of Chicago Press, 1983), 170.

73. Todd Michney, *Surrogate Suburbs: Black Upward Mobility and Neighborhood Change in Cleveland, 1900–1980* (Chapel Hill: University of North Carolina Press, 2017), esp. 178–255.

74. Thomas Hatch, "The Fairfax Community" (second draft), June 5, 1969, Folder "Mayor Stokes' Plan," Cleveland Clinic Archives.

75. Charles L. Hudson to Board of Governors, Cleveland Clinic, March 27, 1967, Folder "Mayor Stokes' Plan," Cleveland Clinic Archives.

76. Moore, *Carl B. Stokes*, 170–72.

77. "Supplemental Information to Document: 'Program for Consolidation-County Health Facilities,'" April 15, 1971; and Cuyahoga County Hospitals Planning Task Force, "Recommended Directions for Cuyahoga County Hospital," ca. April 1971 (from context), both in Series 24 NG1, Box 3, Folder 4, Whitman Papers.

78. Carl Wasmuth to Henry Manning, memorandum on Cleveland Clinic role in east side health center, September 6, 1973, in Folder "68.00–000" [unprocessed], Cleveland Clinic Archives.

79. Arthur S. Holden Jr. to Executive Committee of the Board of Trustees, Cleveland Clinic Foundation, August 28, 1973, Folder "68.00–000" [unprocessed], Cleveland Clinic Archives.

80. Unidentified Fairfax Foundation official, "The East Side Ambulatory Care Center," March 12, 1974, Folder "68.00–000" [unprocessed], Cleveland Clinic Archives.

81. "Who Pays for Care of Poor? Not the Clinic," *Cleveland Press*, February 28, 1976; Fred McGunagle, "Cleveland Clinic: Service to Community Is New," *Cleveland Press*, February 28, 1976.

82. Thomas Hatch to J. H. Nichols, memorandum on "Euclid-105th Business District," January 9, 1968; and Thomas Hatch to J. H. Nichols, memorandum on "Ingleside Hospital & Euclid–East 105th Street Area," November 14, 1968, both in Box 23, Folder 13, Gottron Papers; "Willis Arrested in Harassment at Clinic," *Cleveland Plain-Dealer*, July 16, 1977; William F. Miller, "Doans Corners: E. 105th St. Area Struggles to Rise," *Cleveland Plain-Dealer*, January 10, 1982.

83. For accounts of the Cleveland crisis, see Swanstrom, *Crisis of Growth Politics*; and Davita Silfen Galserg, *The Power of Collective Purse Strings: The Effects of Bank Hegemony on Corporations and the State* (Berkeley: University of California Press, 1989), ch. 5.

84. Robert D. McCreery, James E. Burnett, and William H. Bryant, "Proposal to the Cleveland Foundation for Funding a Program to Cause Further Development of Cleveland as a Health/Medical and High Technology Center," May 11, 1979, Box 19, Folder 551, University Circle Incorporated Papers, Western Reserve Historical Society, Cleveland, Ohio.

85. George Voinovich to Richard Taylor, memorandum on Cleveland Clinic role in East Cleveland development, March 23, 1982; and Office of Public Affairs, "The Cleveland Clinic Foundation: Community Impact Report," July 1982, both in Folder "3-PR20 Community Relations [Neighborhood]," Cleveland Clinic Archives.

86. "The Cleveland Clinic Foundation: Community Impact Report"; Henry D. Ziegler to William Kiser, November 30, 1984, Folder "3-PR20 Community Relations—Clement Center," Cleveland Clinic Archives.

87. Henry D. Ziegler to William Kiser, November 30, 1984; "Minutes of the Meetings of the Board of Governors," January 14, 1987; Henry D. Ziegler to William Kiser, December 24, 1987, all in Folder "3-PR20 Community Relations—Clement Center," Cleveland Clinic Archives.

88. *Annual Report to the Cleveland Metropolitan General Hospital/Highland View Hospital Board of Trustees, 1982–1983*, Folder "68.00–000" [unprocessed], Cleveland Clinic Archives.

89. *Oversight on Financially Distressed Hospitals: Hearing before the Subcommittee on Health and Scientific Research of the Committee on Labor and Human Resources* (Washington, D.C.: U.S. Government Printing Office, 1980), 71–72.

90. Community Advisory Council, Kenneth Clement Center, "Press Conference on the Clement Center," June 18, 1976; and "Community Advisory Council: Its Composition and Responsibilities: East Side Ambulatory Care Center," ca. mid-1970s (from context), both in Folder "68.00–000," Cleveland Clinic Archives.

91. "Memorandum of Understanding [on Hough-Norwood Facility]," August 19, 1968, Container 75, Folder 1426, Stokes Papers; Sidney W. Maurer to David Miller, September 16, 1968, Stokes Papers.

92. "Hough Norwood Family Health Care Center: Grant Application," August 1, 1973— July 31, 1974, Papers of Duncan Neuhaser [semiprocessed], Dittrick Medical History Center, Case Western Reserve University, Cleveland, Ohio.

93. "Hough Norwood Family Health Care Center: Grant Application."

94. Joanne E. Finley, "Progress Report on First Year of Operation of Hough-Norwood Family Health Care Center, Cleveland, Ohio (CG 8897)," March 15, 1968; and "By-Laws of Hough-Norwood Citizens Health Committee," ca. 1967–68 (from context), both in Container 75, Folder 1426, Stokes Papers.

95. Its governance structure is described further in John Campbell, "Working Relationships between Providers and Consumers in a Neighborhood Health Center," *American Journal of Public Health* 61, no. 1 (1971): 97–103.

96. Anna Bell Boiner, notes on door-to-door visits, January 17, 1968, Container 75, Folder 1426, Stokes Papers.

97. Boiner, notes on door-to-door visits.

98. "Hough Norwood Family Health Care Center: Grant Application," 26–28; Hough-Norwood Family Health Care Center, Annual Report (1978), Public Administration Library, Cleveland Public Library, Cleveland, Ohio.

99. Mary Wheeler, "Health Education in the Interagency Approach to Urban Renewal," *American Journal of Public Health* 53, no. 1 (1963): 63.

100. On the Urban League's moralism, see Toure Reed, *Not Alms but Opportunity: The Urban League and the Politics of Racial Uplift, 1910–1950* (Chapel Hill: University of North Carolina Press, 2008).

101. Urban League of Cleveland, "What about Cleveland's Health and Welfare?," June 1963, Public Administration Library, Cleveland Public Library, Cleveland, Ohio.

102. *Health Goals Model for Greater Cleveland: Cleveland Health Goals Project Reports* (Cleveland: Welfare Federation of Cleveland, 1966), 1:8, 10–13.

103. "Profile of Existing Programs for the Prevention and Control of Infectious and Communicable Diseases in Cleveland—Cuyahoga County," in *Health Goals Model for Greater Cleveland: Cleveland Health Goals Project Reports*, vol. 3.

104. "Hough Norwood Family Health Care Center: Grant Application," 18, Appendix A, Tables 2, 3.

105. "Cuyahoga County Hospital: Administrative Problems and Progress, 1962–1977," Series 24NG1, Box 3, Folder 8, Whitman Papers.

106. Author's calculations from U.S. Census data for 1960 and 1970, National Historical Geographical Information Systems database, Minnesota Population Center, University of Minnesota, Minneapolis.

107. "Cuyahoga County Hospital: Administrative Problems and Progress, 1962–1977"; "From the Office of the County Hospital Administrator," ca. mid-1960s (from context), Container 26, Folder "County Hospital," University Circle Incorporated Papers, Western Reserve Historical Society, Cleveland, Ohio.

108. "Recommended Directions for Cuyahoga County Hospital: Report of the Planning Task Force," February 10, 1971, Series 24 NG1, Box 3, Folder 4, Whitman Papers.

109. "Recommended Directions for Cuyahoga County Hospital: Report of the Planning Task Force."

110. Elsewhere, however, county officials strongly implied that Highland View was a candidate for closure. See Henry Manning, speech on consolidation, July 12, 1971, Program for Consolidation 1975; and Seth Taft, "Statement on County Hospital Levy," August 2, 1971, both in Series 24 NG1, Box 3, Folder 4, Whitman Papers.

111. "Strategy," ca. 1971 (from context), Series 24 NG1, Box 3, Folder 4, Whitman Papers; "Cuyahoga County Hospital: Areas of Concern," ca. 1971 (from context), Series 24 NG1, Box 3, Folder 8, Whitman Papers. The latter document, which detailed political opposition to hospitals, contains no author name but was likely written by Samuel Whitman, an associate dean at Case Western Reserve University's medical school.

112. "Strategy"; "Cuyahoga County Hospital: Area of Concern," ca. 1970–71 (from context), Series 24 NG1, Box 3, Folder 8, Whitman Papers.

113. "1,721,300 reasons to vote YES on Issue 7," ca. mid-1971 (from context), Series 24 NG1, Box 3, Folder 4, Whitman Papers.

114. Austin B. Chinn to Henry Manning, memorandum evaluating Metropolitan General Hospital and Highland View Hospital consolidation proposal, February 3, 1971, Series 24 NG1, Box 3, Folder 4, Whitman Papers.

115. Plans for shrinkage of underused and unused beds, in fact, had been in place as early as 1972, though with slight differences in total shift in bed numbers. Henry Manning, "Position Paper: Inpatient Bed Requirements, Program for Consolidation of Cuyahoga County Hospital," May 26, 1972, Dittrick Medical Archives, Case Western Reserve University.

116. Cuyahoga County Hospital System, "Progress Report: Program for Consolidation: County Health Facilities," October 21, 1976, Dittrick Medical Archives, Case Western Reserve University.

117. Davita Silfen Glasberg, "Bank Hegemony and Class Struggle in Cleveland, 1978–1979," in *Fire in the Hearth: The Radical Politics of Place in America*, ed. Mike Davis et al. (New York: Verso Books, 1990); Swanstrom, *Crisis of Growth Politics*, ch. 7.

118. Federation for Community Planning, "Cuyahoga County Health Project: An Agenda for the 1980s: A Report to the Board of County Commissioners of Cuyahoga County," December 1980; and William H. Andrews to Bruce Spitz, October 6, 1980, both in Papers of Duncan Neuhaser [semiprocessed], Dittrick Medical History Center, Case Western Reserve University, Cleveland, Ohio.

119. Committee on Health Care for the Indigent of the Federation for Community Planning, "Resolution on Indigent Health Care," ca. 1982 (from context), Container 18, Greater Cleveland Nurses Association, Series III, Western Reserve Historical Society, Cleveland, Ohio.

120. Frank Kimber, Heather P. Kurent, and Ruth Anna Carlson, "Uncompensated Health Care in Cleveland and Cuyahoga County, Ohio," October 1985, Public Administration Library, Cleveland Public Library, Cleveland, Ohio. As late as 1985, the household income cutoff was 185 percent of the poverty line, with a temporary four-month Medicaid allowance once exceeded (53–55).

121. Regional HMOs had been proposed as early as the start of the 1970s, though with mixed traction or success. See, e.g., "The Planning and Development of a Health Maintenance Organization at the Cleveland Metropolitan General Hospital," December 1, 1972, in Cleveland Health Sciences Library, Allen Memorial Library, Case Western Reserve University, Ohio; "Cleveland Health Care Alternatives: New Health Choices for ADC Recipients," January 30, 1986, Container 10, Greater Cleveland Nurses Association, Series III, Western Reserve Historical Society, Cleveland, Ohio; Hough Area Development Corporation, "New Health Care Systems for Cleveland," November 23, 1971, Container 4, Folder 75, Papers of

the Hough Area Development Corporation, Western Reserve Historical Society, Cleveland, Ohio; Regional HMOs, especially funded by Medicaid, have been understudied and often lumped with those sold by large providers. For an exception, see Lawrence D. Brown, *Politics and Health Care Organization: HMOs as Federal Policy* (Washington, D.C.: Brookings Institution Press, 1983), esp. 44–72.

CHAPTER FIVE

1. For these breakdowns, see Paul Averitt, *Coal Reserves of the United States—A Progress Report* (Washington, D.C.: U.S. Government Printing Office, 1961), 1–32, 60, 82–83.

2. "To the Department of Conservation," petition, ca. 1967, RG 70, Records of the United States Bureau of Mines, Division of Environment, National Surface Mine Study Policy Committee, State Surface Mining Study Files, 1963–1967, Box 9, Folder "Documented Damage: Kentucky," National Archives, College Park, Md.

3. Alice H. Slone to Lyndon Johnson, June 17, 1965, RG 70, Records of the United States Bureau of Mines, Division of Environment, National Surface Mine Study Policy Committee, State Surface Mining Study Files, 1963–1967, Box 9, Folder "Documented Damage: Kentucky," National Archives, College Park, Md.

4. I use the term "Central Appalachia" because this is how scholars in Appalachian studies and government officials referred to this section of the Appalachian belt, which stretches from Alabama to New York in a northeast-southwest direction. For a discussion of geographic definition and labeling, see John Alexander Williams, *Appalachia: A History* (Chapel Hill: University of North Carolina Press, 2001), 1–13.

5. James Currens and Gilbert Smith, "Coal Production in Kentucky, 1790–1975," *Kentucky Geological Survey Information Circular*, 10th ser., 23 (1977): 59–65; *Bureau of Mines Minerals Yearbook: The Mineral Industry of Kentucky* (Washington, D.C.: United States Government Printing Office, 1972). Author's calculations from absolute tonnage figures.

6. "Research Bulletin No. 1," *Appalachian Outlook* 1, no. 1 (1968). On the decline of independent proprietors and the entrance of energy firms into the coal business, see "Principal Mergers and Acquisitions in the Coal Industry, 1963–1975," in *Mergers and Economic Concentration: Hearings before the Subcommittee on Antitrust, Monopoly and Business Rights* (Washington, D.C.: U.S. Government Printing Office, 1979), 441; and *Patterns and Trends in Federal Coal Lease Ownership, 1950–1980* (Washington, D.C.: U.S. Government Printing Office, 1981), 6.

7. August Manifest, "Moving Overburden with Explosives," *Mining Congress Journal* 46 (April 1960); E. F. Eckhardt, "Economics of Large versus Small Haulage Units," *Mining Congress Journal* 47 (May 1961); Henry Rumfelt, "Recent Developments in Surface Mining," *Mining Congress Journal* 51 (September 1965): 77; "Ripping Burden: The Economic Approach," *Coal Age* (July 1965); David G. Lewis, "Application of Contour Stripping Techniques," *Mining Congress Journal* 51 (March 1965); J. H. Wilson, "Auger Mining: Productivity Powers Growth," *Coal Age* (November 1966): 59.

8. Alan Brinkley, *The End of Reform: New Deal Liberalism in Recession and War* (New York: Vintage Books, 1966), 227–64; Nelson Lichtenstein, "The Eclipse of Social Democracy," in *The Rise and Fall of the New Deal Order, 1930–1980*, ed. Steve Fraser and Gary Gerstle (Princeton, N.J.: Princeton University Press, 1989), 130–31.

9. See Landon Storrs, *The Second Red Scare and the Unmaking of the New Deal Left* (Princeton, N.J.: Princeton University Press, 2013).

10. "A Mechanization Study," *United Mine Workers Journal*, February 1, 1962.

11. Chad Montrie, "Expedient Environmentalism: Opposition to Coal Surface Mining in Appalachia and the United Mine Workers of America, 1945–1977," *Environmental History* 5 (2000): 75–98.

12. Paul Nyden, "Rank-and-File Movements in the United Mine Workers of America, Early 1960s–Early 1980s," in *Rebel Rank and File: Labor Militancy and Revolt from Below during the Long 1970s*, ed. Aaron Brenner, Robert Brenner, and Cal Winslow (New York: Verso Books, 2010), 180–84.

13. Ronald Eller, *Uneven Ground: Appalachia since 1945* (Lexington: University Press of Kentucky, 2008), 146–47. For an excellent legal history of key postwar court decisions clarifying coal operators and landowners' respective titles to surface and seams, see Michael V. Withrow, "Broad-Form Deed: Obstacle to Peaceful Co-Existence between Mineral and Surface Owners," *Kentucky Law Journal* 60, no. 3 (1971–72): 742–56. Withrow focuses particularly on Kentucky, where legal decisions were generally more favorable to operators. See, too, Patrick Sheeran and David Wilson, "*Akers v. Baldwin*: The Broad Form Deed Dilemma Revisited," *Journal of Mineral Law and Policy*, 4, no. 1 (1988), esp. 213–18.

14. Four works have influenced my approach to perception and subjectivity in health: Nancy Tomes, *The Gospel of Germs: Men, Women, and the Microbe in American Life* (Chapel Hill: University of North Carolina Press, 1998); David Barnes, *The Great Stink of Paris* (Baltimore: Johns Hopkins University Press, 2006); Javier Auyero and Débora Swistun, *Flammable: Environmental Suffering in an Argentinian Shantytown* (New York: Oxford University Press, 2009); and Conevery Bolton Valenčius, *The Health of the Country: How American Settlers Understood Themselves and Their Land* (New York: Basic Books, 2004).

15. "WHAS Reports: Scars on the Mountainside," July 27, 1961, transcript, Box 403, Folder 4, Cooper Papers. In rare cases, handwriting was ambiguous or illegible. I have denoted these instances with brackets around cryptic words, along with my best guess at what they might be.

16. "WHAS Reports: Scars on the Mountainside."

17. Tom Gish, "Family Flees Strip Mine," *Mountain Eagle* (Whitesburg, Ky.), March 1, 1962.

18. Chad Montrie, *To Save the Land and People: A History of Opposition to Surface Coal Mining in Appalachia* (Chapel Hill: University of North Carolina Press, 2003), 5. Montrie's narrative of escalating awareness and anger toward strip-mining practices parallels my own, though his does not focus on health.

19. Madge and Paul Ashley to Lady Bird Johnson, June 9, 1955, RG 70, Records of the United States Bureau of Mines, Division of Environment, National Surface Mine Study Policy Committee, State Surface Mining Study Files, 1963–1967, Box 9, Folder "Documented Damage: Kentucky," National Archives, College Park, Md.

20. Madge and Paul Ashley to Lady Bird Johnson.

21. Ashley to Lyndon Johnson, July 12, 1965, RG 70, Records of the United States Bureau of Mines, Division of Environment, National Surface Mine Study Policy Committee, State Surface Mining Study Files, 1963–1967, Box 9, Folder "Documented Damage: Kentucky," National Archives, College Park, Md.

22. Ida Vass to Robert Byrd, August 26, 1966, RG 70, Records of the United States Bureau of Mines, Division of Environment, National Surface Mine Study Policy Committee, State Surface Mining Study Files, 1963–1967, West Virginia, Box 20, Folder "West Virginia: Documented Damage," National Archives, College Park, Md.

23. Mrs. Albert Lopeg, February 1, 22, 1967, RG 70, Documented Damage: Kentucky.

24. William Harold Headen to Lyndon Johnson, February 16, 1965, RG 70, Documented Damage: Kentucky.

25. Headen to Lyndon Johnson.

26. Headen to Lyndon Johnson.

27. Kenneth Galyen to John Sherman Cooper, March 11, 1969, Box 492, Folder 1, Cooper Papers.

28. Paul Staton to John Sherman Cooper, February 10, 1972, Box 492, Folder 3, Cooper Papers.

29. Mrs. Roy Fields to John Sherman Cooper, October 7, 1971, Box 492, Folder 4, Cooper Papers.

30. Gerna Campbell and Mrs. Gerna Campbell to John Sherman Cooper, January 3, 1972, Box 492, Folder 4, Cooper Papers.

31. Mr. and Mrs. Harvey Kincaid to Si Galperin, January 28, 1971, reprinted in "Citizens to Abolish Strip Mining," February 1971, Box 22, Folder 1, Papers of Harry Caudill, Special Collections Division, Margaret I. King Library, University of Kentucky, Lexington.

32. Kincaid to Galperin.

33. Kincaid to Galperin.

34. Kincaid to Galperin.

35. Kincaid to Galperin.

36. Kincaid to Galperin.

37. Floyd Davis to Carl Perkins, April 23, 1970, Box D-079, Folder 3, Perkins Papers.

38. For a useful review of internal colonialism and its rising popularity in the region from the mid-1960s onward, see the various essays in Helen Matthews Lewis, Linda Johnson, and Donald Askins, eds., *Colonialism in Modern America: The Appalachian Case* (Boone, N.C.: Appalachian Consortium Press, 1978). On the civil rights movement's uses of the term, see Stokely Carmichael and Charles Hamilton, *Black Power: The Politics of Liberation in America* (New York: Random House, 1967), esp. ch. 1; Robert Allen, *Black Awakening in Capitalist America: An Analytic History* (Garden City, N.Y.: Doubleday, 1969); and Robert Blauner, "Internal Colonialism and Ghetto Revolt," in *Racial Oppression in America* (New York: Harper and Row, 1972).

39. I use the phrase "borders of the fifty states" to acknowledge, as Daniel Immerwahr has argued, that common usage of "the United States" elides territorial holdings that are not considered states—and that were sites of colonial endeavors by another name. See Immerwahr, *How to Hide an Empire: A History of the Greater United States* (New York: Picador, 2019).

40. Although much has been written about Appalachian activism, both surrounding strip mining and a host of other issues, this prior writing rarely mentions activity around environmental health. See, e.g., Montrie, *To Save the Land*; Dwight B. Billings, Gurney Norman, and Katherine Ledford, eds., *Back Talk from Appalachia: Confronting Stereotypes* (Lexington: University Press of Kentucky, 1998); and Stephen L. Fisher, ed., *Fighting Back in Appalachia: Traditions of Resistance and Change* (Philadelphia: Temple University Press, 1992).

41. Petition to Carl Perkins, ca. 1967, Box 492, Folder 1, Cooper Papers.

42. "Resolution concerning Surface Mining, Made and Submitted by the Harlan County Emergency and Rescue Squad, Inc.," February 7, 1972, Box 492, Folder 3, Cooper Papers.

43. "Pond Creek Citizens Petition," ca. 1972, Box D-095, Folder 3, Perkins Papers.

44. "Save Our Kentucky, Inc.," ca. 1971, Box 112, Folder 9, CSM (Part Two) Papers.

45. "EKWRO—Any Problem, They'll Work on It," ca. late 1972, Box 107, Folder 11, CSM (Part Two) Papers.

46. C. R. Collier, R. J. Pickering, and J. J. Musser, eds., *Influences of Strip Mining on the Hydrologic Environment of Parts of Beaver Creek Basin, Kentucky, 1955–1966* (Washington, D.C.: United States Government Printing Office, 1970), C1, C21, C32–C46.

47. Joseph A. Boccary and Willard M. Spaulding Jr., *Effects of Surface Mining on Fish and Wildlife in Appalachia* (Washington, D.C.: United States Government Printing Office, 1968), 12, 17–19.

48. *Surface Mining and the Environment: A Special Report to the Nation* (Washington, D.C.: United States Government Printing Office, 1967), 56, 63–64, 67–70.

49. Currens and Smith, "Coal Production in Kentucky 1790–1975," 60.

50. "Two Killed, 3d Missing; Damage Is in Millions," *Louisville Courier-Journal*, March 13, 1963.

51. Sy Ramsey, "Refugees Mill About in Hard-Hit Misery in Harlan," *Louisville Courier-Journal*, March 13, 1963.

52. "Letcher County Digging Out," *Mountain Eagle* (Whitesburg, Ky.), March 14, 1963.

53. "Down from Sanctified Hill," *Louisville Courier-Journal*, December 16, 1972.

54. "Questions Persist on Strip Mining's Link to Floods," *Louisville Courier-Journal*, May 8, 1977.

55. Willie Curtis, "Surface Mining and the Flood of 1977," *USDA Forest Service Research Note* (1977).

56. Willie Curtis, "Effects of Strip Mining on the Hydrology of Small Mountain Watersheds in Appalachia," in *Ecology and Reclamation of Devastated Land: Proceedings of the International Symposium on Ecology and Revegetation of Drastically Disturbed Areas*, vol. 1, ed. R. J. Hutnik and G. Davis (New York: Gordon and Breach, 1973), 145–57; Willie Curtis, "Strip-Mining Increases Flood Potential for Mountainsheds," *Proceedings of National Symposium on Watersheds in Transition* (Urbana, Ill.: American Water Resources Association, 1972), 360.

57. Curtis, "Strip-Mining Increases Flood Potential for Mountainsheds," 360.

58. "Questions Persist on Strip Mining's Link to Floods," *Louisville Courier-Journal*, May 8, 1977.

59. "Questions Persist on Strip Mining's Link to Floods."

60. Its recommendations were reprinted in Committee on Health and Environmental Effects of Increased Coal Utilization, "Report on Health and Environmental Effects of Increased Coal Utilization," *Environmental Health Perspectives* 36 (November 1980): 136, 139. Despite cataloging a wealth of health risks associated with coal, the Committee recommended increased utilization of coal, in part because of its members' confidence in regulatory tools. I discuss the broader policy climate of this recommendation shortly.

61. Committee on Disposal of Excess Spoil, Board on Mineral and Energy Resources, Commission on Natural Resources, *Disposal of Excess Spoil from Coal Mining and the Surface Mining Control and Reclamation Act of 1977: A Study of Regulatory Requirements, Engineering Practices, and Environmental Protection Objectives* (Washington, D.C.: National Academies Press, 1981), 28.

62. Edmund Faltermayer, "Taming the Strip-Mine Monster," *Life*, October 1, 1971. The classic sociological examination of this episode is Erikson, *Everything in Its Path*.

63. "Statement of Senator John Sherman Cooper before the Subcommittee on Appropriations and Interior and Related Agencies for Fiscal 1967," March 1966, Box 403, Folder 2, Cooper Papers; "Statement of Senator John Sherman Cooper before the Appropriations Subcommittee on Interior and Related Agencies," March 7, 1972, Box 14, Folder 3, Cooper Papers.

64. *Strip Mining and the Flooding in Appalachia: Hearing before a Subcommittee of the Committee on Government Operations* (Washington, D.C.: U.S. Government Printing Office, 1977), 1–8, 36–40.

65. On Science for the People, see Kelly Moore, *Disrupting Science*; Sigrid Schmalzer, Daniel Chard, and Alyssa Botelho, eds., *Documents from America's Movement of Radical Scientists* (Amherst: University of Massachusetts Press, 2018).

66. Jerry Hardt and Albert Fritsch, *Harlan County Flood Report* (Corbin, Ky.: Appalachia—Science in the Public Interest, 1978), 3.

67. Hardt and Fritsch, *Harlan County Flood Report*, ch. 5.

68. "Workshop Announcement: 'Surface Mine Blasting and Public Policy,'" April 1978, Box 117, Folder 11, CSM (Part Two) Papers.

69. Mark Morgan et al., *Citizens' Blasting Handbook* (Corbin, Ky.: Appalachia—Science in the Public Interest, 1978).

70. For a meditation on the evolution of this research, see Phil Brown, "Popular Epidemiology Revisited," *Current Sociology* 45, no. 3 (1997): 137–56.

71. Timothy Mitchell, *Carbon Democracy: Political Power in the Age of Oil* (New York: Verso Books, 2011).

72. "Why Perkins Voted 'No,'" *Kentucky Coal Journal* 3, no. 8 (1977): 1.

73. See "Kentucky's Ravaged Land," *Louisville Courier-Journal*, January 5, 1964.

74. "Eyesore," "Clean Air" (reprints), RG 70, Records of the United States Bureau of Mines, Division of Environment, National Surface Mine Study Policy Committee, General Surface Mining Study Files, 1963–1967, Box 24, Folder "Appalachia-Correspondence-1967," National Archives, College Park, Md.

75. "Our Hottest Client" (reprint), RG 70, Records of the United States Bureau of Mines, Division of Environment, National Surface Mine Study Policy Committee, General Surface Mining Study Files, 1963–1967, Box 24, Folder "Appalachia-Correspondence-1967," National Archives, College Park, Md.

76. "The Invisible Power of Coal" (advertisement), *New York Times*, June 14, 1964.

77. Henry Caulfield to John I. Sweeney, November 12, 1967, RG 70, Records of the United States Bureau of Mines, Division of Environment, National Surface Mine Study Policy Committee, General Surface Mining Study Files, 1963–1967, Box 13, Folder "Appalachian Regional Commission," National Archives, College Park, Md.

78. Walter Hibbard to Charles Moulin, December 20, 1967, RG 70, Records of the United States Bureau of Mines, Division of Environment, National Surface Mine Study Policy Committee, General Surface Mining Study Files, 1963–1967, Box 24, Folder "Appalachia-Correspondence-1967," National Archives, College Park, Md.

79. *Study of Strip and Surface Mining in Appalachia: An Interim Report* (Washington, D.C.: United States Government Printing Office, 1966); *Surface Mining and the Environment: A Special Report to the Nation* (Washington, D.C.: United States Government Printing Office, 1967).

80. *Surface Mining and the Environment*, 84, 90, 96–103.

81. *Surface Mining and the Environment*, 42–43.

82. Earl Hayes to Carl Perkins, April 1, 1970, Box D-079, Folder 3, Perkins Papers.

83. Montrie, *To Save the Land*, 138–39.

84. Constance Nathanson, *Disease Prevention as Social Change: The State, Society, and Public Health in the United States, France, Great Britain, and Canada* (New York: Russell Sage Foundation, 2007), 213.

85. Harry Caudill, *Night Comes to the Cumberlands: A Biography of a Depressed Area* (Boston: Little, Brown, 1963); Michael Harrington, *The Other America: Poverty in the United States* (New York: Macmillan, 1962).

86. Kentucky Area Development Office, "Preliminary Development Outline for Appalachian Kentucky," April 1966, Box 275, Folder 2, ARC Papers.

87. Robert Collins, *More: The Politics of Economic Growth in Postwar America* (New York: Oxford University Press, 2000), chs. 1–2.

88. Eller, *Uneven Ground*, 194.

89. Montrie, "Expedient Environmentalism."

90. On federal energy politics during the 1970s, see Meg Jacobs, *Panic at the Pump: The Energy Crisis and the Transformation of American Politics in the 1970s* (New York: Hill and Wang, 2016), 8, 30.

91. Carl Perkins to Mr. and Mrs. Bill Weinberg, March 5, 1974, Box C-127, Folder 1, Perkins Papers.

92. "Perkins Leads House Fight against Strip Mine Overregulation," press release, September 4, 1980, Box R-098, Folder 30, Perkins Papers.

93. Hilton Davis to Carl Perkins, July 15, 1974, Box C-127, Folder 1, Perkins Papers.

94. Waldo S. La Fon to Carl Perkins, May 27, 1975, Box C-146, Folder 7, Perkins Papers.

95. Carl Bagge to Morris Udall, September 24, 1974, Box C-127, Folder 1, Perkins Papers.

96. Montrie, *To Save the Land*, 169.

97. Gregory Elmes and Trevor Harris, "Industrial Restructuring and the United States Coal-Energy System, 1972–1990: Regulatory Change, Technological Fixes, and Corporate Control," *Annals of the Association of American Geographers* 86, no. 3 (1996): 509–10.

98. *The Acceptable Replacement of Imported Oil with Coal: The Staff Report to the President's Commission on Coal* (Washington, D.C.: U.S. Government Printing Office, 1980); *The President's Commission on Coal: Recommendations and Summary Findings* (Washington, D.C.: U.S. Government Printing Office, 1980), 1–2.

99. *President's Commission on Coal*, 9–10. On the Surface Mining Control and Reclamation Act, see Montrie, *To Save the Land*, 173–80.

100. "Kentucky's Fiscal Year 1978 Appalachian Development Plan," 1978, Box 280, Folder 7, ARC Papers.

101. "Appalachian Data and Development Trends DRAFT 3-4-80," March 4, 1980, Box 281, Folder 2, ARC Papers.

102. Geri Storm to Fred Burks and Alan Lord, "Comments on FY 1980 Addendum to the Kentucky Appalachian Development Plan," January 23, 1980, Box 281, Folder 2, ARC Papers.

103. "Kentucky Appalachia Development Plan, 1983–1987," November 1982, Box 282, Folder 7, ARC Papers.

104. "Kentucky Coal Policy Council," ca. 1980, Box 1, Folder "Coal Policy Council Mailing List," Governor's Office for Coal and Energy Policy Papers [semiprocessed], Kentucky Department of Libraries and Archives, Frankfort.

105. Jennifer Hewlett, "Brown Pushes Coal's Future, Forms Council," *Lexington (Ky.) Herald*, June 25, 1980.

106. "Background of Suggested Legislative and Administrative Action," ca. 1980, Folder "Coal Policy Council," Governor's Office for Coal and Energy Policy Papers [semiprocessed], Kentucky Department of Libraries and Archives, Frankfort.

107. "Background of Suggested Legislative and Administrative Action."

108. For a survey of some of these difficulties, see R. Jeffrey Smith, "Watt Carves up Strip-Mining Policy," *Science* 212, no. 4496 (1981): 759–62; and Donald Menzel and Terry

Edgmon, "The Struggle to Implement a National Surface Mining Policy," *Publius* 10, no. 1 (1980): 81–91.

109. Donald C. Menzel, "Redirecting the Implementation of a Law: The Reagan Administration and Coal Surface Mining Regulation," *Public Administration Review* 43, no. 5 (1983): 414–16.

110. On Reagan's environmental record, see Richard N. L. Andrews, *Managing the Environment, Managing Ourselves: A History of American Environmental Policy* (New Haven, Conn.: Yale University Press, 1999), ch. 13; and George Charles Halverson, "Valuing the Air: The Politics of Environmental Governance from the Clean Air Act to Carbon Trading" (PhD diss., Columbia University, 2017), 276–92.

111. A polemical literature, datable at least to the work of Harry Caudill, has developed along such lines. See Harry Caudill, *My Land Is Dying* (New York: E. P. Dutton, 1973); and, more recently, Jeff Goodell, *Big Coal: The Dirty Secret behind America's Energy Future* (New York: Houghton Mifflin, 2007); Tricia Shapiro, *Mountain Justice: Homegrown Resistance to Mountaintop Removal, for the Future of Us All* (Oakland, Calif.: AK Press, 2010); Michael Shnayerson, *Coal River: How a Few Brave Americans Took on a Powerful Coal Company and the Federal Government to Save the Land They Love* (New York: Farrar, Straus and Giroux, 2008); and Ted Nace, *Climate Hope: On the Front Lines of the Fight Against Coal* (Berkeley, Calif.: Earth Island Institute/CoalSwarm, 2009).

112. Rob Nixon, *Slow Violence and the Environmentalism of the Poor* (Cambridge, Mass.: Harvard University Press, 2011).

CHAPTER SIX

1. Robert J. Batzel, "Health Care: What the Poor People Didn't Get from Kentucky Project," *Science* 172, no. 3982 (1971): 458, 460.

2. Leaflet distributed in Floyd County on Comprehensive Health Services program, March 28, 1971, Box D-093, Folder 7, Perkins Papers.

3. Lewis Jones and Adellea Shields, *Health Care Services and Facilities in the Southern Appalachian Region* (Berea, Ky.: Council of the Southern Mountains, 1955), Berea College Special Collections and Archives, Hutchins Library. The rise and implosion of the system is told in Ivana Krajcinovic, *From Company Doctors to Managed Care: The United Mine Workers' Noble Experiment* (Ithaca, N.Y.: Cornell University Press, 1997); and Richard P. Mulcahy, *A Social Contract for the Coal Fields: The Rise and Fall of the United Mine Workers of America Welfare and Retirement Fund* (Knoxville: University of Tennessee Press, 2000).

4. C. Horace Hamilton, *Health and Health Services in the Southern Appalachians: A Source Book* (Raleigh: North Carolina Agricultural Experiment Station, 1959), Berea College Special Collections and Archives, Hutchins Library. The larger social survey for which Hamilton conducted this research is Rupert Vance and Thomas Ford, *The Southern Appalachian Region: A Survey* (Lexington: University of Kentucky Press, 1962).

5. *Report of the Health Advisory Committee to the Appalachian Regional Commission* (Washington, D.C.: Appalachian Regional Commission, 1966), 23.

6. On the Appalachian Regional Commission generally, see Ronald Eller, *Uneven Ground: Appalachia since 1945* (Lexington: University Press of Kentucky, 2008); and David E. Whisnant, *Modernizing the Mountaineer: People, Power, and Planning in Appalachia*, rev. ed. (Knoxville: University of Tennessee Press, 1994).

7. "Southeastern Kentucky Regional Health Demonstration Project," August 1967, Box 276, Folder 5, ARC Papers; "Kentucky State Department of Health News and Plans: State

'Sets Machinery' for Comprehensive State Health Planning," August 1968; and "Southeastern Kentucky Regional Health Demonstration Project: Health Development Plan for Year 1968–1969," 1968, both in Box 275, Folder 3, ARC Papers.

8. "Appalachian Kentucky Health Program Projects for Implementation in 1967," June 20, 1967, Box 275, Folder 4, ARC Papers; Kentucky Development Plan, December 15, 1967, Box 275, Folder 4, ARC Papers.

9. "Resolution: Hazard-Perry County Jaycees," December 6, 1967, Box D-059, Folder 12, Perkins Papers.

10. Patricia Lee, letter on new hospital, February 2, 1970, Box D-075, Folder 6, Perkins Papers.

11. Mrs. C. M. Brand to Carl Perkins, October 29, 1969, Box D-073, Folder 6, Perkins Papers.

12. "Friends of Jane Cook Hospital," summary of efforts, January 22, 1968, Box D-073, Folder 2, Perkins Papers.

13. T. P. Hipkens, "The Organization of Rural Health Services," June 7–8, 1971, Box 92, Folder 11, CSM (Part Two) Papers; "The ARH Story," 1968, Box 118, Folder 4, CSM (Part Two) Papers.

14. On the Appalachian Volunteers, see Thomas Kiffmeyer, *Reformers to Radicals: The Appalachian Volunteers and the War on Poverty* (Lexington: University Press of Kentucky, 2008).

15. "Red Bird Valley Project," ca. mid-1960s (from context), Box 32, Folder 4, Appalachian Volunteers Papers, Berea College Special Collections and Archives, Hutchins Library, Berea, Ky.

16. "Red Bird Valley Project."

17. "Appalachian Volunteer Summer Project: Health Standards," 1964, Box 80, Folder 6, Appalachian Volunteers Papers, Berea College Special Collections and Archives, Hutchins Library, Berea, Ky.

18. Kenneth Osgood, "The Current Practice of 'Granny' Midwifery in a Rural Southeastern Kentucky County," ca. mid-1960s (from context), Box 40, Folder 6, Papers of the Frontier Nursing Service, Special Collections Division, Margaret I. King Library, University of Kentucky, Lexington.

19. Osgood, "Current Practice of 'Granny' Midwifery."

20. "The First and Second West Virginia Health Consumer Workshops," July 1972, Box 91, Folder 27, CSM (Part Two) Papers; "A Proposal or a Program in Consumer Health Advocacy in Appalachia," ca. 1970, Box 92, Folder 20, CSM (Part Two) Papers.

21. "Southeastern Kentucky Regional Health Demonstration Project"; "Kentucky State Department of Health News and Plans"; "Southeastern Kentucky Regional Health Demonstration Project: Health Development Plan for Year 1968–1969."

22. David Steinman, "Development of a Rural Demonstration Practice," *Journal of the Kentucky Medical Association*, January 1972.

23. David Steinman and J. D. Miller, *Clover Fork Clinic: The Case History of a New Rural Health Center*, Box 398, Folder 4, ARC Papers.

24. On postwar Central Appalachian county-based machines, see Kiffmeyer, *Reformers to Radicals*, which contains a number of examples throughout; and Dwight B. Billings and Kathleen M. Blee, *The Road to Poverty: The Making of Wealth and Hardship in Appalachia* (New York: Cambridge University Press, 2000), 328–36.

25. "The Floyd County Comprehensive Health Program," ca. late 1960s (from context), Box D-078, Folder 2, Perkins Papers; "Health Centers in California, Alabama, Kentucky to

Get $4 Million," July 17, 1969, Box D-078, Folder 2, Perkins Papers; Earl Compton, "Narrative Report," October–December 1968, Box 093, Folder 7, Perkins Papers.

26. "Information on Floyd County Comprehensive Health Services Project," ca. 1969 (from context); Gary D. London to Theodore M. Berry, memorandum on "highlights of the proposed refunding Grant to the Big Sandy Area Community Action Council," July 23, 1968; "Summary of Work Program," 1969 (from context); and "For Delegation of Activities under CAP Grant No. 8986," October 23, 1969, all in Box D-078, Folder 2, Perkins Papers.

27. Accounts of the War on Poverty–era welfare rights movement, written recently and at the time, focus on metropolitan areas, especially New York City. See Felicia Kornbluh, *The Battle over Welfare Rights: Politics and Poverty in Modern America* (Philadelphia: University of Pennsylvania Press, 2007); Premilla Nadasen, *Welfare Warriors: The Welfare Rights Movement in the United States* (New York: Routledge, 2005); and Frances Fox Piven and Richard Cloward, *Poor People's Movements: Why They Succeed, How They Fail* (New York: Viking, 1977), ch. 5.

28. Eastern Kentucky Welfare Rights Organization, "Constitution and By-Laws," ca. late 1960s (from context), Box 107, Folder 9, CSM (Part Two) Papers.

29. Interview with Eula Hall, September 5, 1992, Southern Rural Poverty Collection, Dewitt Wallace Center for Media and Democracy, Duke University.

30. On EKWRO and Hall, see Jessica Wilkerson, *To Live Here, You Have to Fight* (Urbana: University of Illinois Press, 2019), ch. 4.

31. Wilkerson, 103.

32. Interview with Eula Hall, September 5, 1992, Southern Rural Poverty Collection, Dewitt Wallace Center for Media and Democracy, Duke University.

33. University Research Corporation (on behalf of OEO), "Report on Floyd County (Kentucky) Comprehensive Health Services Project," February 5, 1970; and Omar Creeman to E. Austin Jr., memorandum on "Visit to Floyd County Comprehensive Health Services Program," December 16, 1969, both in Box D-094, Folder 1, Perkins Papers.

34. University Research Corporation (on behalf of OEO), "Report on Floyd County (Kentucky) Comprehensive Health Services Project"; and Ernest Hurst to Ernest Glen Hentschel, memorandum on "STAP Assignment with the Floyd County Comprehensive Health Service Program," March 1970, both in Box D-094, Folder 1, Perkins Papers.

35. "EKWRO to Meet with Comprehensive Health," *Hawkeye* (June 1, 1969), 7, Box 150, Folder 1, CSM (Part Two) Papers.

36. University Research Corporation, "Report on Floyd County (Kentucky) Comprehensive Health Services Project"; Creeman to Austin, memorandum on "Visit to Floyd County Comprehensive Health Services Program"; Hurst to Hentschel, memorandum on "STAP Assignment with the Floyd County Comprehensive Health Service Program."

37. University Research Corporation, "Report on Floyd County (Kentucky) Comprehensive Health Services Project"; Creeman to Austin, memorandum on "Visit to Floyd County Comprehensive Health Services Program."

38. Hurst to Hentschel, memorandum on "STAP Assignment with the Floyd County Comprehensive Health Service Program."

39. Floyd County Comprehensive Health Program, meeting minutes, August 13, 1970, Box D-093, Folder 7, Perkins Papers.

40. Floyd County Comprehensive Health Program.

41. Malvina Thomson to Phyllis Pitts, ca. late 1970–early 1971 (from context), Box D-093, Folder 7, Perkins Papers.

42. Clara A. Mays to Phyllis Pitts, February 22, 1971; and Josephine P. Williamson to Phyllis Pitts, February 22, 1971, both in Box D-093, Folder 7, Perkins Papers.

43. Ron Allen et al., "Composite Report: Big Sandy Area Cap, Inc. Painteville, Kentucky," May 20–22, 1970, Box D-093, Folder 7, Perkins Papers; "Questions to Harry Eastburn, Big Sandy C.A.P. Director," *Hawkeye*, ca. early 1970 (from context), Box 150, Folder 1, CSM (Part Two) Papers.

44. "Questions to Harry Eastburn," Big Sandy C.A.P. Director, *Hawkeye*, November 1970, 17, Box 150, Folder 1, CSM (Part Two) Papers.

45. Mud Creek Health Rights Committee to Carl D. Perkins, September 25, 1970, Box D-078, Folder 2, Perkins Papers; Thomas E. Bryant to Carl D. Perkins, October 21, 1970, Box D-078, Folder 2, Perkins Papers.

46. Ernest Glen Hentschel to Stephen Joseph, memorandum on "Meeting between representatives of the Floyd County Comprehensive Health Services Program, Inc. and representatives of the Mud Creek Outpost area," September 1970, Box D-078, Folder 2, Perkins Papers.

47. Russell L. Hall to Carl D. Perkins, October 20, 1970, Box D-078, Folder 2, Perkins Papers.

48. Bill Stumbo to Carl D. Perkins, January 21, 1971, Box D-093, Folder 7, Perkins Papers.

49. William G. Poole to Harry Eastburn, February 3, 1971, Box D-094, Folder 1, Perkins Papers.

50. The relationship was hardly free from friction, particularly at the start, when Cooper attempted to make a number of concessions to the Floyd County group, such as allowing Judge Stumbo to remain on its board. Eula Hall, "Welfare Rights," *Mountain Life and Work*, July–August 1971, 20.

51. Eula Hall to Leon Cooper, March 13, 1971; and Carl Smith to Henry Stumbo and Eleanor Robinson, memorandum on "Notice of Suspension of OEO Grant No. 8986," June 4, 1971, both in Box D-093, Folder 7, Perkins Papers; Eula Hall interview.

52. Thomas E. Bryant, March 1971, memorandum on "OEO Grant NO. 8986," Box D-093, Folder 7, Perkins Papers; EKWRO, "Fact Sheet," April 6, 1971, Box D-093, Folder 7, Perkins Papers.

53. Maxine Kenny, "Mountain Health Care: Politics, Power, and Profits," *Mountain Life and Work*, April 1971, 17.

54. John Burton to Frank Carlucci, February 24, 1971, Box D-093, Folder 7, Perkins Papers.

55. [Elsie—handwriting partially illegible] Whitaker to Henry Stumbo, April 27, 1971, Box D-093, Folder 7, Perkins Papers.

56. Woodrow Rogers and Eula Hall, April 9, 1971, Box D-093, Folder 7, Perkins Papers.

57. Melvina Stumbo Thomson to Carl Perkins, May 24, 1971; Veronica Click to Carl Perkins, May 24, 1971; and "The Entire Staff of Incompetency," note, ca. May–June 1971 (from context), all in Box D-093, Folder 7, Perkins Papers.

58. Smith to Stumbo and Robinson, memorandum on "Notice of Suspension of OEO Grant No. 8986."

59. Thomson to Perkins, May 24, 1971.

60. Ira Katznelson, *When Affirmative Action Was White: An Untold Story of Racial Inequality in Twentieth-Century America* (New York: W. W. Norton, 2005), 22. On segregation of Hill-Burton funds, see Hoffman, *Health Care for Some Rights and Rationing in the United States since 1930* (Chicago: University of Chicago, 2012), ch. 4; and Karen Kruse Thomas, *Deluxe Jim Crow: Civil Rights and American Health Policy, 1935–1954* (Athens: University of Georgia Press, 2011).

61. Batzel, "Health Care," 458, 460.

62. "Why a Health Fair?," *Mountain Life and Work*, July–August 1971, 2; "Model Health Clinic for Mud Creek," ca. early 1970s (from context), Box 107, Folder 11, CSM (Part Two) Papers.

63. EKWRO, "Proposal for a Mud Creek Health Program, Floyd County, KY," ca. 1972 (from context); and "Medical Summary: EKWRO Summer Health Project," June 15–August 15, 1972, both in Box 107, Folder 11, CSM (Part Two) Papers.

64. Eula Hall, "One Thing You Can Tell Them," in *Back Talk from Appalachia: Confronting Stereotypes*, ed. Dwight B. Billings, Gurney Norman, and Katherine Ledford (Lexington: University Press of Kentucky, 1999), 194; Eula Hall, interview with Dorothy Hall Peddle, *Southern Exposure*, March/April 1983, 41.

65. Comprehensive Health Care, Inc., "Establishment of Primary Care Clinics for a Rural Population," August 1, 1974, to July 31, 1975 (in author's possession); Comprehensive Health Care, Inc., Board of Directors, meeting minutes, February 14, 1974, Big Sandy Health Care Archives, Prestonsburg, Ky. The new entity assumed the same name as its predecessor—even though they were formally separate—but changed its name less than a year later.

66. Quentin D. Allen to Joseph E. Coon, November 26, 1974, Box R-098, Folder 7, Perkins Papers.

67. Big Sandy Health Care, Inc., Board of Directors, meeting minutes, January 31, March 14, 1975, Big Sandy Health Care Archives, Prestonsburg, Ky.

68. Interview with Eula Hall, September 5, 1992, Southern Rural Poverty Collection, Dewitt Wallace Center for Media and Democracy, Duke University; Interview with Eula Hall, June 15, 1988, Coal Mining Oral History Project, Louis B. Nunn Center for Oral History, University of Kentucky, Lexington.

69. Big Sandy Health Care, Inc., Board of Directors, meeting minutes, November 9, 1978, October 13, 21, 1977, Big Sandy Health Care Archives, Prestonsburg, Ky.

70. D. J. Schliessmann, F. O. Atchley, M. J. Wilcomb Jr., and S. F. Welch, "Relationship of Environmental Factors to Enteric Disease," *Public Health Monograph No. 54* (Washington, D.C.: U.S. Government Printing Office, 1958), 6, 13, 18–19, 29–30.

71. Schliessmann, Atchley, Wilcomb, and Welch, 19–25.

72. "Medical Summary: EKWRO Summer Health Project."

73. On hookworm in the South, see Margaret Humphreys, "How Four Once Common Diseases Were Eliminated from the American South," *Health Affairs* 28, no. 6 (2009): 1739–42.

74. "Medical Summary: EKWRO Summer Health Project."

75. "Area Health Services Criticized at Public Hearing," May 17, 1975, Box 93, Folder 6, CSM (Part Two) Papers; Simon v. Eastern Kentucky Welfare Rights Organization, Inc. (Simon v. EKWRO), 426 U.S. 26 (1976).

76. "Area Health Services Criticized at Public Hearing."

77. "A Five Year Assessment of the Southeastern Kentucky Regional Health Demonstration Project," October 1974, Box 41, Folder 9, Papers of the Frontier Nursing Service, Special Collections Division, Margaret I. King Library, University of Kentucky, Lexington.

78. Judi Floyd and Doris Gibson, "Hector Health Survey: Family Nursing IV Project," May 1972, Box 41, Folder 8, Papers of the Frontier Nursing Service, Special Collections Division, Margaret I. King Library, University of Kentucky, Lexington.

79. Appalachian Regional Commission, "Staff Draft: Medical Indigency in Central Appalachia," 1978, Box 210, Folder 14, ARC Archives.

80. Appalachian Regional Commission, memorandum on "Proposed Central Appalachia Health System Grants," ca. 1974 (from context), Box 114, Folder 1747, Whisman Papers.

81. Appalachian Regional Commission, "Staff Draft: Medical Indigency in Central Appalachia."

## CONCLUSION

1. David J. Garrow, *Rising Star: The Making of Barack Obama* (New York: William Morrow, 2017), 314.

2. Garrow, 288. This epiphany—and candidate Obama's later ambivalence over community organization's efficacy—is also covered perceptively in John Judis, "Creation Myth," *New Republic*, September 10, 2008.

3. Anna Wilde Matthews, Emily Glazer, and Laura Stevens, "Triple Threat: Amazon, Berkshire, JPMorgan Rattle Health-Care Firms," *Wall Street Journal*, January 30, 2018; Jo Kamp and Anna Wilde Matthews, "New Details of Amazon, Berkshire Hathaway, JPMorgan Health Venture Emerge in Court Testimony," *Wall Street Journal*, February 20, 2019.

4. Sebastian Herrera and Kimberly Chin, "Amazon, Berkshire Hathaway, JPMorgan End Health-Care Venture Haven," *Wall Street Journal*, January 4, 2020.

5. Suhas Gondi and Ziru Song, "Burgeoning Role of Venture Capital in Health Care," *Health Affairs* (blog), January 2, 2019, www.healthaffairs.org/do/10.1377/hblog20181218.956406/full/.

6. David M. Cutler and Fiona Scott Morton, "Hospitals, Market Share, and Consolidation," *JAMA* 310, no. 18 (2013): 1965, 1967.

7. Naomi Klein, *On Fire: The (Burning) Case for a Green New Deal* (New York: Simon and Schuster, 2018), 285.

8. Beth Siegel, Jane Erickson, Bobby Milstein, and Katy Evans Pritchard, "Multisector Partnerships Need Further Development to Fulfill Aspirations for Transforming Regional Health and Well-Being," *Health Affairs* 37, no. 1 (2018): 37. On Health in All Policies at the local level, see *Health in All Policies: Experiences from Local Health Departments* (Washington, D.C.: National Association of County and City Health Officials, 2017); on the Culture of Health more generally, see Robert Wood Johnson Foundation, "Culture of Health Action Framework" (web), 2019, www.rwjf.org/content/rwjf/en/cultureofhealth/taking-action.html.

9. Prabhjot Singh and Dave A. Chokshi, "Community Health Workers—A Local Solution to a Global Problem," *New England Journal of Medicine* 369, no. 10 (2013); Adrienne Lapidos, Jeremy Lapedis, and Michelle Heisler, "Realizing the Value of Community Health Workers—New Opportunities for Sustainable Financing," *New England Journal of Medicine* 380, no. 21 (2019): 895.

10. Anne-Emanuelle Birn, Yogan Pillay, and Timothy H. Holtz, "Towards a Social Justice Approach to Global Health," in *Textbook of Global Health*, 4th ed. (New York: Oxford University Press, 2017), 603–45; World Health Organization, *WHO Guidelines on Health Policy and System Support to Optimize Community Health Worker Programmes* (Geneva: World Health Organization, 2018); Paul Farmer, "Making Human Rights Substantial," in *Partner to the Poor: A Paul Farmer Reader*, ed. Haun Saussy (Berkeley: University of California Press, 2010), 554.

11. Mark Schlesinger, "Paradigms Lost: The Persisting Search for Community in U.S. Health Policy," *Journal of Health Politics, Policy and Law* 22, no. 4 (1997): 937–92.

12. Ban Ki-moon, "Secretary-General's Remarks at Closing of COP21," *United Nations* (web), December 12, 2015, www.un.org/sg/en/content/sg/statement/2015-12-12/secretary-generals-remarks-closing-cop21.

13. Ban Ki-moon, "The U.N.'s Climate Report Exposes How Badly Wrong Leaders Like Trump Have Got Climate Change," *Time* (web), October 8, 2018, https://time.com/5416793/climate-change-ban-ki-moon-trump/.

14. "Endorsing the U.S. Mayors Climate Protection Agreement," United States Conference of Mayors, February 1, 2017, https://world.350.org/spokane/files/2019/01/2007 USMayorsClimateProtectionAgreement.pdf.

15. Richard Orange, "US Mayors Seek to Bypass Trump with Direct Role at UN Climate Talks," *Guardian*, October 10, 2019.

16. Ellen Griffith Spears, *Baptized in PCBs: Race, Pollution, and Justice in an All-American Town* (Chapel Hill: University of North Carolina Press, 2014); David Rosner and Gerald Markowitz, *Deceit and Denial: The Deadly Politics of Industrial Pollution* (Berkeley: University of California Press, 2002), chs. 9, 10; Julie Sze, *Noxious New York: The Racial Politics of Urban Health and Environmental Justice* (Cambridge, Mass.: MIT Press, 2007); David N. Pellow, *Garbage Wars: The Struggle for Environmental Justice in Chicago* (Cambridge, Mass.: MIT Press, 2002); and Robert D. Bullard, *Dumping in Dixie: Race, Class, and Environmental Quality*, 3rd ed. (Boulder, Colo.: Westview, 2003).

17. Naomi Klein, *This Changes Everything: Capitalism vs. the Climate* (New York: Simon and Schuster, 2014), 293–336.

18. H. Res. 109, Recognizing the duty of the Federal Government to create a Green New Deal, 116th Cong., 1st Sess. (2019–20).

19. Derek Thompson, "What's behind South Korea's COVID-19 Exceptionalism?," *Atlantic*, May 6, 2020, www.theatlantic.com/ideas/archive/2020/05/whats-south-koreas -secret/611215/.

20. Aruna Roy and Saba Kohli Davé, "When People and Governments Come Together," *Economic and Political Weekly*, May 2, 2020. On Kerala and health historically, see Sunil Amrith, "Political Culture of Health in India: A Historical Perspective," *Economic and Political Weekly*, January 13, 2007.

21. State of California, Executive Order, N-33-20, March 4, 2020.

22. State of New York, Executive Order, No. 202.8, March 20, 2020.

23. Alan Judd and Greg Bluestein, "Lifting Stay-at-Home Order, Kemp Shifts Focus to Economic Recovery," *Atlanta Journal-Constitution*, April 30, 2020.

24. Malachi Barrett, "Sexist Attacks Cast Michigan Gov. Whitmer as Mothering Tyrant of Coronavirus Dystopia," *MLive*, May 22, 2020, www.mlive.com/public-interest/2020/05 /sexist-attacks-cast-whitmer-as-mothering-tyrant-of-coronavirus-dystopia.html.

25. Eric Bradner, "Georgia Gov. Brian Kemp Faces Resistance over Move to Reopen Economy," *CNN*, April 21, 2020, www.cnn.com/2020/04/21/politics/georgia-governor -coronavirus-backlash/index.html.

26. Khushbu Shahin, "'It Depends on Your Politics': Georgia's Uneven Reopening Breaks along Party Lines," *Guardian*, May 23, 2020.

27. Ana Ceballos, Samantha J. Gross, and Douglas Hanks, "Miami-Dade Bars and Clubs Allowed to Reopen under DeSantis Order, Mask Fines Suspended," *Miami Herald*, September 25, 2020.

28. "Providing Additional Guidance for Empowering a Healthy Georgia in Response to COVID-19," Executive Order No. 08.15.20.01 (State of Georgia), August 15, 2020.

29. Andrew Turner, "Protesters in Huntington Beach Call for Full Reopen of State, Nation," *Los Angeles Times*, May 9, 2020.

30. Luke Money, "Orange County Authorities Won't Enforce Mask Requirement: 'We Are Not the Mask Police,'" *Los Angeles Times*, May 26, 2020.

31. Wei Lyu and George Wehby, "Comparison of Estimated Rates of Coronavirus Disease 2019 (COVID-19) in Border Counties in Iowa without a Stay-at-Home Order and Border Counties in Illinois with a Stay-at-Home Order," *JAMA Network Open* 3, no. 2 (2020): e2011102.

32. "Iowa State Report," White House Coronavirus Task Force, October 18, 2020, www.scribd.com/document/481325291/Iowa-WH-Report-10-18-pdf.

33. Rajib Paul et al., "Progression of COVID-19 from Urban to Rural Areas in the United States: A Spatiotemporal Analysis of Prevalence Rates," *Journal of Rural Health* 36, no. 4 (2020): 591–601.

34. Brystana G. Kaufman et al., "Half of Rural Residents at High Risk of Serious Illness due to COVID-19, Creating Stress on Rural Hospital," *Journal of Rural Health* 36, no. 4 (2020): 584–90; Jacob M. Souch and Jeralynn S. Cossman, "A Commentary on Rural-Urban Disparities in Covid-19 Testing Rates per 100,000 and Risk Factors," *Journal of Rural Health* 37, no. 1 (2021): 188–90.

35. Katie Honan and Paul Berger, "New York City's Ultra-Orthodox Jewish Leaders Decry New Lockdown Measures," *Wall Street Journal*, October 7, 2020; Emma Fitzsimmons and Alexandra Petri, "How N.Y.C.'s Conservative Bastion Became a Virus Hot Spot," *New York Times*, November 11, 2020.

36. Howard Markel, Harvey Lipman, and Alexander Navarro, "Nonpharmaceutical Interventions Implemented by US Cities during the 1918–1919 Influenza Pandemic," *JAMA* 298, no. 6 (2007): 644–54. For an account of why Milwaukee weathered the flu better than any other city of comparable size, see Judith Walzer Leavitt, *The Healthiest City: Milwaukee and the Politics of Health Reform* (Princeton, N.J.: Princeton University Press, 1982), 227–39.

37. Vishnu Varma, "Migrant Workers in Kerala among Most Vulnerable as Covid Caseload Rises," *Indian Express*, November 16, 2020; "Kerala, India's 'Model State' in COVID-19 Fight, Suffers Setback," *Al Jazeera*, October 2, 2020, www.aljazeera.com/news/2020/10/2/kerala-indias-model-state-in-covid-19-fight-sees-cases-surge.

38. The two key intellectual texts undergirding this moment were Michael Hardt and Antonio Negri, *Empire* (Cambridge, Mass.: Harvard University Press, 2000); and Hardt and Negri, *Multitude: War and Democracy in the Age of Empire* (New York: Penguin, 2004). For on-the-ground movements, see Tom Mertes, ed., *A Movement of Movements: Is Another World Really Possible?* (New York: Verso, 2004).

39. Peter N. Funke, "Building Rhizomatic Social Movements? Movement-Building Relays during the Current Epoch of Contention," *Studies in Social Justice* 8, no. 1 (2014): 31.

40. Frances Fox Piven and Richard Cloward, *Poor People's Movements: How They Succeed, Why They Fail* (New York: Viking, 1977), 20.

41. Piven and Cloward, 20.

# Bibliography

ARCHIVES

*California*
  Los Angeles
    Kenneth Hahn Hall of Administration (Los Angeles County)
      Hall of Records
    University of California, Los Angeles
      Library Special Collections, Charles E. Young Research Library
        Augustus Hawkins Papers
      UCLA Archives, Charles E. Young Research Library
        UCLA School of Medicine
  San Marino
    Manuscripts Collection, Huntington Library
      Fletcher Bowron Papers
      John Anson Ford Papers
      Los Angeles County Medical Association Papers
      Papers of Kenneth Hahn
*Connecticut*
  New Haven
    Sterling Memorial Library, Yale University
      Manuscripts and Archives
        Edwin Richard Weinerman Papers
        Papers of John Lindsay (personal)
*Kentucky*
  Berea
    Berea College Special Collections and Archives, Hutchins Library
      Appalachian Volunteers Papers
      Council of Southern Mountains (Part Two) Papers
  Lexington
    Margaret I. King Library, University of Kentucky
      Special Collections Division
        Papers of Harry Caudill
        Papers of John Sherman Cooper

Papers of the Appalachian Regional Commission (ARC)
Papers of the Frontier Nursing Service
Prestonsburg
Big Sandy Health Care Archives
Richmond
Special Collections and Archives, Eastern Kentucky University
Carl Perkins Papers
*Maryland*
College Park
National Archives
Record Group 70, Records of the United States Bureau of Mines
*Minnesota*
Minneapolis
Elmer L. Andersen Library, University of Minnesota
Social Welfare History Archives
Papers of Helen Hall
Papers of the Henry Street Settlement
Minnesota Population Center, University of Minnesota
National Historical Geographical Information Systems database
*New York*
Butler Library, Columbia University
Rare Books, Special Collections and Archives
Papers of Mobilization for Youth
Columbia University Irving Medical Center
Archives and Special Collections, Augustus C. Long Health Sciences Library
Records of the Columbia University Medical Center, Office of the
Vice President for Health Sciences, Dean of the Faculty of Medicine
[semiprocessed]
LaGuardia Community College, City University of New York
LaGuardia and Wagner Archives
Abraham Beame Papers
Edward Koch Papers
John Lindsay Papers (mayoral)
Papers of Ray Trussell
Robert F. Wagner Papers
New York Public Library
Manuscripts and Archives Division, Humanities and Social Sciences Library
Papers of Howard J. Brown
*Ohio*
Beachwood
Cleveland Clinic Archives, Cleveland Clinic
Papers of Richard Gottron [semiprocessed]
Papers of Thomas Hatch [semiprocessed]
Cleveland
Case Western Reserve University Archives, Case Western Reserve University
Papers of Samuel Whitman
Cleveland Public Library
Public Administration Library

Dittrick Medical History Center, Case Western Reserve University
    Papers of Duncan Neuhaser [semiprocessed]
Western Reserve Historical Society
    Anthony J. Celebrezze Papers
    Greater Cleveland Nurses Association, Series III
    Papers of Carl Stokes
    Papers of the Hough Area Development Corporation
    University Circle Incorporated Papers
*Pennsylvania*
  Philadelphia
    Institute for Social Medicine and Community Health
      Howard J. Brown Biographical File
    Van Pelt Library, University of Pennsylvania
      Kislak Center for Special Collections, Rare Books and Manuscripts
        Medical Committee for Human Rights Papers

## PERIODICALS

*Atlanta Journal-Constitution*
*Atlantic*
*Cleveland (Ohio) Plain-Dealer*
*Cleveland (Ohio) Press*
*Daily Trojan* (University of Southern
  California, Los Angeles)
*East Side (N.Y.) News*
*Guardian*
*Lexington (Ky.) Herald*
*Life*
*Los Angeles Herald-Dispatch*

*Los Angeles Sentinel*
*Los Angeles Times*
*Louisville (Ky.) Courier-Journal*
*New York Daily News*
*New York Post*
*New York Times*
*New York World-Telegram and Sun*
*Star Review*
*Time*
*Wall Street Journal*

## BOOKS

Alcaly, Roger, and David Mermelstein, eds. *The Fiscal Crisis of American Cities: Essays on the Political Economy of Urban America with Special Reference to New York*. New York: Vintage Books, 1977.

Alford, Robert. *Health Care Politics: Ideological and Interest Group Barriers to Reform*. Chicago: University of Chicago Press, 1975.

Allen, Robert. *Black Awakening in Capitalist America: An Analytic History*. Garden City, N.Y.: Doubleday, 1969.

Altshuler, Alan. *Community Control: The Black Demand for Participation in Large American Cities*. New York: Pegasus, 1970.

Ammon, Francesca. *Bulldozer: Demolition and Clearance of the Postwar Landscape*. New Haven, Conn.: Yale University Press, 2016.

Amsterdam, Daniel. *The Roaring Metropolis: Businessmen's Campaign for a Civic Welfare State*. Philadelphia: University of Pennsylvania Press, 2016.

Anderson, Martin. *The Federal Bulldozer: A Critical Analysis of Urban Renewal, 1942–1962*. New York: McGraw-Hill, 1967.

Andrews, Richard N. L. *Managing the Environment, Managing Ourselves: A History of American Environmental Policy.* New Haven, Conn.: Yale University Press, 1999.

Andrews, Thomas. *Killing for Coal: America's Deadliest Labor War.* Cambridge, Mass.: Harvard University Press, 2008.

Auyero, Javier, and Débora Alejandra Swistun. *Flammable: Environmental Suffering in an Argentinian Shantytown.* New York: Oxford University Press, 2009.

Avila, Eric. *Popular Culture in the Age of White Flight: Fear and Fantasy in Suburban Los Angeles.* Berkeley: University of California Press, 2004.

Bailey, Robert W. *The Crisis Regime: The MAC, the EFCB, and the Political Impact of the Crisis Regime.* Albany: State University of New York Press, 1984.

Barnes, David S. *The Great Stink of Paris and the Nineteenth-Century Struggle against Filth and Germs.* Baltimore: Johns Hopkins University Press, 2006.

———. *The Making of a Social Disease: Tuberculosis in Nineteenth-Century France.* Berkeley: University of California Press, 1995.

Best, Rachel Kahn. *Common Enemies: Disease Campaigns in America.* New York: Oxford University Press, 2019.

Billings, Dwight B., and Kathleen M. Blee. *The Road to Poverty: The Making of Wealth and Hardship in Appalachia.* New York: Cambridge University Press, 2000.

Billings, Dwight B., Gurney Norman, and Katherine Ledford, eds. *Back Talk from Appalachia: Confronting Stereotypes.* Lexington: University Press of Kentucky, 1998.

Birn, Anne-Emanuelle. *Marriage of Convenience: Rockefeller International Health and Revolutionary Mexico.* Rochester, N.Y.: University of Rochester Press, 2006.

Bottles, Scott. *Los Angeles and the Automobile: The Making of a Modern City.* Berkeley: University of California Press, 1987.

Bouston, Leah. *Competition in the Promised Land.* Princeton, N.J.: Princeton University Press, 2017.

Bradley, Stefan. *Harlem vs. Columbia University: Black Student Power in the Late 1960s.* Urbana: University of Illinois Press, 2009.

Braun, Lundy. *The Surprising Career of the Spirometer from Plantation to Genetics.* Minneapolis: University of Minnesota Press, 2014.

Brinkley, Alan. *The End of Reform: New Deal Liberalism in Recession and War.* New York: Vintage Books, 1966.

Brown, Lawrence D. *Politics and Health Care Organization: HMOs as Federal Policy.* Washington, D.C.: Brookings Institution Press, 1983.

Brown, Phil, Rachel Morello-Frosch, and Stephen Zavestoski, eds. *Contested Illnesses: Citizens, Science, and Health Social Movements.* Berkeley: University of California Press, 2012.

Brown-Nagin, Tomiko. *Courage to Dissent: Atlanta and the Long History of the Civil Rights Movement.* New York: Oxford University Press, 2012.

Bullard, Robert D. *Dumping in Dixie: Race, Class, and Environmental Quality.* 3rd ed. Boulder, Colo.: Westview, 2003.

Burlage, Robb. *New York City's Municipal Hospitals: A Policy Review.* Washington, D.C.: Institute for Policy Studies, 1967.

Cammet, Melani, and Lauren M. MacLean, eds. *The Politics of Non-State Social Welfare.* Ithaca, N.Y.: Cornell University Press, 2014.

Carmichael, Stokely, and Charles Hamilton. *Black Power: The Politics of Liberation in America.* New York: Random House, 1967.

Caro, Robert. *The Power Broker: Robert Moses and the Fall of New York.* New York: Vintage Books, 1987.

Carroll, Tamar. *Mobilizing New York: AIDS, Antipoverty, and Feminist Activism*. Chapel Hill: University of North Carolina Press, 2015.

Caudill, Harry. *My Land Is Dying*. New York: E. P. Dutton, 1973.

———. *Night Comes to the Cumberlands: A Biography of a Depressed Area*. Boston: Little, Brown, 1963.

Chackoway, Barry, ed. *Citizens and Health Care: Participation and Planning for Social Change*. New York: Pergamon, 1981.

Chipkin, Ivor, and Mark Swilling. *Shadow State: The Politics of State Capture*. Johannesburg, South Africa: Wits University Press, 2018.

Clough, John D. *To Act as a Unit: The Story of the Cleveland Clinic*. 4th ed. Cleveland, Ohio: Cleveland Clinic Press, 2005.

Cohen, William. *At Freedom's Edge: Black Mobility and the Southern White Quest for Racial Control, 1861–1915*. Baton Rouge: Louisiana State University Press, 1991.

Coleman, William. *Death Is a Social Disease: Public Health and Political Economy in Early Industrial France*. Madison: University of Wisconsin Press, 1982.

Colgrove, James. *Epidemic City: The Politics of Public Health in New York*. New York: Russell Sage Foundation, 2011.

Colgrove, James, Gerald Markowitz, and David Rosner, eds. *The Contested Boundaries of American Public Health*. New Brunswick, N.J.: Rutgers University Press, 2008.

Collins, Robert. *More: The Politics of Economic Growth in Postwar America*. New York: Oxford University Press, 2000.

Cowie, Jefferson. *Capital Moves: RCA's 70-Year Quest for Cheap Labor*. Ithaca, N.Y.: Cornell University Press, 1999.

Cunningham, Robert, III, and Robert M. Cunningham, Jr. *Blues: A History of the Blue Cross and Blue Shield Systems*. DeKalb: Northern Illinois University Press, 1977.

Davis, Mike. *City of Quartz: Excavating the Future in Los Angeles*. New York: Verso Books, 1990.

———. *Ecology of Fear: Los Angeles and the Imagination of Disaster*. New York: Henry Holt, 1998.

———. *Late Victorian Holocausts: El Niño Famines and the Making of the Third World*. New York: Verso Books, 2000.

Derickson, Alan. *Black Lung: Anatomy of a Public Health Disaster*. Ithaca, N.Y.: Cornell University Press, 1998.

———. *Health Security for All: Dreams of Universal Health Care in America*. Baltimore: Johns Hopkins University Press, 2005.

Dittmer, John. *Local People: The Struggle for Civil Rights in Mississippi*. Urbana: University of Illinois Press, 1994.

DuPuis, E. Melanie, ed. *Smoke and Mirrors: The Politics and Culture of Air Pollution*. New York: New York University Press, 2004.

Duster, Troy. *Backdoor to Eugenics*. New York: Routledge, 1990.

Ehrenreich, Barbara, and John Ehrenreich, eds. *American Health Empire: Power, Profits, and Politics*. New York: Random House, 1970.

Elkind, Sarah. *How Local Politics Shape Federal Policy: Business, Power, and the Environment in Twentieth-Century Los Angeles*. Chapel Hill: University of North Carolina Press, 2011.

Eller, Ronald. *Uneven Ground: Appalachia since 1945*. Lexington: University Press of Kentucky, 2008.

Engel, Jonathan. *Poor People's Medicine: Medicaid and American Charity Care since 1965*. Durham, N.C.: Duke University Press, 2006.

Epstein, Steven. *Impure Science: AIDS, Activism, and the Politics of Knowledge.* Berkeley: University of California Press, 1988.

Evans, Richard J. *Death in Hamburg: Society and Politics in the Cholera Years, 1830–1910.* New York: Penguin, 1987.

Eyler, John. *Victorian Social Medicine: The Ideas and Methods of William Farr.* Baltimore: Johns Hopkins University Press, 1979.

Fernández, Johanna. *The Young Lords: A Radical History.* Chapel Hill: University of North Carolina Press, 2020.

Fink, Leon, and Brian Greenberg. *Upheaval in the Quiet Zone: A History of Hospital Workers' Union, Local 1199.* Urbana: University of Illinois Press, 1989.

Fisher, Stephen L., ed. *Fighting Back in Appalachia: Traditions of Resistance and Change.* Philadelphia: Temple University Press, 1992.

Fleck, Ludwik. *Genesis and Development of a Scientific Fact.* Chicago: University of Chicago Press, 1998.

Frazier, Nishani. *Harambee City: The Congress of Racial Equality in Cleveland and the Rise of Black Power Populism.* Fayetteville: University of Arkansas Press, 2017.

Freeman, Joshua. *Working-Class New York: Life and Labor since World War II.* New York: New Press, 2000.

Fuchs, Ester R. *Mayors and Money: Fiscal Policy in New York and Chicago.* Chicago: University of Chicago Press, 1992.

Gamble, Vanessa. *Making a Place for Ourselves: The Black Hospital Movement, 1920–1945.* New York: Oxford University Press, 1995.

Gans, Herbert J. *The Urban Villagers: Group and Class in the Life of Italian-Americans.* New York: Free Press, 1962.

Garrow, David J. *Rising Star: The Making of Barack Obama.* New York: William Morrow, 2017.

Geismer, Lily. *Don't Blame Us: Suburban Liberals and the Transformation of the Democratic Party.* Princeton, N.J.: Princeton University Press, 2014.

Germany, Kent. *New Orleans after the Promises: Poverty, Citizenship, and the Search for the Great Society.* Athens: University of Georgia Press, 2007.

Goldberg, David, and Trevor Griffey, eds. *Black Power at Work: Community Control, Affirmative Action, and the Construction Industry.* Ithaca, N.Y.: Cornell University Press, 2011.

Goodell, Jeff. *Big Coal: The Dirty Secret behind America's Energy Future.* New York: Houghton Mifflin, 2007.

Gordon, Colin. *Dead on Arrival: The Politics of Health Care in Twentieth-Century America.* Princeton, N.J.: Princeton University Press, 2003.

Gostin, Lawrence O. *Public Health Law: Power, Duty, Restraint.* Berkeley: University of California Press, 2008.

Grossman, James. *Land of Hope: Chicago, Black Southerners, and the Great Migration.* Chicago: University of Chicago Press, 1991.

Hacker, Jacob S. *The Divided Welfare State: The Battle over Public and Private Benefits in the United States.* New York: Cambridge University Press, 2002.

Hamlin, Christopher. *Public Health and Social Justice in the Age of Chadwick: Britain, 1800–1854.* New York: Cambridge University Press, 1998.

Hammonds, Evelyn. *Childhood's Deadly Scourge: The Campaign to Control Diphtheria in New York City, 1880–1930.* Baltimore: Johns Hopkins University Press, 2002.

Hardt, Jerry, and Albert Fritsch. *Harlan County Flood Report.* Corbin, Ky.: Appalachia—Science in the Public Interest, 1978.

Hardt, Michael, and Antonio Negri. *Empire*. Cambridge, Mass.: Harvard University Press, 2000.

———. *Multitude: War and Democracy in the Age of Empire*. New York: Penguin, 2004.

Harrington, Michael. *The Other America: Poverty in the United States*. New York: Macmillan, 1962.

Hecht, Susannah, and Alexander Cockburn. *The Fate of the Forest: Developers, Destroyers, and Defenders of the Amazon*. 2nd ed. Chicago: University of Chicago Press, 2010.

Hendricks, Ricky. *A Model for National Health Care: The History of Kaiser Permanente*. New Brunswick, N.J.: Rutgers University Press, 1993.

Highsmith, Andrew. *Demolition Means Progress: Flint, Michigan, and the Fate of the American Metropolis*. Chicago: University of Chicago Press, 2015.

Hirsch, Arnold. *Making the Second Ghetto: Race and Housing in Chicago, 1940–1960*. Chicago: University of Chicago Press, 1983.

Horace, C. Hamilton. *Health and Health Services in the Southern Appalachians: A Source Book*. Raleigh: North Carolina Agricultural Experiment Station, 1959.

Horne, Gerald. *The Fire This Time: The Watts Uprising and the 1960s*. Charlottesville: University of Virginia Press, 1995.

Horwitt, Sanford. *Let Them Call Me Rebel: Saul Alinsky, His Life and Legacy*. New York: Vintage Books, 1992.

Howell, Joel. *Technology in the Hospital: Transforming Patient Care in the Early Twentieth Century*. Baltimore: Johns Hopkins University Press, 1995.

Immerwahr, Daniel. *How to Hide an Empire: A History of the Greater United States*. New York: Picador, 2019.

———. *Thinking Small: The United States and the Lure of Community Development*. Cambridge, Mass.: Harvard University Press, 2015.

Jacobs, Jane. *Life and Death of Great American Cities*. New York: Random House, 1961.

Jacobs, Meg. *Panic at the Pump: The Energy Crisis and the Transformation of American Politics in the 1970s*. New York: Hill and Wang, 2016.

Joseph, Miranda. *Against the Romance of Community*. Minneapolis: University of Minnesota Press, 2002.

Katz, Michael B. *Improving Poor People: The Welfare State, the "Underclass," and Urban Schools as History*. Princeton, N.J.: Princeton University Press, 1997.

———. *In the Shadow of the Poorhouse: A Social History of Welfare in America*. New York: Basic Books, 1986.

Katznelson, Ira. *City Trenches: Urban Politics and the Patterning of Class in the United States*. Chicago: University of Chicago Press, 1981.

———. *When Affirmative Action Was White: An Untold Story of Racial Inequality in Twentieth-Century America*. New York: W. W. Norton, 2005.

Kerr, Daniel R. *Derelict Paradise, Homelessness, and Urban Development in Cleveland, Ohio*. Amherst: University of Massachusetts Press, 2011.

Kiffmeyer, Thomas. *Reformers to Radicals: The Appalachian Volunteers and the War on Poverty*. Lexington: University Press of Kentucky, 2008.

Klein, Jennifer. *For All These Rights: Business, Labor, and the Shaping of America's Public-Private Welfare State*. Princeton, N.J.: Princeton University Press, 2003.

Klein, Naomi. *This Changes Everything: Capitalism vs. the Climate*. New York: Simon and Schuster, 2014.

———. *On Fire: The (Burning) Case for a Green New Deal*. New York: Simon and Schuster, 2018.

Kornbluh, Felicia. *The Battle over Welfare Rights: Politics and Poverty in Modern America.* Philadelphia: University of Pennsylvania Press, 2007.

Korstad, Robert, and James Lelouis. *To Right These Wrongs: The North Carolina Fund and the Battle to End Poverty and Inequality in 1960s America.* Chapel Hill: University of North Carolina Press, 2010.

Krajcinovic, Ivana. *From Company Doctors to Managed Care: The United Mine Workers' Noble Experiment.* Ithaca, N.Y.: Cornell University Press, 1997.

Kurashige, Scott. *The Shifting Grounds of Race: Black and Japanese Americans in the Making of Multiethnic Los Angeles.* Princeton, N.J.: Princeton University Press, 2008.

Kusmer, Kenneth. *A Ghetto Takes Shape: Black Cleveland, 1870–1930.* Urbana: University of Illinois Press, 1978.

Langston, Nancy. *Toxic Bodies: Hormone Disruptors and the Legacy of DES.* New Haven, Conn.: Yale University Press, 2011.

Leavitt, Judith Walzer. *The Healthiest City: Milwaukee and the Politics of Health Reform.* Princeton, N.J.: Princeton University Press, 1982.

Lefkowitz, Bonnie. *Community Health Centers: A Movement and the People Who Made It Happen.* New Brunswick, N.J.: Rutgers University Press, 1997.

Lewis, Helen Matthews, Linda Johnson, and Donald Askins, eds. *Colonialism in Modern America: The Appalachian Case.* Boone, N.C.: Appalachian Consortium Press, 1978.

Lo, Clarence Y. H. *Small Property versus Big Government: Social Origins of the Property Tax Revolt.* Berkeley: University of California Press, 1990.

Love, Spencie. *One Blood: The Death and Resurrection of Charles R. Drew.* Chapel Hill: University of North Carolina Press, 1997.

Loyd, Jenna. *Health Rights Are Civil Rights: Peace and Justice Activism in Los Angeles, 1963–1978.* Minneapolis: University of Minnesota Press, 2014.

Marris, Peter, and Martin Rein. *Dilemmas of Social Reform: Poverty and Community Action.* 2nd ed. Chicago: Aldine, 1973.

Martin, Helen Eastman. *The History of the Los Angeles County Hospital, 1878–1968, and the Los Angeles County–University of Southern California Medical Center, 1968–1978.* Los Angeles: University of Southern California Press, 1979.

McBride, David. *Integrating the City of Medicine: Blacks in Philadelphia Health Care, 1910–1965.* Philadelphia: Temple University Press, 1989.

McCaughhey, Robert. *Stand, Columbia: A History of Columbia University.* New York: Columbia University Press, 2003.

McGirr, Lisa. *Suburban Warriors: The Origins of the New American Right.* Princeton, N.J.: Princeton University Press, 2001.

McKee, Guian. *The Problem of Jobs: Liberalism, Race, and Deindustrialization in Philadelphia.* Chicago: University of Chicago Press, 2008.

McKeown, Thomas. *The Modern Rise of Population.* New York: Academic Press, 1976.

———. *The Role of Medicine: Dream, Mirage, or Nemesis.* Oxford: Blackwell, 1979.

Mertes, Tom, ed. *A Movement of Movements: Is Another World Really Possible?* New York: Verso Books, 2004.

Metzl, Jonathan. *The Protest Psychosis: How Schizophrenia Became a Black Disease.* Boston: Beacon, 2010.

Michener, Jamila. *Fragmented Democracy: Medicaid, Federalism and Unequal Politics.* New York: Cambridge University Press, 2012.

Michney, Todd. *Surrogate Suburbs: Black Upward Mobility and Neighborhood Change in Cleveland, 1900–1980.* Chapel Hill: University of North Carolina Press, 2017.

Mitchell, Timothy. *Carbon Democracy: Political Power in the Age of Oil*. New York: Verso Books, 2011.

Mittman, Gregg. *Breathing Space: How Allergies Shape Our Lives and Landscapes*. New Haven, Conn.: Yale University Press, 2008.

Molina, Natalia. *Fit to Be Citizens? Public Health and Race in Los Angeles, 1879–1939*. Berkeley: University of California Press, 2006.

Montrie, Chad. *To Save the Land and People: A History of Opposition to Surface Coal Mining in Appalachia*. Chapel Hill: University of North Carolina Press, 2003.

Moore, Kelly. *Disrupting Science: Social Movements, American Scientists, and the Politics of the Military, 1945–1975*. Princeton, N.J.: Princeton University Press, 2008.

Moore, Leonard. *Carl B. Stokes and the Rise of Black Power*. Urbana: University of Illinois Press, 2002.

Mulcahy, Richard P. *A Social Contract for the Coal Fields: The Rise and Fall of the United Mine Workers of America Welfare and Retirement Fund*. Knoxville: University of Tennessee Press, 2000.

Nace, Ted. *Climate Hope: On the Front Lines of the Fight against Coal*. Berkeley, Calif.: Earth Island Institute/CoalSwarm, 2009.

Nadasen, Premilla. *Welfare Warriors: The Welfare Rights Movement in the United States*. New York: Routledge, 2005.

Nathanson, Constance. *Disease Prevention as Social Change: The State, Society, and Public Health in the United States, France, Great Britain, and Canada*. New York: Russell Sage Foundation, 2007.

Nelson, Alondra. *Body and Soul: The Black Panther Party and the Fight against Medical Discrimination*. Minneapolis: University of Minnesota Press, 2011.

Nelson, Nicole C. *Model Behavior: Animal Experiments, Complexity, and the Genetics of Psychiatric Disorders*. Chicago: University of Chicago Press, 2018.

Newfield, Jack, and Paul DuBrul. *The Abuse of Power: The Permanent Government and the Fall of New York*. New York: Viking, 1977.

Nixon, Rob. *Slow Violence and the Environmentalism of the Poor*. Cambridge, Mass.: Harvard University Press, 2011.

Oberlander, Jonathan. *The Political Life of Medicare*. Chicago: University of Chicago Press, 2003.

O'Connor, Alice. *Poverty Knowledge: Social Science, Social Policy, and the Poor in Twentieth-Century U.S. History*. Princeton, N.J.: Princeton University Press, 2001.

O'Connor, James. *Natural Causes: Essays in Ecological Marxism*. New York: Guilford, 1998.

Offner, Amy. *Sorting Out the Mixed Economy: The Rise and Fall of Welfare and Development States in the Americas*. Princeton, N.J.: Princeton University Press, 2019.

O'Neill, Tip. *All Politics Is Local and Other Rules of the Game*. New York: Random House, 1994.

Opdycke, Sandra. *No One Was Turned Away: The Role of Public Hospitals in New York City since 1900*. New York: Oxford University Press, 2000.

Oreskes, Naomi, and Erik M. M. Conway. *Merchants of Doubt: How a Handful of Scientists Obscured the Truth on Issues from Tobacco Smoke to Global Warming*. New York: Bloomsbury, 2011.

Orleck, Annelise. *Storming Caesar's Palace: How Black Mothers Fought Their Own War on Poverty*. Boston: Beacon, 2006.

Orleck, Annelise, and Lisa Gayle Hazirjian, eds. *The War on Poverty: A New Grassroots History, 1964–1980*. Athens: University of Georgia Press, 2011.

Parks, Robert B., ed. *Community Health Services for New York City: A Case Study in Urban Medical Delivery*. New York: Praeger, 1968.

Patterson, James T. *America's Struggle against Poverty, 1900–1994*. Cambridge, Mass.: Harvard University Press, 1994.

Payne, Charles. *I've Got the Light of Freedom: The Organizing Tradition and the Mississippi Freedom Struggle*. Berkeley: University of California Press, 1995.

Pellow, David N. *Garbage Wars: The Struggle for Environmental Justice in Chicago*. Cambridge, Mass.: MIT Press, 2002.

Phillips, Kimberley. *Alabama North: African-American Migrants, Community, and Working-Class Activism in Cleveland, 1915–1945*. Urbana: University of Illinois Press, 1999.

Phillips-Fein, Kim. *Fear City: New York's Fiscal Crisis and the Rise of Austerity Politics*. New York: Metropolitan Books, 2017.

Piven, Frances Fox, and Richard Cloward. *Poor People's Movements: Why They Succeed, How They Fail*. New York: Viking, 1977.

Proctor, Robert. *Cancer Wars: How Politics Shapes What We Know and Don't Know about Cancer*. New York: Basic Books, 1995.

Pulido, Laura. *Black, Brown, Yellow, and Left: Radical Activism in Los Angeles*. Berkeley: University of California Press, 2006.

Quadagno, Jill. *One Nation, Uninsured: Why the U.S. Has No National Health Insurance*. New York: Oxford University Press, 2005.

Reed, Touré F. *Not Alms but Opportunity: The Urban League and the Politics of Racial Uplift, 1910–1950*. Chapel Hill: University of North Carolina Press, 2008.

Reverby, Susan. *Examining Tuskegee: The Infamous Syphilis Study and Its Legacy*. Chapel Hill: University of North Carolina Press, 2009.

Roberts, Dorothy. *Fatal Invention: How Science, Politics, and Big Business Re-Create Race in the Twenty-First Century*. New York: New Press, 2011.

Roberts, Samuel K. *Infectious Fear: Politics, Disease, and the Health Effects of Segregation*. Chapel Hill: University of North Carolina Press, 2009.

Rosenberg, Charles. *The Care of Strangers: The Rise of America's Hospital System*. New York: Basic Books, 1987.

Rosenberg, Charles, and Janet Golden, eds. *Framing Disease: Studies in Cultural History*. New Brunswick, N.J.: Rutgers University Press, 1987.

Rosner, David. *A Once Charitable Enterprise: Hospitals and Health Care in Brooklyn and New York, 1885–1915*. New York: Cambridge University Press, 1982.

Rosner, David, and Gerald Markowitz. *Deadly Dust: Silicosis and the Politics of Occupational Disease in Twentieth-Century America*. Princeton, N.J.: Princeton University Press, 1991.

———. *Deceit and Denial: The Deadly Politics of Industrial Pollution*. Berkeley: University of California Press, 2003.

Rothman, David J. *Strangers at the Bedside: A History of How Law and Bioethics Transformed Medical Decision Making*. New York: Basic Books, 1991.

Sabin, Paul. *Crude Politics: The California Oil Market, 1900–1940*. Berkeley: University of California Press, 2005.

Sanders, Crystal. *A Chance for Change: Head Start and Mississippi's Black Freedom Struggle*. Chapel Hill: University of North Carolina Press, 2016.

Sardell, Alice. *The U.S. Experiment in Social Medicine: The Community Health Center Program, 1965–1986*. Pittsburgh: University of Pittsburgh Press, 1989.

Scala, Charles. *Report on Status of Fordham Hospital and Hospital Situation in the Bronx*. New York: Fordham Hospital Alumni Association, 1961.

Schmalzer, Sigrid, Daniel S. Chard, and Alyssa Botelho, eds. *Science for the People: Documents from America's Movement of Radical Scientists*. Amherst: University of Massachusetts Press, 2018.

Schmidt, David. *Citizen Lawmakers: The Ballot Initiative Revolution*. Philadelphia: Temple University Press, 1989.

Schrader, Stuart. *Badges without Borders: How Global Counterinsurgency Transformed American Policing*. Berkeley: University of California Press, 2019.

Schrag, Peter. *Paradise Lost: California's Experience, America's Future*. Berkeley: University of California Press, 1998.

Self, Robert O. *American Babylon: Race and the Struggle for Postwar Oakland*. Princeton, N.J.: Princeton University Press, 2003.

Sellers, Christopher C. *Crabgrass Crucible: Suburban Nature and the Rise of Environmentalism in Twentieth-Century America*. Chapel Hill: University of North Carolina Press, 2012.

———. *Hazards of the Job: From Industrial Disease to Environmental Health Science*. Chapel Hill: University of North Carolina Press, 1997.

Shah, Nayan. *Contagious Divides: Epidemics and Race in San Francisco's Chinatown*. Berkeley: University of California Press, 2001.

Shapiro, Tricia. *Mountain Justice: Homegrown Resistance to Mountaintop Removal, for the Future of Us All*. Oakland, Calif.: AK Press, 2010.

Shnayerson, Michael. *Coal River: How a Few Brave Americans Took on a Powerful Coal Company and the Federal Government to Save the Land They Love*. New York: Farrar, Straus and Giroux, 2008.

Sides, Josh. *L.A. City Limits: African American Los Angeles from the Great Depression to the Present*. Berkeley: University of California Press, 2003.

Simpson, Andrew. *The Medical Metropolis Health Care and Economic Transformation in Pittsburgh and Houston*. Philadelphia: University of Pennsylvania Press, 2019.

Smil, Vaclav. *China's Environmental Crisis: An Inquiry into the Limits of National Development*. Armonk, N.Y.: M. E. Sharpe, 1993.

Smith, David Barton. *Health Care Divided: Race and Healing a Nation*. Ann Arbor: University of Michigan Press, 1999.

Soffer, Jonathan. *Ed Koch and the Rebuilding of New York City*. New York: Columbia University Press, 2012.

Souther, J. Mark. *Believing in Cleveland: Managing Decline in "The Best Location in the Nation."* Philadelphia: Temple University Press, 2017.

Sparer, Michael. *Medicaid and the Limits of State Health Reform*. Philadelphia: Temple University Press, 1996.

Spears, Ellen Griffith. *Baptized in PCBs: Race, Pollution, and Justice in an All-American Town*. Chapel Hill: University of North Carolina Press, 2014.

Starr, Paul. *The Social Transformation of Medicine: The Rise of a Sovereign Profession and the Making of a Vast Industry*. New York: Basic Books, 1984.

Stein, Judith. *Running Steel, Running America: Race, Economic Policy, and the Decline of American Liberalism*. Chapel Hill: University of North Carolina Press, 1998.

Stevens, Rosemary. *American Medicine and the Public Interest*. New Haven, Conn.: Yale University Press, 1971.

———. *In Sickness and in Wealth: American Hospitals in the Twentieth Century*. New York: Basic Books, 1989.

Stokes, Carl. *Promises of Power: A Political Autobiography*. New York: Simon and Schuster, 1973.

Stradling, David, and Richard Stradling. *Where the River Burned: Carl Stokes and the Struggle to Save Cleveland*. Ithaca, N.Y.: Cornell University Press, 2017.

Sugrue, Thomas. *Sweet Land of Liberty: The Forgotten Struggle for Civil Rights in the North*. New York: Random House, 2008.

Swanstrom, Todd. *The Crisis of Growth Politics: Cleveland, Kucinich, and the Challenge of Urban Populism*. Philadelphia: Temple University Press, 1985.

Sze, Julie. *Noxious New York: The Racial Politics of Urban Health and Environmental Justice*. Cambridge, Mass.: MIT Press, 2007.

Tabb, William K. *The Long Default: New York City and the Urban Fiscal Crisis*. New York: Month Review, 1982.

Thomas, Karen Kruse. *Deluxe Jim Crow: Civil Rights and American Health Policy, 1935–1954*. Athens: University of Georgia Press, 2011.

Tomes, Nancy. *The Gospel of Germs: Men, Women, and the Microbe in American Life*. Chapel Hill: University of North Carolina Press, 1998.

———. *Remaking the American Patient: How Madison Avenue and Modern Medicine Turned Patients into Consumers*. Chapel Hill: University of North Carolina Press, 2016.

Valenčius, Conevery Bolton. *The Health of the Century: How American Settlers Understood Themselves and Their Land*. New York: Basic Books, 2004.

Vance, Rupert, and Thomas Ford. *The Southern Appalachian Region: A Survey*. Lexington: University of Kentucky Press, 1962.

Vogel, Sara. *BPA and the Struggle to Define the Safety of Chemicals*. Berkeley: University of California Press, 2012.

Wailoo, Keith. *Dying in the City of Blues: Sickle Cell Anemia and the Politics of Race and Health*. Chapel Hill: University of North Carolina Press, 2000.

Warren, Christian. *Brush with Death: A Social History of Lead Poisoning*. New Haven, Conn.: Yale University Press, 2011.

Weaver, Timothy P. R. *Blazing the Neoliberal Trail: Urban Political Development in the United States and the United Kingdom*. Philadelphia: University of Pennsylvania Press, 2016.

Whisnant, David. *Modernizing the Mountaineer: People, Power, and Planning in Appalachia*. Rev. ed. Knoxville: University of Tennessee Press, 1994.

Wilkerson, Jessica. *To Live Here, You Have to Fight: How Women Led Appalachian Movements for Social Justice*. Urbana: University of Illinois Press, 2019.

Williams, Greer. *Western Reserve's Experiment in Medical Education and Its Outcome*. New York: Oxford University Press, 1980.

Williams, John Alexander. *Appalachia: A History*. Chapel Hill: University of North Carolina Press, 2001.

Winant, Gabriel. *The Next Shift: The Fall of Industry and the Rise of Health Care in Rust Belt America*. Cambridge, Mass.: Harvard University Press, 2021.

Yudell, Michael. *Race Unmasked: Biology and Race in the 20th Century*. New York: Columbia University Press.

Zelizer, Julian. *The Fierce Urgency of Now: Lyndon Johnson, Congress, and the Battle for the Great Society*. New York: Penguin, 2015.

Zipp, Samuel. *Manhattan Projects: The Rise and Fall of Urban Renewal in Cold War New York*. New York: Oxford University Press, 2010.

ARTICLES, CHAPTERS, THESES, AND DISSERTATIONS

Abel, Emily, Elizabeth Fee, and Theodore Brown. "Milton I. Roemer: Advocate of Social Medicine, International Health, and National Health Insurance." *American Journal of Public Health* 98, no. 9 (2008): 1596–97.

Alam, Eram. "Cold War Crises: Foreign Medical Graduates Respond to US Doctor Short-ages, 1965–1975." *Social History of Medicine* 33, no. 1 (2020): 132–51.

Allswang, John M. "Tom Bradley of Los Angeles." *Southern California Quarterly* 74, no. 1 (1992): 55–105.

Amrith, Sunil. "Political Culture of Health in India: A Historical Perspective." *Economic and Political Weekly* 42, no. 2 (2007): 114–21.

Anderson, Elmer A. "The Watts Health Miracle." *California Medicine* 115, no. 5 (1971): 65.

Aronowitz, Robert. "Lyme Disease: The Social Construction of a Disease and Its Social Consequences." In *Making Sense of Illness: Science, Society, and Disease*, 57–83. New York: Cambridge University Press, 1998.

Aub, Joseph C. "Comparison of Organic and Inorganic Lead Poisoning." In *Proceedings of the Third Day of the Fourth Air Pollution Medical Conference*, 52–61. Berkeley: California State Department of Health, 1960.

Barnes, David S. "The Rise or Fall of Tuberculosis in Belle-Epoque France: A Reply to Allan Mitchell." *Social History of Medicine* 5 (1992): 279–90.

Batzel, Robert J. "Health Care: What the Poor People Didn't Get from Kentucky Project." *Science* 172, no. 3982 (1971): 458–60.

Bayer, Ronald, David Merritt Johns, and Sandro Galea. "Salt and Public Health: Contested Science and the Challenge of Evidence-Based Decision Making." *Health Affairs* 31, no. 12 (2012): 2738–46.

Birn, Anne-Emanuelle. "Gates's Grandest Challenge: Transcending Technology as Public Health Ideology." *Lancet* 366, no. 9484 (2005): 514–19.

Birn, Anne-Emanuelle, Yogan Pillay, and Timothy H. Holtz. "Towards a Social Justice Approach to Global Health." In *Textbook of Global Health*, 4th ed., 603–45. New York: Oxford University Press, 2017.

Blackmar, Elizabeth. "Accountability for Public Health: Regulating the Housing Market in New York City." In *Hives of Sickness: Public Health and Epidemics in New York City*, edited by David Rosner, 42–64. New Brunswick, N.J.: Rutgers University Press, 1995.

Blauner, Robert. "Internal Colonialism and Ghetto Revolt." In *Racial Oppression in America*, 82–110. New York: Harper and Row, 1972.

Boone, Christopher G. "Zoning and Environmental Inequity in the Industrial East Side." In *Land of Sunshine: An Environmental History of Metropolitan Los Angeles*, edited by William Deverell and Greg Hise, 167–78. Pittsburgh: University of Pittsburgh Press, 2006.

Brandt, Allan M., and Martha Gardner. "Antagonism and Accommodation: Interpreting the Relationship between Public Health and Medicine in the United States during the 20th Century." *American Journal of Public Health* 90, no. 5 (2000): 711–12.

Brecher, Charles. "Historical Evolution of HHC." In *Public Hospital Systems in New York and Paris*, edited by Victor G. Rodwin, Charles Brecher, Dominique Jolly, and Raymond J. Baxter, 59–83. New York: New York University Press, 1992.

Breslow, Lester, and John Goldsmith. "Health Effects of Air Pollution." *American Journal of Public Health* 48, no. 7 (1958): 913–17.

Brown, Harold J., and Raymond S. Alexander. "The Gouverneur Ambulatory Care Unit: A New Approach to Ambulatory Care." *American Journal of Public Health* 54, no. 10 (1944): 1663.

Brown, Phil. "Popular Epidemiology Revisited." *Current Sociology* 45, no. 3 (1997): 137–56.

Brubaker, Rogers. "Ethnicity without Groups." In *Ethnicity without Groups*, 7–27. Cambridge, Mass.: Harvard University Press, 2004.

Campbell, John. "Working Relationships between Providers and Consumers in a Neighborhood Health Center." *American Journal of Public Health* 61, no. 1 (1971): 97–103.

Chowkwanyun, Merlin. "Biocitizenship on the Ground: Health Activism and the Medical Governance Revolution." In *Biocitizenship: The Politics of Bodies, Governance, and Power*, 178–99. New York: New York University Press, 2018.

———. "'The Neurosis That Has Possessed Us': Political Repression in the Cold War Medical Profession." *Journal of the History of Medicine and Allied Sciences* 73, no. 3 (2018): 255–73.

———. "The New Left and Public Health: The Health Policy Advisory Center, Community Organizing, and the Big Business of Health, 1967–1975." *American Journal of Public Health* 101, no. 2 (2011): 238–49.

Chowkwanyun, M., G. Markowitz, and D. Rosner. *Toxic Docs: Version 1.0* (database). New York: Columbia University and City University of New York, 2020. www.toxicdocs .org/d/jy5kvGqvo52w1x88MRDbZBkk5?lightbox=1.

Colgrove, James. "The McKeown Thesis: A Historical Controversy and Its Enduring Influence." *American Journal of Public Health* 92, no. 5 (2002): 725–29.

Committee on Health and Environmental Effects of Increased Coal Utilization. "Report on Health and Environmental Effects of Increased Coal Utilization." *Environmental Health Perspectives* 36 (November 1980): 135–53.

Currens, James C., and Gilbert E. Smith. "Coal Production in Kentucky, 1790–1975." *Kentucky Geological Survey Information Circular*, 10th ser., 23 (1977).

Curtin, Mike. "The O'Neill-DiSalle Years, 1957–1963." In *Ohio Politics*, edited by Alexander P. Lamis and Mary Anne Sharkey, 42–58. Kent, Ohio: Kent State University Press, 1958.

Curtis, Willie. "Effects of Strip Mining on the Hydrology of Small Mountain Watersheds in Appalachia." In *Ecology and Reclamation of Devastated Land: Proceedings of the International Symposium on Ecology and Revegetation of Drastically Disturbed Areas*, vol. 1, edited by R. J. Hutnik and G. Davis, 145–57. New York: Gordon and Breach, 1973.

———. "Strip-Mining Increases Flood Potential for Mountainsheds." *Proceedings of National Symposium on Watersheds in Transition*, 357–60. Urbana, Ill.: American Water Resources Association, 1972.

Cutler, David M., and Fiona Scott Morton. "Hospitals, Market Share, and Consolidation." *JAMA* 310, no. 18 (2013): 1964–70.

Cutler, David, Allison Rosen, and Sandeep Vijan. "The Value of Medical Spending in the United States, 1960–2000." *New England Journal of Medicine* 355, no. 9 (2006): 920–27.

Dasgupta, Aniruddha, and Victoria A. Beard. "Community Driven Development, Collective Action and Elite Capture in Indonesia." *Development and Change* 38 (2007): 229–49.

De Jong, Greta. "Plantation Politics: The Tufts-Delta Health Center and Intraracial Class Conflict in Misssissippi, 1965–1972." In *The War on Poverty: A New Grassroots History, 1964–1980*, edited by Annelise Orleck and Lisa Gayle Hazirjian, 256–79. Athens, GA: University of Georgia Press, 2011.

Eckhardt, E. F. "Economics of Large versus Small Haulage Units." *Mining Congress Journal* 47 (May 1961): 56–58.

Elmes, Gregory A., and Trevor M. Harris. "Industrial Restructuring and the United States Coal-Energy System, 1972–1990: Regulatory Change, Technological Fixes, and Corporate Control." *Annals of the Association of American Geographers* 86, no. 3 (1996): 507–29.

Epstein, Steven. "The Construction of Lay Expertise: AIDS Activism and the Forging of Credibility in the Reform of Clinical Trials." *Science, Technology, and Human Values* 20, no. 4 (1995): 408–37.

"E. Richard Weinerman, M.D." *American Journal of Public Health* 60, no. 5 (1970): 797–99.

Fairchild, Amy L., David Rosner, James Colgrove, Ronald Bayer, and Linda P. Fried. "The EXODUS of Public Health: What History Can Tell Us about the Future." *American Journal of Public Health* 100, no. 1 (2010): 54–63.

Farmer, Paul. "Making Human Rights Substantial." In *Partner to the Poor: A Paul Farmer Reader*, edited by Haun Saussy, 545–59. Berkeley: University of California Press, 2010.

Fuchs, Victor. "The Basic Forces Influencing Costs of Medical Care." In *Essays in the Economics of Health and Medical Care*, 39–50. New York: National Bureau of Economic Research/Columbia University Press, 1972.

Funke, Peter N. "Building Rhizomatic Social Movements? Movement-Building Relays during the Current Epoch of Contention." *Studies in Social Justice* 8, no. 1 (2014): 27–44.

Glasberg, Davita Silfen. "Bank Hegemony and Class Struggle in Cleveland, 1978–1979." In *Fire in the Hearth: The Radical Politics of Place in America*, edited by Mike Davis, Steven Hiatt, Marie Kennedy, Susan Ruddick, and Michael Sprinkler, 195–218. New York: Verso Books, 1990.

Goldsmith, John, and Lester Breslow. "Epidemiological Aspects of Air Pollution." *Journal of the Air Pollution Control Association* 9, no. 3 (1959): 129–32.

Gondi, Suhas, and Zirui Song. "Burgeoning Role of Venture Capital in Health Care." *Health Affairs* (blog), January 2, 2019. www.healthaffairs.org/do/10.1377/hblog20181218.956406/full/.

Gostin, Lawrence O. "*Jacobson v. Massachusetts* at 100 Years: Police Power and Civil Liberties in Tension." *American Journal of Public Health* 95, no. 4 (2005): 576–81.

Gottschalk, Marie. "The Elusive Goal of Universal Health Care: Organized Labor and the Institutional Straightjacket of the Private Welfare State." *Journal of Policy History* 11, no. 4 (1999): 367–98.

Green, Laurie B. "Saving Babies in Memphis: The Politics of Race, Health, and Hunger during the War on Poverty." In *The War on Poverty: A New Grassroots History, 1964–1980*, edited by Annelise Orleck and Lisa Gayle Hazirjian, 133–58. Athens: University of Georgia Press, 2011.

Gutiérrez, Ramón A. "Internal Colonialism: An American Theory of Race." *Du Bois Review* 1, no. 2 (2004): 281–95.

Haagen-Smit, A. J. "The Air Pollution Problem in Los Angeles." *Engineering and Science* 14 (December 1950): 7–13.

———. "Chemistry and Physiology of Los Angeles Smog." *Industrial and Engineering Chemistry* 44, no. 6 (1952): 1342–46.

———. "A Lesson from the Smog Capital of the World." *Proceedings from the National Academy of Sciences of the United States of America* 67, no. 2 (1970): 887–97.

Haagen-Smit, A. J., Ellis F. Darley, Milton Zaitlin, Herbert Hull, and Wilfred Noble. "Investigation on Injury to Plants from Air Pollution in the Los Angeles Area." *Plant Physiology* 27, no. 1 (1952): 18–19.

Hendricks, Rickey. "Medical Practice Embattled: Kaiser Permanente, the American Medical Association, and Henry J. Kaiser on the West Coast, 1945–1955." *Pacific Historical Review* 60, no. 4 (1991): 439–73.

Hershman, Ellyn Adrienne. "California Legislation on Air Contaminant Emissions from Stationary Sources." *California Law Review* 58, no. 6 (1970): 1474–98.

Hoffman, Beatrix. "Emergency Rooms: The Reluctant Safety Net." In *History and Health Policy in the United States: Putting the Past Back*, edited by Rosemary A. Stevens, Charles E. Rosenberg, and Lawton R. Burns, 250–72. New Brunswick, N.J.: Rutgers University Press, 2006.

Hufford, Harry Lee. "City-County Health Department Mergers in Los Angeles County, July 1, 1964: A Case Study." MSc thesis, University of Southern California, 1966.

Humphreys, Margaret. "How Four Once Common Diseases Were Eliminated from the American South." *Health Affairs* 28, no. 6 (2009): 1734–44.

Hunt, Darnell, and Ana-Christina Ramón. "Killing 'Killer King': The *Los Angeles Times* and a 'Troubled' Hospital in the 'Hood.'" In *Black Los Angeles: American Dreams and Racial Realities*, edited by Darnell Hunt and Ana-Christina Ramón, 283–320. New York: New York University Press, 2010.

Juravich, Nick. "'Harlem Sophistication': Community-Based Paraprofessional Educators in Harlem and East Harlem." In *Harlem: A Century of Schooling and Resistance in a Black Community*, edited by Ansley T. Erickson and Ernest Morrell, 234–56. New York: Columbia University Press, 2020.

Katznelson, Ira. *City Trenches: Urban Politics and the Patterning of Class in the United States.* Chicago: University of Chicago Press, 1981.

Kaufman, Brystana G., et al. "Half of Rural Residents at High Risk of Serious Illness due to COVID-19, Creating Stress on Rural Hospital." *Journal of Rural Health* 36, no. 4 (2020): 584–90.

Kennedy, Howard W. "Legislative and Regulatory Action in Air Pollution Control." *Public Health Reports* 78, no. 9 (1963): 799–806.

Kenny, Michael G. "A Question of Blood, Race, and Politics." *Journal of the History of Medicine and Allied Sciences* 61, no. 4 (2006).

Kindig, David. "Understanding Population Health Terminology." *Milbank Quarterly* 85, no. 1 (2007): 139–61.

Kindig, David, and Greg Stoddart. "What Is Population Health?" *American Journal of Public Health* 93, no. 3 (2003): 380–93.

Kotin, Paul. "The Role of Atmospheric Pollution in the Pathogenesis of Pulmonary Cancer: A Review." *Cancer Research* 16, no. 5 (1956): 375–93.

Kotin, Paul, Hans L. Falk, Paul Mader, and Marilyn Thomas. "Aromatic Hydrocarbons: I. Presence in the Los Angeles Atmosphere and the Carcinogenicity of Atmospheric Extracts." *A.M.A. Archives of Industrial Hygiene and Occupational Medicine* 9, no. 2 (1954): 154–63.

Kotin, Paul, Hans L. Falk, and Marilyn Thomas. "Aromatic Hydrocarbons: II. Presence in the Particulate Phase of Gasoline-Engine Exhausts and the Carcinogenicity of Exhaust Extracts." *A.M.A. Archives of Industrial Hygiene and Occupational Medicine* 9, no. 2 (1954): 164–77.

————. "Aromatic Hydrocarbons: III. Presence in the Particulate Phase of Diesel-Engine Exhausts and the Carcinogenicity of Exhaust Extracts." *A.M.A. Archives of Industrial Hygiene and Occupational Medicine* 11, no. 2 (1955): 113–20.

Kotin, Paul, and W. C. Hueper. "Relationship of Industrial Carcinogens to Cancer in the General Population." *Public Health Reports* 70, no. 3 (1955): 331–33.

Krieger, Nancy. "Does Racism Harm Health? Did Child Abuse Exist before 1962? On Explicit Questions, Critical Science, and Current Controversies: An Ecosocial Perspective." *American Journal of Public Health* 93, no. 2 (2003): 194–99.

Landrigan, Philip, Richard Fuller, Nereus J. R. Acosta, Olusoji Adeyu, Robert Arnold, Niladri Basu, Abdoulaye Bibi Baldé, et al. "The *Lancet* Commission on Pollution and Health." *Lancet* 391, no. 10119 (2017): 462–512.

Lapidos, Adrienne, Jeremy Lapedis, and Michelle Heisler. "Realizing the Value of Community Health Workers—New Opportunities for Sustainable Financing." *New England Journal of Medicine* 380, no. 21 (2019): 1990–92.

Lear, Linda. "Rachel Carson's 'Silent Spring.'" *Environmental History Review* 17, no. 2 (1993): 23–48.

Levidow, Les. "Precautionary Uncertainty: Regulating GM Crops in Europe." *Social Studies of Science* 31, no. 5 (2001): 842–74.

Lewis, David G. "Application of Contour Stripping Techniques." *Mining Congress Journal* 51 (March 1965): 59–64.

Lichtenstein, Nelson. "From Corporatism to Collective Bargaining: The Eclipse of Social Democracy." In *The Rise and Fall of the New Deal Order, 1930–1980*, edited by Steve Fraser and Gary Gerstle, 122–52. Princeton, N.J.: Princeton University Press, 1989.

Light, Harold L., and Harold J. Brown. "The Gouverneur Health Services Program: A Historical View." *Milbank Memorial Quarterly* 45, no. 4 (1967): 375–90.

Link, Bruce, and Jo Phelan. "McKeown and the Idea That Social Conditions Are Fundamental Causes of Disease." *American Journal of Public Health* 92, no. 5 (2002): 730–32.

Lipsky, Michael, and Morris Lounds. "Citizen Participation and Health Care: Problems of Government Induced Participation." *Journal of Health Politics, Policy and Law* 1, no. 1 (1976): 85–111.

Lopez, Russ. "Public Health, the APHA, and Urban Renewal." *American Journal of Public Health* 99, no. 9 (2009): 1603–11.

Lyu, Wei, and George Wehby. "Comparison of Estimated Rates of Coronavirus Disease 2019 (COVID-19) in Border Counties in Iowa without a Stay-at-Home Order and Border Counties in Illinois with a Stay-at-Home Order." *JAMA Network Open* 3, no. 2 (2020): e2011102.

Mader, Paul, Joseph Gliksman, Marcel Eye, and Leslie A. Chambers. "Photochemical Formation of Air Contaminants from Automobile Exhaust Vapors. Effects of Different Motor Fuels." *Industrial and Engineering Chemistry* 50, no. 8 (1958): 1173–74.

Mader, Paul, Merlyn Heddon, Marcel Eye, and Walter Hamming. "Effects of Present-Day Fuels on Air Pollution." *Industrial and Engineering Chemistry* 48, no. 9 (1956): 1508–11.

Manifest, August. "Moving Overburden with Explosives." *Mining Congress Journal* 46 (April 1960): 64–65.

Markel, Howard, Harvey Lipman, J. Alexander Navarro, Alexandra Sloan, Joseph R. Michalsen, Alexandra Minna Stern, and Martin S. Cetron. "Nonpharmaceutical Interventions Implemented by US Cities during the 1918–1919 Influenza Pandemic." *JAMA* 298, no. 6 (2007): 644–54.

Mayeux, Sara, and Karen Tani. "Federalism Anew." *American Journal of Legal History* 56, no. 1 (2016): 128–38.

"A Mechanization Study." *United Mine Workers Journal*, February 1, 1962.

"Medical Empires: Who Controls?" *Health/PAC Bulletin*, November–December 1968.

Menzel, Donald C. "Redirecting the Implementation of a Law: The Reagan Administration and Coal Surface Mining Regulation." *Public Administration Review* 43, no. 5 (1983): 411–20.

Menzel, Donald C., and Terry D. Edgmon. "The Struggle to Implement a National Surface Mining Policy." *Publius* 10, no. 1 (1980): 81–91.

Mills, Clarence A. "Air Pollution and Community Health." *American Journal of the Medical Sciences* 224, no. 4 (1952): 403–7.

Mitchell, Allan. "An Inexact Science: The Statistics of Tuberculosis in Late 19th-Century France." *Social History of Medicine* 3, no. 3 (1990): 387–403.

———. "Tuberculosis Statistics and the McKeown Thesis: A Rebuttal to David Barnes." *Social History of Medicine* 5, no. 2 (1992): 291–96.

Montrie, Chad. "Expedient Environmentalism: Opposition to Coal Surface Mining in Appalachia and the United Mine Workers of America, 1945–1977." *Environmental History* 5, no. 1 (2000): 75–98.

Nyden, Paul. "Rank-and-File Movements in the United Mine Workers of America, Early 1960s–Early 1980s." In *Rebel Rank and File: Labor Militancy and Revolt from Below during the Long 1970s*, edited by Aaron Brenner, Robert Brenner, and Cal Winslow, 173–97. New York: Verso Books, 2010.

Oltman, Adele. "Liberalism and the Crisis of Health Care in Harlem in the 1960s." *Social History of Medicine* 29, no. 1 (2015): 44–65.

Osman, Suleiman. "'We're Doing It Ourselves': The Unexpected Origins of New York City's Public-Private Parks during the 1970s Fiscal Crisis." *Journal of Planning History* 16, no. 2 (2017): 162–74.

Patel, Sejal. "The Eclipse of the Community Study: The Roseto Study in Historical Context." PhD diss., University of Pennsylvania, 2007.

Paul, Rajib, et al. "Progression of COVID-19 from Urban to Rural Areas in the United States: A Spatiotemporal Analysis of Prevalence Rates." *Journal of Rural Health* 36, no. 4 (2020): 591–601.

Phelan, Jo, Bruce Link, Ana Diez-Roux, Ichiro Kawachi, and Bruce Levin. "'Fundamental Causes' of Social Inequalities in Mortality: A Test of the Theory." *Journal of Health and Social Behavior* 45, no. 3 (2004): 265–85.

Platteau, Jean-Phillippe. "Monitoring Elite Capture in Community-Driven Development." *Development and Change* 35, no. 2 (2004): 223–46.

Platteau, Jean-Phillippe, and Anita Abraham. "Participatory Development in the Presence of Endogenous Community Imperfections." *Journal of Development Studies* 39, no. 2 (2002): 104–36.

Powell, Rodney. "What Has Happened in the Watts-Willowbrook Program." In *Medicine in the Ghetto*, edited by John C. Norman, 73–85. New York: Appleton-Century-Crofts, 1969.

Reed, Adolph, Jr. "The Curse of Community." In *Class Notes: Posing as Politics and Other Thoughts on the American Scene*. New York: New Press, 2000.

———. "Sources of De-Mobilization in the New Black Political Regime: Incorporation, Ideological Capitulation, and Radical Failure in the Post-Segregation Era." In *Stirrings in the Jug: Black Politics in the Post-Segregation Era*, 117–59. Minneapolis: University of Minnesota Press, 1999.

"Ripping Burden: The Economic Approach." *Coal Age*, July 1965.

Rodriguez-Trias, Helen. "The Medical Staff and the Hospital." *Bulletin of the New York Academy of Medicine* 48, no. 11 (1972): 1423–27.

Rosen, Christine Meisner. "'Knowing' Industrial Pollution: Nuisance Law and the Power of Tradition in a Time of Rapid Economic Change, 1840–1865." *Environmental History* 8, no. 4 (2003): 565–97.

Ross, Steven J. "How Hollywood Became Hollywood: Money, Politics, and Movies." In *Metropolis in the Making: Los Angeles in the 1920s*, edited by Tom Sitton and William Deverell, 255–76. Berkeley: University of California Press, 2001.

Roy, Aruna, and Saba Kohli Davé. "When People and Governments Come Together: Analysing Kerala's Response to the COVID-19 Pandemic." *Economic and Political Weekly*, May 2, 2020.

Rumfelt, Henry. "Recent Developments in Surface Mining." *Mining Congress Journal* 51 (September 1965): 77–98.

Schlesinger, Mark. "Paradigms Lost: The Persisting Search for Community in U.S. Health Policy." *Journal of Health Politics, Policy and Law* 22, no. 4 (1997): 937–92.

Sheeran, Patrick, and David Wilson. "*Akers v. Baldwin*: The Broad Form Deed Dilemma Revisited." *Journal of Mineral Law and Policy* 4, no. 1 (1988): 213–34.

Shermer, Elizabeth Tandy. "'Is Freedom of the Individual Un-American?' Right-to-Work Campaigns and Anti-Union Conservatism, 1943–1958." In *The Right and Labor in America: Politics, Ideology, and Imagination*, edited by Nelson Lichtestein and Shermer, 114–36. Philadelphia: University of Pennsylvania Press, 2012.

Shonick, William, and Walter Price. "Reorganizations of Health Agencies by Local Government in American Urban Centers: What Do They Portend for 'Public Health'?" *Milbank Memorial Fund Quarterly: Health and Society* 55, no. 2 (1977): 233–71.

Siegel, Beth, Jane Erickson, Bobby Milstein, and Katy Evans Pritchard. "Multisector Partnerships Need Further Development to Fulfill Aspirations for Transforming Regional Health and Well-Being." *Health Affairs* 37, no. 1 (2018): 30–37.

Singh, Prabhjot, and Dave A. Chokshi. "Community Health Workers—A Local Solution to a Global Problem." *New England Journal of Medicine* 369, no. 10 (2013): 894–96.

Smith, Nathan, Peter Rogatz, and Martin Cherkasky. "The Case for Voluntary and Municipal Hospital Affiliation." *American Journal of Public Health* 52, no. 12 (1963): 1989.

Smith, R. Jeffrey. "Watt Carves Up Strip-Mining Policy." *Science* 212, no. 4496 (1981): 759–60, 762.

Snyder, Lynne Page. "'The Death-Dealing Smog over Donora, Pennsylvania': Industrial Air Pollution, Public Health Policy, and the Politics of Expertise, 1948–1949." *Environmental History Review* 18, no. 1 (1994): 117–39.

Souch, Jacob M., and Jeralynn S. Cossman. "A Commentary on Rural-Urban Disparities in COVID-19 Testing Rates per 100,000 and Risk Factors." *Journal of Rural Health* 37, no. 1 (2021): 188–90.

Starr, Paul. "Rebounding with Medicare: Reform and Counterreform in American Health Policy." *Journal of Health Politics, Policy and Law* 43, no. 4 (2018): 707–30.

Sugrue, Thomas. "All Politics Is Local." In *The Democratic Experiment: New Directions in American Political History*, edited by Meg Jacobs, William J. Novak, and Julian E. Zelizer, 301–26. Princeton, N.J.: Princeton University Press, 2003.

———. "Crabgrass-Roots Politics: Race, Rights, and the Reaction against Liberalism in the Urban North, 1940–1964." *Journal of American History* 82, no. 2 (1995): 551–78.

Steinman, David. "Development of a Rural Demonstration Practice." *Journal of the Kentucky Medical Association* 70, no. 1 (1972): 28–33.

Szreter, Simon. "The Importance of Social Intervention in Britain's Mortality Decline, c. 1850–1914: A Re-Interpretation of the Role of Public Health." *Social History of Medicine* 1, no. 1 (1988): 1–38.

———. "Rethinking McKeown: The Relationship between Public Health and Social Change." *American Journal of Public Health* 92, no. 5 (2002): 722–25.

Tapp, Jesse W., Rena Gazaway, and Kurt Deuschle. "Community Health in a Mountain Neighborhood." *Archives of Environmental Health* 8 (April 1964): 516–17.

Taylor, Clarence. "Race, Rights, Empowerment." In *Summer in the City: John Lindsay, New York, and the American Dream*, edited by Joseph P. Viteritti, 61–78. Baltimore: Johns Hopkins University Press, 2014.

Thomas, A. James, and R. L. Peterson. "City-County Health Department Mergers." *Public Health Reports* 77, no. 4 (1962): 341–48.

Thorsheim, Peter. "Interpreting the London Fog Disaster of 1952." In *Smoke and Mirrors: The Politics and Culture of Air Pollution*, edited by E. Melanie DuPuis, 154–69. New York: New York University Press, 2004.

Tobbell, Dominique. "Plow, Town, and Gown: The Politics of Family Practice in 1960s America." *Bulletin of the History of Medicine* 87, no. 4 (2013): 648–80.

Tranquada, Robert. "Participation of the Poverty Community in Health Planning." *Social Science and Medicine* 7, no. 9 (1973): 719–28.

Trussell, Ray. "The Municipal Hospital System in Transition." *Bulletin of the New York Academy of Medicine* 38, no. 4 (1962): 221–36.

Tuchman, Lester. "Immediate and Long-Range Problems in the Municipal Hospitals of New York City." *Bulletin of the New York Academy of Medicine* 37, no. 8 (1961): 537–41.

Vayda, Eugene. "Changing Patterns of Medical Care." *Bulletin of the Academy of Medicine of Cleveland* 50, no. 6 (1965): 10–12.

Wainess, Flint J. "The Ways and Means of National Health Care Reform, 1974 and Beyond." *Journal of Health Politics, Policy and Law* 24, no. 2 (1991): 305–33.

Warner, John Harley. "Grand Narrative and Its Discontents: Medical History and the Social Transformation of American Medicine." *Journal of Health Politics, Policy and Law* 29, no. 4–5 (2004): 757–80.

Wheeler, Mary P. "Health Education in the Interagency Approach to Urban Renewal." *American Journal of Public Health* 53, no. 1 (1963): 63–66.

"Why Perkins Voted No." *Kentucky Coal Journal* 3, no. 8 (1977): 1.

Williams, David R., and Chiquita Collins. "US Socioeconomic and Racial Differences in Health: Patterns and Explanations." *Annual Review of Sociology* 21 (1995): 349–86.

Wilson, J. H. "Auger Mining: Productivity Powers Growth." *Coal Age* (November 1966): 56–62.

Withrow, Michael V. "Broad-Form Deed: Obstacle to Peaceful Co-Existence between Mineral and Surface Owners." *Kentucky Law Journal* 60, no. 3 (1972): 742–56.

## PUBLISHED REPORTS AND HEARINGS

*The Acceptable Replacement of Imported Oil with Coal: The Staff Report to the President's Commission on Coal.* Washington, D.C.: United States Government Printing Office, 1980.

*Air Quality Criteria for Sulfur Oxides.* Washington, D.C.: United States Government Printing Office, 1969.

Averitt, Paul. *Coal Reserves of the United States—A Progress Report.* Washington, D.C.: United States Government Printing Office, 1961.

Boccary, Joseph A., and Willard M. Spaulding Jr. *Effects of Surface Mining on Fish and Wildlife in Appalachia.* Washington, D.C.: United States Government Printing Office, 1968.

*Bureau of Mines Minerals Yearbook: The Mineral Industry of Kentucky.* Washington, D.C.: United States Government Printing Office, 1972.

California Governor's Commission on the Los Angeles Riots. *Violence in the City: An End or a Beginning? A Report* (1965).

Collier, C. R., R. J. Pickering, and J. J. Musser, eds. *Influences of Strip Mining on the Hydrologic Environment of Parts of Beaver Creek Basin, Kentucky, 1955–1966.* Washington, D.C.: United States Government Printing Office, 1970.

Committee on Disposal of Excess Spoil, Board on Mineral and Energy Resources, Commission on Natural Resources. *Disposal of Excess Spoil from Coal Mining and the Surface Mining Control and Reclamation Act of 1977: A Study of Regulatory Requirements, Engineering*

*Practices, and Environmental Protection Objectives.* Washington, D.C.: National Academies Press, 1981.

*The Comprehensive Neighborhood Health Services Program, Guidelines.* Washington, D.C.: Office of Economic Opportunity, 1968.

Curtis, Willie. "Surface Mining and the Flood of 1977." *USDA Forest Service Research Note* (1977).

Danielson, John A. *Air Pollution Engineering Manual: Air Pollution Control District of Los Angeles.* Research Triangle Park, N.C.: Environmental Protection Agency, 1973.

*Federal Role in Urban Affairs: Hearings before the Subcommittee on Executive Reorganization of the Committee on Government Operations, United States Senate, Eighty-Ninth Congress, Second Session, Part 4.* Washington, D.C.: U.S. Government Printing Office, 1966.

*First Technical Progress Report Covering Work Done in 1954.* Los Angeles: Air Pollution Foundation, 1955.

*Health Consequences of Sulfur Oxides: A Report from CHESS, 1970–1971.* Research Triangle Park, N.C.: Environmental Protection Agency, 1974.

*Health Goals Model for Greater Cleveland: Cleveland Health Goals Project Reports.* Vols. 1, 3. Cleveland, Ohio: Welfare Foundation of Cleveland, 1966.

*Health in All Policies: Experiences from Local Health Departments.* Washington, D.C.: National Association of County and City Health Officials, 2017.

Johnson, Lyndon B. Annual message to Congress on the State of the Union (speech, Washington, D.C., January 8, 1964). University of California, Santa Barbara, American Presidency Project, www.presidency.ucsb.edu/documents/annual -message-the-congress-the-state-the-union-25.

Morgan, Mark L., and Edwin A. Moss. *Citizens' Blasting Handbook.* Corbin, Ky.: Appalachia— Science in the Public Interest, 1978.

*Oversight on Financially Distressed Hospitals: Hearing before the Subcommittee on Health and Scientific Research of the Committee on Labor and Human Resources.* Washington, D.C.: U.S. Government Printing Office, 1980.

*Patterns and Trends in Federal Coal Lease Ownership, 1950–1980.* Washington, D.C.: United States Government Printing Office, 1981.

*Plan and Policies for Future Development of Western Reserve University School of Medicine and University Hospitals of Cleveland.* Cleveland, Ohio: Committee on Plans and Development, 1954.

*The President's Commission on Coal: Recommendations and Summary Findings.* Washington, D.C.: United States Government Printing Office, 1980.

"Principal Mergers and Acquisitions in the Coal Industry, 1963–1975." In *Mergers and Economic Concentration: Hearings before the Subcommittee on Antitrust, Monopoly and Business Rights.* Washington, D.C.: United States Government Printing Office, 1979.

*Proceedings of the Second Southern California Conference on Elimination of Air Pollution, Ambassador Hotel, Los Angeles, November 14, 1956: Twelve Months' Progress—and the Year Ahead.* California State Chamber of Commerce, 1956.

Reed, Thomas H., and Doris H. Reed. *The Organization of the Cleveland City Hospital: A Report to the Cleveland Bureau of Governmental Research.* New York: National Municipal League, 1949.

*Report of the Blue Ribbon Panel to Governor Nelson A. Rockefeller on Municipal Hospitals of New York City.* Albany: New York State Department of Health, 1967.

*Report of the Health Advisory Committee to the Appalachian Regional Commission.* Washington, D.C.: Appalachian Regional Commission, 1966.

"Research Bulletin No. 1." *Appalachian Outlook* 1, no. 1 (1968).

Roemer, Milton. "Health Services in the Los Angeles Riot Area." In *Transcripts, Depositions, Consultants' Reports, and Selected Documents of the Governor's Commission on the Los Angeles Riots* [microfilm]. California: Governor's Commission on the Los Angeles Riots, 1966.

Sawicki, Carole R. *Seminar Summary: Sampling and Analysis of the Various Forms of Atmospheric Lead*. Research Triangle, N.C.: United States Environmental Protection Agency, 1975.

Schliessmann, D. J., F. O. Atchley, M. J. Wilcomb Jr., and S. F. Welch. "Relationship of Environmental Factors to Enteric Diseases in Areas of Eastern Kentucky." *Public Health Monograph No. 54*. Washington, D.C.: United States Government Printing Office, 1958.

State of New York Commission of Investigation. *Recommendations of the New York State Commission of Investigation concerning New York City's Municipal Hospitals and the Affiliation Program*. New York: Community Council of Greater New York, 1968.

*Strip Mining and the Flooding in Appalachia: Hearing before a Subcommittee of the Committee on Government Operations*. Washington, D.C.: United States Government Printing Office, 1977.

*A Study of Community Health Services in Cleveland and Cuyahoga County, Ohio: Report of Study Team to Public Health Study Group of Cleveland Metropolitan Services Commission*. Cleveland, Ohio: Cleveland Metropolitan Services Corporation [METRO], 1957.

*Study of Strip and Surface Mining in Appalachia: An Interim Report*. Washington, D.C.: United States Government Printing Office, 1966.

*Surface Mining and the Environment: A Special Report to the Nation*. Washington, D.C.: United States Government Printing Office, 1967.

Traffic Survey Committee. *Street Traffic Management for Los Angeles: Appraisal and Recommendations Prepared for the City of Los Angeles*. Los Angeles: Traffic Survey Committee, 1948.

*Transportation in the Los Angeles Area*. Los Angeles: Citizens Traffic and Transportation Committee for the Extended Los Angeles Area, 1957.

Trussell, Ray, and Frank Van Dyke. *Prepayment for Hospital Care in New York State: A Report on the Eight Blue Cross Plans Serving New York Residents*. New York: School of Public Health and Administrative Medicine, Columbia University, 1961.

U.S. Census Bureau. *Census of Population: 1950*. Vol. 2, *Characteristics of the Population, Part 35, Ohio*. Washington, D.C.: U.S. Government Printing Office, 1952.

U.S. Census Bureau. *Census of Population: 1960*. Vol. 1, *Characteristics of the Population, Part 37, Ohio*. Washington, D.C.: U.S. Government Printing Office, 1961.

Viseltear, Arthur, Arnold I. Kisch, and Milton Roemer. *The Watts Hospital: A Health Facility Is Planned for a Metropolitan Slum Area*. Arlington, Va.: United States Department of Health, Education, and Welfare, 1967.

# Index

Ackerman, Laura, 44
affiliation between public facilities and
    voluntary hospitals: and ad hoc nature
    in Los Angeles, 97–98; in Cleveland,
    142; early deliberations about in
    New York City, 15–19; and eventual
    entrenchment in New York City, 51–56;
    high-profile critiques of, 31–37; protest
    against, 22–28, 116–19, 134–35
air pollution, 58–95
Air Pollution Control District
    (Los Angeles), 65–66, 73–75, 78–79,
    83–86
Alinsky, Saul, 1, 39. *See also* Industrial Areas
    Foundation
Allen, Quentin, 219, 222
Allen, Wayne, 98
Amazon, 227
American Smelting and Refining
    Company, 65–66
APCD. *See* Air Pollution Control District
Appalachian Regional Commission, 193,
    199, 203, 205, 223–24
Appalachian Regional Hospitals (ARH),
    205, 222
Appalachian Volunteers, 206, 219
ASPI (Appalachia: Science in the Public
    Interest), 189–90
Aub, Joseph, 92–93
austerity, 47–57, 136–38, 161
automobiles: and challenges in regulation
    of, 83–86, 89–90; and contribution to
    smog, 71–78 passim

Ban Ki-moon, 229
Bates, Jim, 112–18
Beckman, Arnold O., 78
Beefhyde Hollow (Ky.), 177–78
Bell County (Ky.), 174
Bellevue Hospital, 19, 29, 53
Bellin, Lowell, 51–52
Berkshire Hathaway, 227
Beth Israel Medical Center, 30, 40–46
    passim
Bethlehem Steel, 61, 74–75
Big Sandy Community Action Program,
    211–15 passim
Big Sandy Health Care, Inc., 219
Black Grassroots Caucus (Los Angeles),
    134–35
Black nationalism, 108, 114
Black Panthers, 41
Black physicians, 104, 107
"blight," 155
bonds, 49–50, 100, 108–10, 132, 161, 168–69
Bottoms, Keisha Lance, 232
Bowron, Fletcher, 62
Boyle, Tony, 205
Breathitt County (Ky.), 186
Breslow, Lester, 86, 88–89. *See also*
    Goldsmith, John
broad form deed, 177
Bronx, 22–26, 49, 55
Brooklyn, 49, 55–56
Brooklyn Hospital, 55
Brown, Edmund, 131
Brown, Howard J., 30–31, 144

budgets, 18, 47–57, 136–38, 161

Buffalo Creek mining disaster (W.Va.), 188, 195

Bullock, Sandra, 58

bureaucracy, 35–48, 113–16, 119–23, 217–18

Burlage, Robb, 34–35. *See also* Health Policy Advisory Center; Rubin, Samuel

Byrd, Robert, 191

California, 58–139: and adoption of lead standard, 93; and committee on air pollution, 78–79, 83–84; and formation of statewide air pollution control agency, 94–95

California Air Resources Board, 94

California Institute of Technology, 75–78, 83–84, 91

Caltech (California Institute of Technology), 75–78, 83–84, 91

CAP. *See* Community Action Program

CARB (California Air Resources Board), 94

cartography: arguments made with, 102–4, 203

Case Western Reserve University, 140

Caudill, Harry, 197

Cedars of Lebanon Hospital, 100, 112

Cedars-Sinai Medical Center, 100, 112

Celebrezze, Anthony, 142

Central Appalachia, 173–225; definition of, 174; demands for medical care in, 205; early studies of medical care in, 203

Chambers, Leslie, 157

Charles R. Drew Medical Society, 116–19

Charles R. Drew Postgraduate School of Medicine, 132, 135–36

Cherkasky, Martin, 17, 19, 24–25, 52, 55

Citizens Committee on Air Pollution (Los Angeles), 84

city-county relations: in Los Angeles, 61–63, 99, in Cleveland, 141–43, 168–71.

City Hospital (Cleveland). *See* Metropolitan General Hospital

City Hospital at Elmhurst (New York), 19, 26–28, 31, 162

civil rights, 8, 101

Clay County (Ky.), 174, 206

Clean Air Act, 12, 94, 200

Cleveland, 140–72; East Side landscape of, 140; fiscal crisis of 1978's impact on, 161; history of civil rights activism in, 151; Hough riot in, 150–51; population change in, 168; racial politics of, 155–57; and strong organized labor traditions of, 144

Cleveland Clinic, 140, 152–63

*Cleveland Now!*, 157

climate change, 228; and local politics, 229–30

Clover Fork Clinic, 207

coal, 173–201

coal industry: hegemony of, 190–201; public relations efforts of, 191–95; and relationship to larger growth imperatives, 198–201; and role in energy independence imperatives, 198–99

colonialism, as analogy for public hospitals and private academic medical centers, 34–35

Columbia University, 20–22, 51

Commission on California State Government Organization and Economy, 127

Committee on Interns and Residents, 16

Community Action Program, 38, 113, 211. *See also* lay participation in medicine; maximum feasible participation

community health: attempts to implement localist vision of, 30–31, 38–40, 111–25, 144–50, 164–66, 207, 218–20; as defense of sanctified goods or commons, 22–28, 178; different conceptions of, 6–7; as means of democratizing medicine, 38–48, 113–16, 119–23, 207; as rooted in circumscribed populations, 113–16, 119–23, 136, 144–50; universalist rhetoric of, 12, 57, 64, 66, 72, 85, 109–10. *See also* localism

Community Health Council (Watts), 113–16, 119–23

Community Health Foundation (Cleveland), 144–50, 167

community health workers, 31, 39–41, 111–18, 163–66, 221, 228–29

Community Medical Foundation (Los Angeles), 103–4, 144

community organizing, 1–2, 38–40, 112–18, 164–67, 208–25 passim
Compton, Earl, 211
Congress of Racial Equality (Cleveland), 151
consolidation: in contemporary health care landscape, 227–28; of public hospitals in Cuyahoga County, 168–71; of public hospitals in New York City via affiliation, 15–19, 51–56
Cooper, John Sherman, 181, 188
Cooper, Leon, 214
County General Hospital (Los Angeles), 97–98, 100, 109, 125–26, 128–31, 133
County-USC Medical Center (Los Angeles). *See* County General Hospital (Los Angeles)
Covid-19, 230–34; and variation in local-level responses, 232–34; and variation in state-level responses, 231–32
Craggett, Daisy, 151
Culture of Health, 228
Cumberland Hospital (New York), 55
Curtis, Willie, 186–90
Cuyahoga County (Ohio), 142–43, 159, 162, 168–71
Cruz, Gloria, 41–43. *See also* Health Revolutionary Unity Movement

Daugherty, R. L., 75, 83–84, 91
decentralization, 9; and core structure of OEO neighborhood health centers program, 28–31, 38–47, 111–25, 207–18; Cuyahoga County plans for, 159; Los Angeles County discussions about, 131
deep (underground) mining: decline of, 174, 188
DeSantis, Ron, 232
Deukmejian, George, 138
Deutsch, I. A., 58–59, 63
DeValasco, Gustavo, 55
*Dilemmas of Social Reform* (Marris and Rein), 3–4
District Council 37 (New York), 54
Downstate Medical School, 56
Drew, Charles, 116
Dummett, Clifton, 121

Eastern Kentucky Welfare Rights Organization, 184, 202, 208–25 passim
Edelman, Edmund, 136
Egeberg, Roger, 100, 112
Eisenhower, Dwight, 95
EKWRO (Eastern Kentucky Welfare Rights Organization), 184, 202, 208–25 passim
Elmhurst, 26–28, 31
Emergency Financial Control Board (New York), 50–51
energy independence, 197–99
English, Joseph, 45, 49, 120
environmental health activism, 59–61, 72–73, 79–82, 93, 177–90, 230
Environmental Protection Agency, 59, 94
Ervin, Frank, 135
Evarts (Ky.), 207

Fairfax, 158–59
Fairfax Foundation, 160
federalism, 9; and distribution of OEO health program funds, 40–46, 111–25, 217–18; and impact on Medicaid reliability, 48, 126–28, 224
Federation for Community Planning (Cleveland), 171
fiscal crisis: and 1978 impact on Cleveland, 161; and 1975 impact on New York City, 47–57
flooding, 186–88
Florence-Firestone, 109
Flower Fifth Avenue Hospital, 33
Floyd County (Ky.), 175, 182, 202–25; and political machines in, 207–8
Floyd County Comprehensive Health Program, 207–18; and structure of, 208, 210
Ford, Gerald, 48, 50, 199
Ford, John Anson, 62–63, 79–80, 100
Fordham Hospital, 18, 22–26, 31, 55
foreign medical graduates, 16, 20, 23
Frankel, John, 119
freeways, 94
Fritchman, Stephen H., 104
Frontier Nursing Service, 223
Future Outlook League, 151

Gans, Herbert J., 27
Garcetti, Eric, 230
Gilbert, Roy, 103
Giorgi, Elsie, 112–20 passim
Glenville (Cleveland), 155, 157
Golden State Medical Society, 107
Goldsmith, John, 86. *See also* Breslow, Lester
Goodrich (Cleveland), 164
Gouverneur Health Services Program, 18, 28–31, 38–47, 55
governance, 11–12; Gouverneur Health Services Program battles about, 38–47; Martin Luther King, Jr. Hospital battles about, 132, 134–36; and relative absence of rancor about in Cleveland; Watts health center battles about, 111–23
grassroots health activism: 22–31, 38–47, 59–61, 72–73, 79–82, 93, 111–25, 134–35, 177–90
Graves, Joseph, 132
Greater Cleveland Growth Association, 149, 161
Great Migration, 101
Great Society, 6, 38
Greene, Callie, 134–35
Green New Deal, 230
Greenpoint Hospital (New York), 32–33, 55
Griswold, Smith, 90
growth liberalism, 197–201

Haagen-Smit, Arie, 75–78, 84, 86, 94
Hahn, Kenneth, 75, 90, 104, 108–11
Hall, Eula, 209, 214–16, 218–20, 222, 224
Hall, Russell D., 209–10
Hamilton, James, 99; warning about racial exclusion, 101
Harbor General Hospital, 98, 126
Harlan County (Ky.), 173, 189
Harlan County Emergency and Rescue Squad, 184
Harlem Hospital, 19, 20–22, 54
Harrington, Michael, 197
Hawkins, Augustus, 115, 119–20
Hayes, Frank, 136
Haynes, Alfred, M., 135–36
Health and Hospitals Corporations, 45–46, 47–51, 120

health care consolidation, 227–28
health care costs, 11, 144
health care crisis: three notions of, 10–12. *See also* governance; medical maldistribution; sustainability
health care teams, 147–48, 162
Health in All Policies, 228
Health Insurance Plan of New York, 30
health maintenance, 147–48
health maintenance organization, 137, 288n121
Health Policy Advisory Center (Health/PAC), 34–35. *See also* Burlage, Robb; Rubin, Samuel
Health Revolutionary Unity Movement, 41–44. *See also* Cruz, Gloria
Health Services Administration (New York), 49
Hechler, Ken, 195
Hentschel, Glen, 212
Heyman, David, 15. *See also* Heyman Commission
Heyman Commission, 15–19
HHC (Health and Hospitals Corporations), 45–46, 47–51, 120
HiAP (Health in All Policies), 228
Highland View Hospital (Cleveland), 168–71
Hill-Burton Hospital Survey and Construction Act, 101
HIP (Health Insurance Plan of New York), 30
HMO (health maintenance organization), 137, 288n121
Holloman, Mike, 50–51
Hoover Redevelopment Project, 112
Hospital Advisory Commission (Los Angeles), 104, 108
Hospital Council of Greater New York, 29
Hough, 150–67; 1966 riot in, 150; overcrowded housing in, 166; segregation in, 152–53
Hough Area Council (Cleveland), 151
Hough-Norwood Family Health Care Center (Cleveland), 164–67, 171
House Un-American Activities Committee, 104

HRUM (Health Revolutionary Unity Movement), 41–44. *See also* Cruz, Gloria
hydrocarbons: and contribution to smog, 75–78; later regulation of, 79, 83–94
hydrologic pollution: 181, 184–5

Industrial Areas Foundation (IAF), 1, 39. *See also* Alinsky, Saul
industrial-ecological accord, 61–66, 71–72, 74, 78–79, 85, 89
Institute for Policy Studies, 34

Jackson, Leo, 155, 157
Jackson County (Ky.), 174
Jacobs, Jane, 27
Johnson, Lyndon B., 3–6 passim, 38, 173, 181, 202
Johnston, H. F., 70–71
John Wesley County Hospital (Los Angeles), 99, 109
J. P. Morgan Chase, 227

Kaiser Permanente Health Plan, 144, 149
Karkus, Harvey, 42–43
Kehoe, Robert, 92–93
Kemp, Brian, 232
Kennedy, Harold W., 62
Kennedy, Ted, 133
Kenneth Clement Center (Cleveland), initial planning of, 157–58, 160–63, 167, 171
Kentucky, 173–25; state-level energy policy in, 199–201; surveys of maldistribution in, 203–6
Kentucky Coal Policy Council, 200
Kerala (India), 231, 234
Kerner report, 105
Kings County Hospital (New York), 32–33
Kings County Physicians Guild (New York), 27
Kirk, Grayson, 21
Knight, Goodwin: and Special Committee on Air Pollution, 78–79, 83–84
Knott County (Ky.), 178, 184
Koch, Ed, 51, 55

Kotin, Paul: and claims about smog and lung cancer, 87–88, 91; and funding by tobacco industry, 91
Kucinich, Dennis, 161

labor unions: and influence on medical care innovation, 30–31, 144–50; and political strength in Ohio, 143; and protests and strikes against cuts and lack of resources, 54, 100; and tensions with community groups, 43
LACMA (Los Angeles County Medical Association), 82, 88
lay participation in medicine, 8, 38–48 passim, 111–16, 218–20. *See also* maximum feasible participation
lay perceptions of risk, 72–73, 79–82, 177–90
Legg, Herbert, 84
Letcher County (Ky.), 174, 177
Lewis, John L., 176, 205
Light, Harold L., 31
Lincoln Hospital (New York), 19, 49–51
Lindsay, John, 32, 46
Local 347 (Los Angeles), 100
Local 1199 (New York), 43–44
local hiring, 30, 111, 161–62, 219
localism: in health policy and public health research, 4–5; historical specificity of, 6; limits and promise of, 12–13, 123–25, 166–67, 220–25, 226–36; and notions of "community health," 6–7; and recent American historical writing, 2. *See also* community health
Locher, Ralph, 157
London: 1952 smog attack in, 86
Los Angeles: business cooperation with air pollution control of, 61–66, 71–72, 74, 78–79, 85, 89; effect of 1970s economics on, 125–38; and lack of comprehensive industrial zoning, 93; midcentury public hospital boom in, 97–100; population change in, 85; segregation in, 101, 102–4; unique county governance of 61–63; unique topography of, 58–59; various business factions in, 63–64; Watts riot in, 96–97

Los Angeles County Board of Supervisors, 60–63, 72–75, 80–82, 86, 96
Los Angeles County Medical Association, 82, 88
Los Angeles County Welfare Planning Council, 101
Lower East Side (New York), 28–31, 38–47, 55
Lower East Side Neighborhood Health Council–South (New York), 38–46
Lower East Side Neighborhoods Association (New York), 28

Magruder, P. S., 84–86
Manning, Henry, 162
Mark, Vernon, 135
Marris, Peter, 3–4
Martin County (Ky.), 202
Martin Luther King, Jr. Hospital, 108–11, 131–38; initial debate about construction and financing of, 108–11; opening of, 131–32; and relationship with UCLA, 132; and unexpected pressures experienced by, 132–34
maximum feasible participation, 6, 38–48 passim, 111–16, 208–19. See also lay participation in medicine; War on Poverty
McCabe, Louis, 72–73
McCarthyism, 104, 107, 148–49, 176
McCone, John, 96–97, 108
McCone Commission, 96–97, 108
McGovern, George, 195
Medicaid: Cleveland Clinic concerns about new patients resulting from, 158; exodus from public hospital system as a result of, 52, 109; and outsize presence in health policy scholarship, 6; passage of, 38; and rerouting in Floyd County Comprehensive Health Program, 208; and role as potential inflator of health care costs, 11; unreliable finances of, 48, 126–28, 224
Medi-Cal (Calif.), 126–28, 130, 133, 137
medical care and relative contribution to population health improvement, 9–10, 35–37, 39–40, 123–25, 166–67, 220–25

medical maldistribution, 11; as a problem in Central Appalachia, 203–6, 222–23; as a problem in Hough, 151–53, 157–58; as a problem on the Lower East Side, 28–30; as a problem in Watts, 100–107
Medicare: exodus from public hospital system as a result of, 52, 109; and outsize presence in health policy scholarship, 6; passage of, 38; and re-routing in Floyd County Comprehensive Health Program, 208; and role as potential inflator of health care costs, 11
Merritt, Houston, 21
Metropolitan General Hospital (Cleveland), 141–43, 157, 168–71; and consolidation with Highland View Hospital (Cleveland), 168–71. See also Highland View Hospital (Cleveland)
Metropolitan Hospital (New York), 19, 33
Metzenbaum, Howard, 163
Mize, James, 128
Mizrahi, Terry, 39, 43, 45
Mobilization for Youth, 45–46
Montefiore Medical Center (New York), 17, 20, 53
Morrisania Hospital (New York), 17, 20
Moses, Robert, 22–23, 57
Mountain People's Rights, 214
Mount Sinai Medical Center (New York), 26–28, 55
Mud Creek Clinic, 218–20
Mud Creek Health Rights Committee, 212
Municipal Assistance Corporation (New York), 50

NAACP (Cleveland), 151
NAACP (Los Angeles), 108
National Coal Association, 193, 198
National Commission on Civil Disorders, 105
National Municipal League, 141
Neiburger, Morris, 66–68
New Federalism, 48
New Left: and influence on critiques of affiliation, 34–35. See also Burlage, Robb; Health Policy Advisory Center
Newsom, Gavin, 232

New York: 14–58; and investigations of affiliation in New York City, 32–34; and unreliability of Medicaid funds in, 48

New York City: 14–57; population change in, 49; presence of neighborhood health centers program in, 28–31, 38–47; rise of hospital affiliation in, 15–19, 51–56

New York Medical College, 33

*Night Comes to the Cumberlands* (Caudill), 197

nitrogen, 75–78

Nixon, Richard, 48, 133, 217

North Central Bronx Hospital (New York), 49, 53, 55

Norwood (Cleveland), 165

Obama, Barack, 1–2, 226–27

Ocasio-Cortez, Alexandria, 230

OEO. *See* Office of Economic Opportunity

Office of Air Pollution Control (Los Angeles), 62–65

Office of Economic Opportunity: and neighborhood health centers program, 28–31, 38–47, 111–25, 120–22, 164; and participatory governance, 38, 40, 43, 164, 208–19; role in adjudicating community disputes, 43, 115–16, 121, 208–19

Office of Surface Mining, 200

Ohio: 140–72; and labor politics in, 143

Ohio American Federation of Labor and Congress of Industrial Organizations (AFL-CIO), 143

Ohio State Medical Association, 143

oil shocks of the 1970s, 197–98

Olive View Hospital (Los Angeles), 98

O'Neill, Tip, 2, 6

OSM (Office of Surface Mining), 200

*Other America, The* (Harrington), 197

ozone, 75–78

Palm Lane Housing Project, 110–11

Paris climate agreement, 229

participatory democracy, 34–35

patient dumping, 32–33

patient empowerment, 28–31, 147–48

patient experience: in Central Appalachia, 209–10; in Cleveland, 146–48; in Los Angeles, 99–100, 125–26, 128–31; in New York City, 19–20, 29–30, 46–47

Patterson, Basil, 54

People's Lobby, 93

Perk, Ralph, 161

Perkins, Carl D., 184, 191, 198, 211

Piel, Gerald, 35–37

police power to promote public health, 62

Pond Creek Citizens, 184

Powell, Rodney, 121–25, 222

prepaid group practice, 30, 103–4, 144–50

Proposition 13 (California), 136–37

public hospitals: impact of 1975 New York City fiscal crisis on, 47–57; and initial crisis of sustainability in New York City, 15–16; and patient discontent before affiliation in New York City, 19–20; and various crises of sustainability in Cleveland, 141–43, 168–71; and various crises of sustainability in Los Angeles, 125–26, 128–38

public nuisance law, 62

public-private sector relations, 7, 15–19, 51–56, 97–98, 142

Pure Air Committee, 84–86

Queens (New York), 26–27

racial uprisings. *See* riots

racism: and invocation against new infrastructure, 110, 149–50, 169–70; in invocation of stereotypes by officials, 103, 156; in medicine, 8, 105–7, 152–63, 135

residential segregation, 101, 152–53

residents: and exodus from New York City public hospitals, 15–16; and protests and strikes against cuts and lack of resources, 125, 134

Reagan, Ronald, 93, 127–29, 131, 200

Reed, Doris, 141–42

Reed, Thomas, 141–42

Rein, Martin, 3–4

Retail Workers and Meat Cutters union (Ohio), 143

riots: and fears of more protest in Cleveland, 155–56; and immediate causes in Cleveland, 150;

riots (*continued*)
and immediate causes in Watts, 105;
as nationwide phenomenon, 96–97;
and official commissions to study
roots in Cleveland, 150–51; and official
commission to study roots in Los
Angeles, 105–7; proper terminology
to describe, 97, 271n3; sociological
deprivation as root of, 105–7, 150–52;
and unofficial commission to study
roots in Cleveland, 151
Robinson, Eleanor, 214, 219
Rockefeller, John D., IV, 198–99
Rockefeller, Nelson: and blue-ribbon
report on affiliations, 32
Roemer, Milton, 105–7
Rogers, Alex, 109, 126
Roth, Herman, 68–70. *See also* Swenson,
Engelbrekt
Rubin, Samuel, 26, 34. *See also* Burlage,
Robb, Health Policy Advisory Center
Ryan, Leo, 189

Save Our Kentucky, 184
Scala, Charles, 23–26
Schechter, Arnold, 212
Science for the People, 189
scientific uncertainty, 8, 71–75, 184–90
SDS (Students for a Democratic Society),
34–35
Seeley, John R., 136
Shriver, Sargent, 111, 119–20
smog: constraints on regulation of, 89–95;
debates over health effects of, 79–82,
86–91; discovery of hydrocarbon
contribution to, 75–78; early attacks
of, 59–61; early elastic definitions of,
62; early regulation of, 64–66; early
scientific investigation of, 66–71; impact
of petrochemical industry on, 65–66,
72, 83–86; later regulation of, 65–66,
73–75, 79, 83–86, 89–90; in popular
culture about Los Angeles, 58
South-Central Multi-Purpose Service
Health Center (Watts center),
111–25, 137
Southeastern Kentucky Regional Health
Demonstration Project, 205, 207, 222–23

Southern California Air Pollution
Foundation, 84
Southern Christian Leadership Conference
(Los Angeles), 138
Spellman, Mitchell, 135
Stanford Research Institute, 88
State Advisory Hospital Council
(California), 107–8
Stokes, Carl, 157–59, 161
Students for a Democratic Society,
34–35
Stumbo, Henry, 210, 216
Sturgill, William B., 200
sulfur: early regulation of, 65–66; and
reconsideration of role in smog, 75–78;
and scientific inquiry on contribution
to smog, 70–71, 74
surface (strip) mining: everyday lay
experience of, 177–84; forced relocation
resulting from, 178, 182; and growing
interpretation as a threat to health
and well-being, 177–84, 186–90; noise
pollution from, 178; rise of, 174–77; role
of anti-labor imperative in, 176–77; role
of technological innovation in, 175–76;
scientific investigation of, 184–90
Surface Mining Control and Reclamation
Act, 199
sustainability, 10–11; in Central Appalachia,
205, 219, 222; in Cleveland, 142; in Los
Angeles, 125–31, 133, 136–38; in New
York City, 15–19, 47–57
Swartout, H. O, 64
Swenson, Engelbrekt, 68–70. *See also* Roth,
Herman
Sydenham Hospital, 18, 53–56

Taft-Hartley Act, 176
tetraethyl lead, 91–93
Thaler, Seymour, 32–34
Third Worldism, 34–35
Tranquada, Robert, 112–21
Trump, Donald, 232
Trussell, Ray: as architect of affiliation,
15–29; as head of Beth Israel, 40–46,
56–57; as target of antiaffiliation protest,
21–22, 27–28
Tuchman, Lester, 27–28

Udall, Morris, 198
UMWA. *See* United Mine Workers of America
Union Eye Care Center, 144
United Auto Workers, 30, 144
United Mine Workers of America (UMWA), 144, 176–77; and Miners Memorial Hospitals, 205, 219, 224
United States Bureau of Mines, 194–95
United States Department of Health, Education, and Welfare, 48, 137, 219
United States Department of the Interior, 173
United States Forest Service, 186–88
United States Public Health Service: and studies of potential for group practice in Cleveland, 143–44; and studies of southeastern Kentucky health problems, 220–21
University Circle (Cleveland), 151–52, 161
University of California at Los Angeles (UCLA), 108, 136
University-Euclid urban renewal project, 153–55
University Hospitals, 140
University of Southern California (USC), 97–98, 108, 111–25 passim
Urban League (Cleveland), 166–67
Urban League (Los Angeles), 103
urban renewal, 22–23, 94, 110–12, 151–54
USPHS. *See* United States Public Health Service

Vance, Rupert, 203.
vapor control, 79, 83–85, 89
Vayda, Eugene, 146
Vernon (Los Angeles), 68, 74, 87, 93, 101

*Violence and the Brain* (Mark and Ervin), 135
Voinovich, George, 161

Wagner, Robert, 16, 19, 30
War on Poverty: common critiques of, 123; and lay empowerment, 3–4, 6; and neighborhood health centers program, 38–47, 111–25, 164–67, 207–18. *See also* lay participation in medicine; maximum feasible participation
water pollution, 180–81
Watts, 95–124; 1965 riot in, 96–97; segregation in, 101
Watts Community Labor Action Committee, 108
Watts Health Advisory Committee, 108
Watts Medical, Dental and Pharmaceutical Society, 117
Weinberger, Caspar, 127
Weinerman, Richard, 144
Welfare Foundation of Cleveland, 143, 167
Western Oil and Gas Association, 65–66, 84–86
Western Reserve University, 140
White, Sol, 104–5, 107, 119–21
Whitesburg (Ky.), 178
Whitmer, Gretchen, 232
Will, Arthur J., 99
Willis, Winston, 160–61
Willowbrook, 101
Wilson, Glenn, 144
Witherill, Liston, 133–34
Wolfe, Samuel, 51–53
Woodhull Hospital, 49, 55–56

Yedidia, Avram, 144
Young, John, 200
Young, Robert, 220, 222
Young Lords Party, 41–42

# Studies in Social Medicine

Nancy M. P. King, Gail E. Henderson, and Jane Stein, eds., *Beyond Regulations: Ethics in Human Subjects Research* (1999).

Laurie Zoloth, *Health Care and the Ethics of Encounter: A Jewish Discussion of Social Justice* (1999).

Susan M. Reverby, ed., *Tuskegee's Truths: Rethinking the Tuskegee Syphilis Study* (2000).

Beatrix Hoffman, *The Wages of Sickness: The Politics of Health Insurance in Progressive America* (2000).

Margarete Sandelowski, *Devices and Desires: Gender, Technology, and American Nursing* (2000).

Keith Wailoo, *Dying in the City of the Blues: Sickle Cell Anemia and the Politics of Race and Health* (2001).

Judith Andre, *Bioethics as Practice* (2002).

Chris Feudtner, *Bittersweet: Diabetes, Insulin, and the Transformation of Illness* (2003).

Ann Folwell Stanford, *Bodies in a Broken World: Women Novelists of Color and the Politics of Medicine* (2003).

Lawrence O. Gostin, *The AIDS Pandemic: Complacency, Injustice, and Unfulfilled Expectations* (2004).

Arthur A. Daemmrich, *Pharmacopolitics: Drug Regulation in the United States and Germany* (2004).

Carl Elliott and Tod Chambers, eds., *Prozac as a Way of Life* (2004).

Steven M. Stowe, *Doctoring the South: Southern Physicians and Everyday Medicine in the Mid-Nineteenth Century* (2004).

Arleen Marcia Tuchman, *Science Has No Sex: The Life of Marie Zakrzewska, M.D.* (2006).

Michael H. Cohen, *Healing at the Borderland of Medicine and Religion* (2006).

Keith Wailoo, Julie Livingston, and Peter Guarnaccia, eds., *A Death Retold: Jesica Santillan, the Bungled Transplant, and Paradoxes of Medical Citizenship* (2006).

Michelle T. Moran, *Colonizing Leprosy: Imperialism and the Politics of Public Health in the United States* (2007).

Karey Harwood, *The Infertility Treadmill: Feminist Ethics, Personal Choice, and the Use of Reproductive Technologies* (2007).

Carla Bittel, *Mary Putnam Jacobi and the Politics of Medicine in Nineteenth-Century America* (2009).

Samuel Kelton Roberts Jr., *Infectious Fear: Politics, Disease, and the Health Effects of Segregation* (2009).

Lois Shepherd, *If That Ever Happens to Me: Making Life and Death Decisions after Terri Schiavo* (2009).

Mical Raz, *What's Wrong with the Poor? Psychiatry, Race, and the War on Poverty* (2013).

Johanna Schoen, *Abortion after Roe* (2015).

Nancy Tomes, *Remaking the American Patient: How Madison Avenue and Modern Medicine Turned Patients into Consumers* (2016).

Mara Buchbinder, Michele Rivkin-Fish, and Rebecca L. Walker, eds., *Understanding Health Inequalities and Justice: New Conversations across the Disciplines* (2016).

Muriel R. Gillick, *Old and Sick in America: The Journey through the Health Care System* (2017).

Michael E. Staub, *The Mismeasure of Minds: Debating Race and Intelligence between Brown and "The Bell Curve"* (2018).

Mari Armstrong-Hough, *Biomedicalization and the Practice of Culture: Globalization and Type 2 Diabetes in the United States and Japan* (2018).

Kathleen Bachynski, *No Game for Boys to Play: The History of Youth Football and the Origins of a Public Health Crisis* (2019).

Mical Raz, *Abusive Policies: How the American Child Welfare System Lost Its Way* (2020).

Emily K. Abel, *Sick and Tired: An Intimate History of Fatigue* (2021).

Merlin Chowkwanyun, *All Health Politics Is Local: Community Battles for Medical Care and Environmental Health* (2022).